Caregiving

Research • Practice • Policy

Ronda C. Talley, Series Editor

An official publication of
The Rosalynn Carter Institute for Caregiving

For further volumes:
http://www.springer.com/series/8274

Ronda C. Talley • Shirley S. Travis
Editors

Multidisciplinary Coordinated Caregiving

Research • Practice • Policy

Rosalynn Carter
INSTITUTE
FOR CAREGIVING

Springer

Editors
Ronda C. Talley
College of Education and Behavioral Sciences
Western Kentucky University
Bowling Green
Kentucky
USA

Shirley S. Travis
College of Health and Human Services
George Mason University
Fairfax
Virginia
USA

ISSN 2192-340X ISSN 2192-3418 (electronic)
ISBN 978-1-4614-8972-6 ISBN 978-1-4614-8973-3 (eBook)
DOI 10.1007/978-1-4614-8973-3
Springer New York Heidelberg Dordrecht London

Library of Congress Control Number: 2013951818

Printed on acid-free paper

Springer is part of Springer Science+Business Media (www.springer.com)

To those who taught me life's most important lessons—my family.

And to the mentors and special colleagues from many disciplines who shared their knowledge and friendship with me throughout my professional career:
Dr. Jane R. Mercer, Dr. Joseph P. Cangemi,
Dr. Sylvia Rosenfield, Dr. Sam Guskin,
Dr. Michael Tracy, Dr. Sue Eklund,
Dr. Mrytle Scott, Mr. Robert Weenolsen,
Ms. Linda Hamilton, Mr. "Mac",
and Ms. Sarah Taylor.

Ronda C. Talley

To William J. (Jim) McAuley,
loving husband, father, and son.

Shirley S. Travis

Editorial Board

Series Foreword

From its inception in 1987, the Rosalynn Carter Institute for Caregiving (RCI) has sought to bring attention to the extraordinary contributions made by caregivers to their loved ones. I grew up in a home that was regularly transformed into a caregiving household when members of my family became seriously ill, disabled, or frail with age, so my interest in the issue is personal. In my hometown of Plains, Georgia, as in most communities across our country, it was expected that family members and neighbors would take on the responsibility of providing care whenever illness struck close to home. Delivering such care with the love, respect, and attention it deserves is both labor-intensive and personally demanding. Those who do so represent one of this nation's most significant yet underappreciated assets in our health delivery system.

When the RCI began, "caregiving" was found nowhere in the nation's health lexicon. Its existence was not a secret but rather simply accepted as a fact of life. In deciding on the direction and priorities of the new institute, we convened groups of family and professional caregivers from around the region to tell their personal stories. As I listened to neighbors describe caring for aged and/or chronically ill or disabled family members, I recognized that their experiences reflected mine. They testified that while caregiving for them was full of personal meaning and significance and could be extremely rewarding, it could also be fraught with anxiety, stress, and feelings of isolation. Many felt unprepared and most were overwhelmed at times. A critical issue in the "field" of caregiving, I realized, was the need to better understand the kinds of policies and programs necessary to support those who quietly and consistently care for loved ones.

With the aging of America's baby boomers expected to double the elderly population in the next 20 years, deinstitutionalization of individuals with chronic mental illnesses and developmental disabilities, a rising percentage of women in the workforce, smaller and more dispersed families, changes in the role of hospitals, and a range of other factors, caregiving has become one of the most significant issues of our time. Caregiving as an area of research, as a focus and concern of policy making, and as an area of professional training and practice has reached a new and unparalleled level of importance in our society and indeed globally.

As we survey the field of caregiving today, we now recognize that it is an essential component of long-term care in the community, yet also a potential health risk for those who provide care. The basic features of a public health approach have emerged: a focus on populations of caregivers and recipients, tracking and surveillance of health risks, understanding the factors associated with risk status, and the development and testing of the effectiveness of various interventions to maximize benefits for both the recipients of care and their providers.

The accumulated wisdom from this work is represented in the volumes that make up the Springer Caregiving Series. This series presents a broad portrait of the nature of caregiving in the USA in the twenty-first century. Most Americans have been, are now, or will be caregivers. With our society's increasing demands for care, we cannot expect a high quality of life for our seniors and others living with limitations due to illness or disability unless we understand and support the work of caregivers. Without thoughtful planning, intelligent policies, and sensitive interventions, there is the risk that the work of family, paraprofessional, and professional caregivers will become intolerably difficult and burdensome. We cannot let this happen.

The current volume builds on previous volumes in the RCI series. What becomes apparent as one scans this volume's content is that no single discipline holds proprietary rights to caregiving. This is not, however, to suggest that it therefore belongs to many disciplines. Rather the message conveyed within and across the volume's chapters is that caregiving by definition is most effective when disciplines collaborate. By having many human service and health service professions appreciate the power of caregiving for both providers and recipients—as well as costs to providers—we increase significantly the pace at which caregiving happens in a manner coordinated with other health providers. But the real power of caregiving occurs when those providing services escape their disciplinary shackles and work together to identify caregiving needs; appreciate how together they can support both caregiver and provider, thus magnifying the power of caregiving to improve the lives of those with acute or chronic disorders and improve the quality of life within their families.

Readers of this series will find hope and evidence that improved support for family and professional caregivers lies within our reach. The field of caregiving has matured and, as evidenced in these volumes, has generated rigorous and practical research findings to guide effective and enlightened policy and program options. My hope is that these volumes will play an important role in documenting the research base, guiding practice, and moving our nation toward effective polices to support all of America's caregivers.

Rosalynn Carter

Contents

Contributors

Laura M. Arnstein College of Medicine, Genetics & Developmental Pediatrics, Medical University of South Carolina, Charleston, USA

K. Leigh Baldwin Department of Defense, Ft. Campbell, KY, USA

Frances K. Barg Department of Family Medicine and Community Health, University of Pennsylvania School of Medicine, Philadelphia, USA

Ronald T. Brown University of North Texas at Dallas, Dallas, USA

Miae Chun Department of Social Work, Chongshin University, Seoul, South Korea

Wendy Shiekman Cohen Philadelphia, USA

John E. Crews Division of Human Development and Disability, National Center on Birth Defects and Developmental Disabilities, Centers for Disease Control and Prevention, Atlanta, USA

Martha R. Crowther Department of Psychology, University of Alabama, Tuscaloosa, USA

Diane Elmore American Psychological Association, Washington, USA

National Center For Child Traumatic Stress, Duke University Medical Center, Durham, NC, USA

Rebecca Henderson Philadelphia, USA

Nancy R. Hooyman CSWE National Center on Gerontological Social Work Education, School of Social Work, University of Washington, Seattle, USA

Shannon E. Jarrott Department of Human Development, Virginia Polytechnic Institute and State University, Blacksburg, USA

Shimrit Keddem University of Pennsylvania, Philadelphia, USA

Bob G. Knight University of Southern California, Los Angeles, USA

Lewina O. Lee Department of Epidemiology, Boston University School of Public Health, Boston, USA

Department of Veterans Affairs Boston Healthcare System, Boston, MA, USA

Donald Lollar Oregon Institute on Disability and Development, Portland, USA

Division of Human Development and Disability, National Center on Birth Defects and Developmental Disabilities, Centers for Disease Control and Prevention, Atlanta, USA

Karen A. Roberto Center for Gerontology and the Institute for Society, Culture and Environment, Virginia Polytechnic Institute and State University, Blacksburg, USA

Katherine Morton Robinson University of North Florida, Jacksonville, USA

Lisa Sparks M.S. Health and Strategic Communication, Chapman University, Orange, USA

Chao Family Comprehensive Cancer Center, NCI Designated, University of California, Irvine, USA

Nora Super U.S. Department of Health & Human Services, Washington, USA

George Washington University, Washington, USA

Ronda C. Talley College of Education and Behavioral Sciences, Western Kentucky University, Bowling Green, USA

Division of Human Development and Disability, National Center on Birth Defects and Developmental Disabilities, Centers for Disease Control and Prevention, Atlanta, USA

Shirley S. Travis College of Health and Human Services, George Mason University, Fairfax, USA

Janet Valluzzi Division of Human Development and Disability, National Center on Birth Defects and Developmental Disabilities, Centers for Disease Control and Prevention, Atlanta, USA

About the Editors

Ronda C. Talley, PhD, MPH is Professor of Psychology at Western Kentucky University. Dr. Talley's professional experience includes providing national leadership on caregiving issues and organizational development as Executive Director of the Rosalynn Carter Institute for Caregiving and the National Quality Caregiving Coalition; working with federal government groups to promote caregiving issues as Associate Director of Legislation, Policy, and Planning/Health Scientist for the Centers for Disease Control and Prevention, U.S. Department of Health and Human Services, in Atlanta, GA; and promoting the science and practice of psychology in the schools as Associate Executive Director of Education and Director of School Policy and Practice at the American Psychological Association in Washington, DC. Dr. Talley taught ethics and legal issues in school psychology at the University of Maryland, College Park, and clinical, counseling, and school psychology students at Spalding University in Louisville, KY. Prior to that time, Dr. Talley worked a teacher of students with special needs and school administrator for almost 20 years in the Jefferson County (KY) Public Schools where she supervised a multi-disciplinary private practice.

Dr. Talley received the Outstanding Alumni Award from Indiana University and the Jack Bardon Distinguished Service Award from the Division of School Psychology of the American Psychological Association. She serves on the national board of the American Association of Caregiving Youth, the Indiana University School of Education Board of Visitors, and the Western Kentucky University National Alumni Advisory Board. Dr. Talley is Editor-in-Chief of the Springer CARE book series on diverse caregiving issues. Dr. Talley may be reached at 1906 College Heights Boulevard, GRH 3023, Bowling Green, KY 42101; by telephone at (270) 745-2780; or via e-mail: Ronda.Talley@wku.edu.

Shirley S. Travis, PhD, APRN, FAAN was the founding Dean of the College of Health and Human Services at George Mason University. Her research and publications address the patterns of care that dependent older adults and their family caregivers require over time. Her awards and honors include the Janssen Eldercare Lifetime Achievement Award for contributions to the healthcare of older Americans, Academic Gerontologist of the Year by the Southern Gerontological

Society for her record of applied research in long-term care, and the Springer Geriatric/Gerontological Nursing Research Award for her end of life research. From 2001 to 2004, Dr. Travis was an Eminent Scholar of the Rosalynn Carter Institute for Caregiving and served on the Institute Board of Directors from 2004 to 2008. Dr. Travis has authored or co-authored more than 100 articles, books, and book chapters on aging and long-term care.

She is a Past President of the National Gerontological Nursing Association and a former Chair of the Clinical Medicine Section (now Health Sciences Section)/Vice President of the Gerontological Society of America. During her career she was an elected fellow of the Association for Gerontology in Higher Education, the Gerontological Society of America, the National Gerontological Nursing Association, and the American Academy of Nursing. Dr. Travis served as Dean of College of Health and Human Services at George Mason University from 2005 to 2012, and is the founding dean of the college. She is currently a Senior Administrative faculty member in the college, as she completes her transition to retirement.

About the Authors

K. Leigh Baldwin, PhD, MS, EdS, MAEd, NCSP is dually credentialed in Clinical and School Psychology. She is a Ph.D. graduate of the University of Kentucky and subsequently completed a post-Doctoral Masters degree in Education. Dr. Baldwin has served as a consultant to national organizations and presents on a variety of topics, including ethics in practice, the recovery philosophy of care, family caregiving, and psycheducational consultation. During her tenure in public schools, Dr. Baldwin led grand-funded initiatives promoting literacy as well as integrating technology in curricula. Subsequently, as a faculty member she was recognized with distinguished faculty honors for excellence in teaching and program development. In addition, Dr. Baldwin was the founding director of The Recovery Mall, an award-winning hospital treatment program in Western Kentucky, She has served on the Board of Directors of several community organizations, including chairing fundraising campaigns for youth organizations and helping to improve housing options for individuals who have mental illness. Dr. Baldwin currently works for the Department of Defense at Fr. Campbell, KY, leading a multidisciplinary team focused on soldier care and recovery. Dr. Baldwin has both personal and professional experience as a caregiver and is dedicated to advancing knowledge of caregiving-related concerns.

Frances K. Barg, PhD, MEd is Associate Professor of Family Medicine and Community Health at the Hospital of the University of Pennsylvania and Co-Director of the Mixed Methods Research Lab.

Ronald T. Brown PhD is the second president of the University of North Texas at Dallas. Previously, he served as the provost and senior vice president for academic affairs at Wayne State University in Detroit, MI, and as dean of the College of Health Professions and Social Work as well as interim dean of the School of Dentistry at Temple University in Philadelphia, PA. Dr. Brown held the position of associate dean of the College of Health Sciences at the Medical University of South Carolina where he received the Scholar of the Year Award and the Mitchell I. Rubin Award for Distinguished Contributions to the Advancement of Medical Science in the Field of Health Care in Pediatrics at the Medical University of South Carolina. Dr. Brown has directed a pre- and post-doctoral clinical psychology program and served as a consultant to attorneys, universities and the federal government.

Dr. Brown has been a member of the Council of Representatives of the American Psychological Association, where he served as president of the Society of Pediatric Psychology of the American Psychological Association. He received the society's Martin P. Levin Award for Mentorship and the Logan Wright Distinguished Research Award. He has been a member of the Behavioral Medicine Interventions and Outcomes study section at the National Institutes of Health (NIH). He chaired several special panels at NIH, including one that conducted an intramural review of the Pediatric Oncology Branch, the Pioneers research program for early career scientists and the advisory board of the Heart Lung and Blood Institute, Sickle Cell Branch. A licensed and board-certified psychologist, Dr. Brown is President-elect of the Association of Psychologists in Academic Health Centers of the American Psychological Association. Other boards of which he is a member include the American Academy of Pediatrics, Psychosocial Committee; Detroit Receiving Hospital; and the Center on Work and Family at Claremont McKenna College.

Dr. Brown is editor of *Professional Psychology: Research and Practice* and past editor of *The Journal of Pediatric Psychology* and is. He has served on the editorial board of over 15 journals in the field of health care and child psychology and has published nine books and more than 300 articles and chapters.

Laura Arnstein Carpenter, PhD, BCBA Dr. Carpenter's professional interests include autism spectrum disorders, developmental disabilities, and learning disabilities.

Miae Chun is an assistant professor in the Department of Social Work, Chongshin University, South Korea. She also serves as the editor for the Journal of the Korean Gerontological Society, and as a Deputy Secretary-General of the Organizing Committee for the 20th IAGG World Congress of Gerontology and Geriatrics being held in 2013 in Seoul, Korea. In addition, she is serving her community as a chairperson of Seoul Ganganm-gu District Social Welfare Practical Affairs Consultation Services, and a member of the Long-Term Care Insurance Development Forum of the Ministry of Health and Welfare in South Korea.

Wendy Shiekman Cohen is currently a Manager in Accenture's Management Consultant practice, specializing in the areas of Human Capital Strategy, Organization Effectiveness, Talent, and Change Management. Her career has been focused on the intersection of organizational psychology and anthropology, corporate cultures, and business. Wendy received her MBA from The Wharton School in Management and Organizational Behavior in 2010, and her BA from University of Pennsylvania in English and Anthropology in 2002.

John E. Crews, DPA is a Health Scientist with the Vision Health Initiative in the Division of Diabetes Translation of the National Center for Chronic Disease Prevention and Health Promotion, Centers for Disease Control and Prevention in Atlanta, GA. Dr. Crews' specialties are vision impairment and aging, caregiving, and disability; his research interests also include health disparities among people with disabilities and aging with a disability.

Dr. Crews has more than 30 years of experience in vision rehabilitation and disability research. He managed a clinical program for older people with visual impairments in Michigan between 1977 and 1992. He then became the Acting Director of the Rehabilitation Research and Development Center on Aging at the Department of Veterans Affairs in Atlanta. In 1998, he joined the Centers for Disease Control and Prevention.

Dr. Crews received his BA from Franklin College in Franklin, IN. He received two Master of Arts degrees, one from Indiana University in Bloomington, IN, and another from Western Michigan University in Kalamazoo, MI. He received his DPA from Western Michigan University. He has written numerous peer-reviewed scientific articles and two books, *Vision Loss in an Aging Society* and *The Multiple Dimensions of Caregiving and Disability*. Dr. Crews served on the Board of Trustees of the American Foundation for the Blind and on board committees of Lighthouse International. He was board chair of the National Literacy Center of the American Foundation for the Blind in Atlanta. He serves on the editorial board of the *Journal of Visual Impairment and Blindness*, and also serves on the National Commission on Vision and Health.

Martha R. Crowther, PhD, MPH is Associate Professor in the Department of Psychology at The University of Alabama. She may be reached at PO Box 870348, Tuscaloosa, AL 35487; by telephone at 205-348-7802; or via e-mail at mrcrowther@as.ua.edu.

Dr. Elmore has worked as a policy advisor, advocate, and congressional staff member, using her psychology and public health training to analyze and inform the debate on a variety of important health policy issues, including health reform, violence against women, human trafficking, hate crime, emergency preparedness and response, military service member and veteran health care, and funding for scientific research and mental health services. She currently serves as Director of the Policy Program for the UCLA-Duke University National Center for Child Traumatic Stress and is an Adjunct Professor in the School of Public Affairs at American University. Previously, she served as the Associate Executive Director of the American Psychological Association's (APA) Public Interest Government Relations Office, Director of the APA Congressional Fellowship Program, and coordinator of APA activities related to military service members, Veterans, and their families. She also worked as the Society for the Psychological Study of Social Issues (SPSSI) James Marshall Public Policy Scholar in the APA Public Policy Office, working on policy initiatives related to trauma, violence, and abuse and aging issues.

Prior to her work at APA, Dr. Elmore served as an AAAS/APA Health Policy Fellow in the office of then-Senator Hillary Rodham Clinton, where she was a member of a legislative team responsible for policy issues including health care, mental and behavioral health, aging, trauma and abuse, and military service member and veteran health care.

Dr. Elmore earned her PhD in Counseling Psychology from the University of Houston and completed the doctoral internship at the National Center for PTSD, Pacific Islands Division/Honolulu VA Medical Center. She holds a Master of Public Health degree from Johns Hopkins University with a dual concentration in public health policy and public health preparedness.

Rebecca Henderson currently assists with research in the University of Pennsylvania's Department of Family Medicine. She holds a BA in Anthropology and Linguistics from the University of Mary Washington.

Dr. Nancy R. Hooyman Professor in Gerontology and Dean Emeritus at the University of Washington School of Social Work, received her Ph.D. in Sociology and Social Work from the University of Michigan. She is recipient of the School's first endowed professorship in gerontology, the Nancy R. Hooyman Professorship. She served as Principal Investigator of the Hartford Geriatric Enrichment in Social Work Education Project (GeroRich), a national curriculum change initiative (2001–2004); co-PI of the Hartford-funded Planning Grant National Center for Family Care Initiatives (2007–2009); and PI of the Hartford Practicum Partnership Project at the School of Social Work (2006–2009). She is co-Principal Investigator of the CSWE National Center on Gerontological Social Work Education (2004–2012); and a Co-Investigator on Caregiving with Pride, funded by NIA (Dr. Karen Fredriksen-Goldsen, PI). She is author of 11 books and over 130 peer review articles and book chapters related to gerontology and women's issues, and is a frequent presenter on multigenerational policy and practice, gender inequities in family caregiving, feminist gerontology, end-of-life care, and gerontological curricular change. Her co-authored books include a widely used text, Social Gerontology: A Multidisciplinary Perspective (9th edition); Transforming Social Work Education: The First Decade of the Hartford Geriatric Social Work Initiative; Living through Loss: Interventions across the Lifespan; Achieving Curricular and Organizational Change; Feminist Perspectives on Family Care: Policies toward Gender Justice; and Taking Care of Older Relatives, one of the first widely used books on family caregiving.

She is the recipient of the 2009 CSWE Lifetime Achievement Award in Social Work Education and the 1998 Lifetime Achievement Award from the Association for Gerontology Education in Social Work Education, and was inducted into the American Academy of Social Work and Social Welfare in 2011. She is a Fellow and past-chair of the Social Research Policy and Practice (SRPP) Section of GSA; Past-President of SSWR; Past-President of the National Association of Deans and Directors of Social Work; past-Board member of the National Institute for the Advancement of Social Work Research; and Past Chairperson of the Action Network for Social Work Education and Research. She has served on the Advisory Boards for all the Hartford Foundation Geriatric Initiatives, has been a National Mentor five times, and is a member of the Hartford Scholars selection committee. She chairs the interdisciplinary Elder Friendly Future Partnership at UW. In Seattle, she is immediate past-President of the Board of Senior Services and chaired the United Way Impact Council on Older Adults.

Shannon Jarrott is Associate Professor and Director of Intergenerational Programs in the department of Human Development. After completing graduate studies at Penn State, she joined Virginia Tech in 1999 as a faculty member and the first Director of Research at the department's Adult Day Services (ADS) program. Her research focuses on intergenerational community building with a specialization in shared site intergenerational programs serving frail elders. She leads the Neighbors Growing Together program, which consists of Adult Day Services and the Child

Development Center for Learning and Research. This award-winning group is the oldest university-based shared site intergenerational program in the US. Dr. Jarrott has been invited to contribute to United Nations and other international efforts to promote intergenerational theory, research, and practice.

Shimrit Keddem, MS is the manager of the Mixed Methods Research Lab in the Perelman School of Medicine at the University of Pennsylvania. Ms. Keddem received a BA in Psychology from McGill University and a Masters in Urban Spatial Analysis from the University of Pennsylvania.

Bob G. Knight, PhD is the Merle H. Bensinger Professor of Gerontology, Psychology, and Counseling Psychology at the Andrus Gerontology Center, University of Southern California, where he also serves as Director of the Tingstad Older Adult Counseling Center.

Lewina O. Lee, PhD is a Research Fellow at the Department of Epidemiology, Boston University School of Public Health and the Department of Veterans Affairs Boston Healthcare System. She may be reached at 150 South Huntington Avenue (151MAV), Boston, MA 02130; by telephone at (857) 364-6364; or via email at lol@bu.edu.

Donald Lollar, EdD is Director, Oregon Center for Disability and Development at the Oregon Health and Science University. The Oregon Institute on Disability & Development (OIDD) at the Child Development and Rehabilitation Center is one of 67 US University Centers for Excellence in Developmental Disabilities. He is also Professor, Department of Public Health and Preventive Medicine at OHSU and Associate Director for Academic Affairs at the Child Development and Rehabilitation Center of OHSU. Dr. Lollar is an initiator and member of the World Health Organization task force to adapt the international classification (ICF) for children and youth with disabilities. He serves on the ICF-CY Task Force, an ongoing international activity related to disability classification for children and youth.

Don Lollar served as Senior Research Scientist, Division for Human Development and Disability, National Center on Birth Defects and Developmental Disabilities (NCBDDD) at the Centers for Disease Control and Prevention in Atlanta. Prior to joining CDC, Dr. Lollar practiced rehabilitation psychology for 25 years, providing assessment and therapy services to children, adults, and families across the lifespan. His advanced degrees are from Indiana University, and his most recent writings include co-editing an Archives of Physical Medicine and Rehabilitation supplement on the *Science of Disability Outcomes*, and articles for the *Annual Review of Public Health, Public Health Reports*, and the *Journal of Developmental and Behavioral Pediatrics*. He spent seven years developing public health science and programs to increase participation in society among people with disabilities by promoting health and preventing secondary conditions, and directed NCBDDD's Office of Extramural Research, leading the mental health workgroup. He served as the co-lead of the HEALTHY PEOPLE 2010 workgroup on Disability and Secondary Conditions (Chapter 6 of HP 2010), and served as CDC representative to the advisory committee for the Child and Adolescent Measurement of Health Initiative and the Surgeon General's Task Force on Children's Mental Health.

Karen A. Roberto, PhD is Professor and Director of the Center for Gerontology and the Institute for Society, Culture and Environment at Virginia Tech. Her research program focuses on health and social support in late life and includes studies of the health of rural older women, family relationships and caregiving, and elder abuse. Dr. Roberto is a fellow of the Gerontological Society of America, the Association for Gerontology in Higher Education, the National Council on Family Relations, and the World Demographic Association.

Katherine Morton Robinson, PhD, RN is an Associate Professor of Nursing at the University of North Florida, in Jacksonville, Florida. Dr. Robinson specializes in issues related to family caregiving, nursing theory and the history of nursing. Her clinical interests are critical care and adult health acute care nursing. This work was completed when she was a Brook's Scholar for the College of Health at the University of North Florida.

Lisa Sparks, MS, PhD is Foster and Mary McGaw Endowed Professor in Behavioral Sciences at Chapman University in Orange, California where she serves as Head/Director of the Master of Science graduate program in Health and Strategic Communication in the Schmid College of Science and Technology. Dr. Sparks also serves as Full Member of the Chao Family/NCI Designated Comprehensive Cancer Center at the University of California, Irvine in the School of Medicine, Division of Population Sciences; and Adjunct Professor in the Department of Population Health and Disease Prevention, Program in Public Health. Prior to joining Chapman in 2006, Dr. Sparks occupied faculty positions at George Mason University in Fairfax, Virginia and the University of Texas at San Antonio.

Dr. Sparks is a highly regarded teacher-scholar whose published work spans more than 100 research articles and scholarly book chapters, and is the author and editor of more than ten books in the areas of communication, health, and aging with a distinct focus on intersections of provider-patient interaction and family decision-making as related to cancer communication science. Check out Dr. Sparks' invited talk on Health Risk Messages and Decision-Making at 2011 TEDx OrangeCoast event: http://www.youtube.com/watch?v=d4JNyyuonko.

Dr. Sparks has served as Principal Investigator (PI) and Co-PI on a number of research grants including the ASCO-Komen Improving Cancer Care Grant, funded by Susan G. Komen for the Cure (2011–2012): An intervention trial of text messaging to improve patient adherence to adjuvant hormonal therapy (with PI Neugut; Co-PI's Hershman); California Mental Health Services Authority (CalMHSA) Grant Award: Statewide Stigma and Discrimination Reduction: Partnering with Media and the Entertainment Industry (2011–2014); and Robert Wood Johnson Foundation (RWJF) Grant Award: Hablamos juntos: Improving patient-provider communication for Latinos. Dr. Sparks has also served as a scientific consultant and advisor to the National Institutes of Health/National Cancer Institute, Institute for Healthcare Advancement, American Medical Association, American Medical Student Association, Educational Testing Service, Southwest Oncology Group, American Association of Cancer Research, Entertainment Industries Council and the United States House of Representatives at the Library of Congress on Capitol Hill in Washington, DC.

She is a Founding Senior Scientific Research Fellow for the Entertainment Industries Council (EIC), Burbank, CA/Reston, VA and a National Scientific Advisor for the Entertainment and Media Communication Institute, Center for Sun Safety and Skin Cancer Prevention in partnership with the Sun Safety Alliance. Dr. Sparks is a former Cancer Communication Research Fellow for the Health Communication and Informatics Research Branch, Behavioral Research Program, Division of Cancer Control and Population Sciences, National Cancer Institute, National Institutes of Health, Bethesda, MD and has served as an External Scientific Reviewer for NIH. Dr. Sparks' recent books include Patient-Provider Interaction: A Global Health Communication Perspective (Polity Press, 2010 with M. Villagran), Health Communication in the 21st Century (Blackwell, 2008 with K. B. Wright and H. D. O'Hair) 2nd edition (2012), Handbook of Communication and Cancer Care (Hampton Press, 2007 with H. D. O'Hair and G. L. Kreps), Cancer, Communication and Aging (Hampton Press, 2008 with H. D. O'Hair and G. L. Kreps), La Comunicación en el Cancer: Comunicación y apoyo emocional en el laberinto del cancer (Aresta, 2009 with M. Villagran). Dr. Sparks has served as Editor of Communication Research Reports; Guest Editor of Patient Education and Counseling, Health Communication and Communication Education and serves on several editorial boards including Health Communication, Journal of Applied Communication Research, Journal of Computer-Mediated Communication, and Communication Quarterly.

Dr. Sparks' research goal is to understand and create evidence based health messages that effectively change health behavior resulting in better health outcomes by applying social science theory and methods to the continuum of cancer care surrounding issues of health promotion, disease prevention, survivorship, and health disparities. Dr. Sparks' research and teaching interests in intergroup (intergenerational, intercultural) communication and aging approaches merge with her research in health, risk, and crisis communication domains including provider-patient interaction, family caregiving, health information and decision-making, patient-centered communication, breaking bad news, health literacy, health organizations, interpersonal based public health campaigns, communicating about crises, and communicating relevant messages with vulnerable populations when information is uncertain during periods of health risk. Her achievements, leadership qualities, and strong commitment to advance the intersections of Communication, Health, Aging and Cancer Communication Sciences are significant as evidenced by: (a) the number of publications (over 100) most of which are peer-reviewed; (b) the obtainment and consistent effort to obtain competitive peer-reviewed research grants and contracts; (c) the recognition of her scientific stature; (d) her collaborations with the top national and international scientists in communication and related scientific fields such as public health, medicine, and gerontology; (e) her teaching and mentoring of numerous undergraduate and graduate students and junior faculty; and (f) her demonstrated leadership and administrative roles as Head/Director of the Health and Strategic Communication Graduate Program at Chapman University, Editor of Communication Research Reports, Guest Editor of Health Communication, Patient Education and Counseling, and Communication Education as well as her editorial service for a number of peer-reviewed journals and continued service on several executive boards and associations.

Lisa Sparks (PhD, University of Oklahoma, 1998) is Foster and Mary McGaw Endowed Professor in Behavioral Sciences at Chapman University and Full Member of Chao Family Comprehensive/NCI Designated Cancer Center and Adjunct Professor of Public Health, University of California, Irvine. Requests for reprints should be sent to Lisa Sparks, Chapman University, Schmid College of Science, One University Drive, Orange, CA, 92866, sparks@chapman.edu; University of California, Irvine, Program in Public Health, AIRB 2081, Irvine, CA, 92697, lsparks1@uci.edu.

Nora Super serves as Director, Public Affairs, for the Office of the National Coordinator of the Office of Health Information Technology. In this role, she is responsible for stakeholder engagement activities to hospitals, physicians, consumers, vendors, and policymakers. Nora directs all ONC interactions with stakeholders at the policy, programmatic, and regulatory levels. ONC employs an array of communication channels to engage them, including: in-person meetings between the National Coordinator and other key HHS officials and stakeholder organizations; speaking and exhibiting at conferences and forums; and web-based roundtables with various stakeholder groups, to share electronic health record (EHR) adoption updates; key successes and challenges; and to learn about stakeholder issues and experiences. Nora also serves as ONC's primary liaison with Congress and the White House.

Prior to joining ONC, Nora Super served as Director, Federal Government Relations, Health and Long-Term Care at AARP. In this role, she was responsible for managing AARP's government relations activities regarding health care reform, Medicare, Medicaid, long-term care, and prescription drugs. Before AARP, Nora represented the political and health policy interests of Kaiser Permanente's eight regional Permanente Medical Groups as the Permanente Federation's Director of Public Policy and Government Relations.

Nora has more than 20 years of experience working in Washington, DC, with an expansive background in a wide range of health policy issues, including Medicare, Medicaid, HIPAA, ERISA, and other federal and state health programs. She has worked in academia and in the private sector, including the GWU Medical School, the National Health Policy Forum, the Washington Business Group on Health, and the Employee Benefit Research Institute. She has also served in government at the local, state, and congressional level. Nora has published several papers and issue briefs on a wide variety of health policy topics.

A native of New Orleans, Nora studied political science at Tulane University and completed her masters' work in public administration, with a concentration on health policy, at George Washington University.

Dr. Janet Valluzzi serves in the Center for Medicare & Medicaid Services in the U.S. Department of Health and Human Services (DHHS/CMS/OA/CMMI/PFP/REG). She has also researched caregiving issues at the Centers for Disease Control and Prevention.

Part I
Introduction

The Status of Professional Caregiving in America

Shirley S. Travis and Ronda C. Talley

To care for others is as old as human existence. To provide care, or caregiving, is about the needs of those who are dependent on others for some aspect of their life and well-being and their relationships to those who are fit and able to provide assistance. It is about accepting responsibility to care for those in need and about being willing to accept care that is offered.

In recent decades, dramatic shifts in the social and economic fabric of life in the United States have created what some consider a crisis in family life and the social support and public policies needed to support caregiving in the twenty-first century. Data on labor force participation, the current aging of the massive baby boom generation, the care the baby boomers are providing to their aging parents, and the care the baby boomers will need in the future are all forces that are challenging and transforming our notions about how we will care for ourselves and for each other in America (Gillon 2004; Macunovich 2002).

In a world that has moved rapidly toward multidisciplinary and interdisciplinary thinking to solve some of the most pressing social problems of this century, it seemed almost "retro" to spend time studying caregiving issues in discipline-specific chapters. We knew that those individuals who embrace collaborative study or practice might argue that studying the complexities of caregiving is done best when the issues are understood from multidisciplinary or interdisciplinary perspectives. We also made that argument (Travis and Duer 2000). However, in conceptualizing this text we came to believe that without some appreciation for the thinking, methodological and interventional nuances of the discrete disciplines collaborative models of either type will be lacking.

S. S. Travis (✉)
College of Health and Human Services, George Mason University,
4400 University Drive, Fairfax, VA 22030-4444, USA

R. C. Talley
Western Kentucky University, 1906 College Heights Boulevard,
GRH 3023, Bowling Green, KY 42101, USA
e-mail: Ronda.Talley@wku.edu

R. C. Talley, S. S. Travis (eds.), *Multidisciplinary Coordinated Caregiving*,
Caregiving: Research • Practice • Policy, DOI 10.1007/978-1-4614-8973-3_1,

Our ultimate goal was to raise an individual and collective call to the professions for greater involvement in caregiving research, education, advocacy, policy, and practice and to create a point of departure for future collaborative efforts. We sought to develop a resource that would be respectful of the expertise that individual disciplines have contributed so mightily to direct care and to our current understanding of caregiving, while also providing a resource for those will ultimately create collaborative approaches to contemporary caregiving issues. Thus, the decision was made to present a set of interesting and relevant professions with the expectation that understanding discipline specific progress, problems, and concerns will educate those who are unfamiliar with a discipline and facilitate future dialogue about multidisciplinary and interdisciplinary perspectives on and interventions for complex caregiving in America.

Genesis of the Caregiving Book Series

Efforts to develop this book began in 2000, when Johnson & Johnson, an international health care business leader, and Dr. Ronda Talley, executive director of the Rosalynn Carter Institute for Caregiving, began discussions that led to the development of the Johnson & Johnson/Rosalynn Carter Institute Caregivers Program. Through this program, the Rosalynn Carter Institute convened a series of ten expert panels over a period of several years to address a wide variety of caregiving issues. These included disability, Alzheimer's disease, cancer, mental health, life span caregiving, rural caregiving, intergenerational caregiving, education and support for caregivers, building community caregiving capacity, and the topic of this volume, interdisciplinary professional caregiving. With Springer as our partner, the RCI books were integrated into the Springer caregiving book series, *Caregiving: Research, Policy, and Practice* with Dr. Talley as Editor-in-Chief.

Definitions

For the purpose of consistency throughout this book, several concepts will be defined here.

Caregiving means many things to individuals across different disciplines. Some disciplines are largely direct care providers or work closely with those who provide direct care, others study professional (formal) and nonprofessional (informal) caregivers and caregiving environments and services, and still others advocate for and create policy about caregivers and caregiving services and resources. We wondered what it would be like to ask authors of representative disciplines to describe their discipline-specific perspectives and contributions to caregiving in America. This chapter provides insight into how we addressed the question.

For our purposes, throughout our chapters we use the term *multidisciplinary* when we are referring to several individuals from different disciplines who share common goals, but are working independent of each other in discipline specific roles and functions (Antai-Otong 1997; Robertson 1992; Tuchman 1996). In contrast, *interdisciplinary* teams intentionally blur disciplinary boundaries in order to arrive at shared understanding of a problem and to bring their collective knowledge and skill to bear in achieving common goals (Robertson 1992; Tuchman 1996).

Throughout the book, we use the term *professional caregivers* to refer to paid care providers such as physicians, nurses, social workers, psychologists, case managers, hospice workers, home health aides, and many others. The designation as professional caregiver excludes those family caregivers who receive funds to provide care from new and emerging sources, such as the Medicaid Cash and Counseling Demonstration Program (Talley and Crews 2013).

Since professional caregivers and family caregivers work collaboratively to provide coordinated care, we feel that it is important to further address the definition of family caregivers as it is used in this book. To do so, we turned to several of the well-known caregiving researchers and advocacy groups.

The National Alliance for Caregiving and the American Association of Retired Persons (NAC-AARP, n.d.) define *caregiving* as "caring for an adult family member or friend." A second definition of caregiving, promoted by the National Family Caregivers Association (NFCA), is "offering the necessary physical and mental health support to care for a family member." Among the descriptions of informal or family caregiving, one that has been widely accepted over time was offered in 1985 by Horowitz, who indicated that informal care involves four dimensions: *direct care* (helping to dress, managing medications), *emotional care* (i.e., providing social support and encouragement), *mediation care* (i.e., negotiating with others on behalf of the care receiver), and *financial care* (i.e., through managing fiscal resources, including gifts or service purchases) (Horowitz, 1985).

The Administration on Aging (n.d.) defines a *caregiver* as "anyone who provides assistance to another in need."

Family caregiver is defined by the Health Plan of New York and NAC (n.d.) as "a person who cares for relatives and loved ones." Metlife and NAC (2006) expand on this by offering additional qualifiers; they state that a family caregiver is "a person who cares for relatives and loved ones who are frail, elderly, or who have a physical or mental disability." Similarly, the National Family Caregivers Association (NFCA, n.d.) adds that family caregivers provide a vast array of emotional, financial, nursing, social, homemaking, and other services on a daily or intermittent basis. The NFCA advocates for the term *family caregiver* to be defined broadly to include friends and neighbors who assist with care by providing respite, running errands, or a whole host of other tasks that support the caregiver and care recipient. In this volume, we use the terms informal caregiver and family caregiver interchangeably and employ the comprehensive definition of family caregiver that refers to caring relatives, friends, and neighbors.

Professional Caregiving Issues

We asked three questions to help us decide on the final selection of chapters. First, does the discipline value caregiving? We looked for this evidence in the volume of published articles, books, monographs, and reports on caregiving issues and the presence of caregiving topics on the programs of national or regional meetings. Second, what are the discipline-specific contributions to caregiving issues? Are the professional contributions largely in practice, research, education and training, policy and advocacy, or some combination of these areas? Since we asked our authors to address all of these areas, we sought chapters about professions that were concerned with most if not all aspects of these caregiving interests. Finally, what are the new disciplines that are becoming heavily engaged in contemporary caregiving related work? The affiliation of authors in published works and at various professional meetings provided some clues about new or up and coming involvement. The configuration and backgrounds of the members of special interest and advocacy groups, community coalitions, and demonstration projects also gave us important insights into their collaborative interests.

Early in our discussions, health communication and public health were clear contenders for selection along with the more traditional groups, such as gerontology, nursing, psychology, and social work. We looked at law, ethics, and environmental design, all of which have a place in a call to the professions around caregiving. But in the final analysis, we tried to select chapters that would meet our goal of creating the most valuable framework for the greatest number of people to engage in meaningful and important future collaborations around and initiatives targeted to caregiving issues and concerns. As you will see in the chapters that follow, we allowed some flexibility in the issues and content the authors decided to present about their disciplinary contributions to caregiving.

Another group of chapter in Part includes rather extensive chapters for human development, health communication, anthropology, public health, and public policy. These are all very broad and complex fields of disciplinary study that have the potential to significantly inform collaborative work with and about caregiving.

Human development comes from the field of home economics and draws heavily from the behavioral and social sciences, especially psychology and sociology. We included this chapter because so much of what is known about aging studies and family caregiving can be attributed to scholars with a human development and aging orientation. Life span development provides the integrated framework for the members of this discipline. The tenets of the life span development perspective are presented in this highly instructive chapter on caregiving and the caregiving experience. Many readers will likely find the sections on education and intervention practices to be informative and making a unique contribution to the whole of this text.

Health communication, we are told, includes two elements: message production and processing, and the creation of shared meaning about health issues and relationships. These frameworks are especially useful in health communication, health education, and health behavior study and practice. Although some of this work will be familiar to those readers from other disciplines, this chapter offers several excellent discussions of the applicability of the models for such activities as campaign designs and health risk assessments.

Our anthropology colleagues opted to focus on medical anthropology, as a subdiscipline within anthropology, in order to present an anthropology of caregiving. This is a very elegant chapter that will likely resonate well across most professions. It touches on gender and ethnicity issues and the cultural concepts of health and illness. If you have ever wondered how people learn the role of caregiver, this is a chapter you will read with great interest.

Public health is not a discipline that immediately comes to mind when thinking about caregiving. However, recently a group of colleagues argued that within a public health model, caregiving is an essential function involving family caregivers, care recipients, and professional caregivers. These collaborative partnerships are essential for effective management of disability and disease in vulnerable populations. The chapter defines public health caregiving and details the federal, state, department, scientific, and professional organizations that have influenced public health caregiving.

The final chapter in this group on public policy and caregiving describes the many challenges associated with designing and evaluating relevant and affordable social programs. It is a fitting closure to the discourse of the previous chapters because the author uses the critically important Medicaid and Medicare programs, to explain how policy professionals affect caregiving practice, education and training, research, public policy, and advocacy. This chapter provides an important overview of the relevant problems and issues to be addressed in all future discussions and deliberations.

Part I offers information about theoretical approaches and practice roles that tend to be identified with one discipline. Each author attributes his or her discipline with making significant contributions to the current state of caregiving in the USA, as viewed by the discipline. In reality, none of these authors believes that a single discipline or professional group has acted alone. This is the somewhat artificial environment in which we asked them to write their chapters. What we think readers will get out of these chapters is a better appreciation of the contributions that each discipline can bring to collaborative work and the strong professional identities they bring to caregiving collaborations. If you are in public policy, for example, a richer and deeper understanding of the discipline-specific theoretical contributions of individuals in social work will likely inform your future collective thinking about the economics and policy of caregiving and long-term care in ways that may redirect multidisciplinary and interdisciplinary scholarly inquiry.

Chapters 2, 4, and 6 in Part I represent a group of professions often classified as direct care providers. This includes nursing, social work, and occupational therapy, respectively. Each chapter provides some history of the profession and discipline specific orientations to care recipients and their informal caregivers. Chapter 2 describes family nursing practice. Chapter 4 introduces the social work perspective of person-in-environment. Chapter 6 describes the occupational therapy framework for client-centered care. In their own way, these disciplines articulate the value of holistic care for their clients. They also approach care with the similar goal of providing for the health and well-being of a client and his or her family, with full participation in decision making by the client and family caregivers. Although there is substantial evidence that these professions are committed to caregiving involvement, each chapter lays out a series of recommendations that range from organizational change within the profession to value change and educational reform that will position the groups for greater and more effective collaborative inquiry and discovery.

Chaps. 3, 5, and 7 in Part I present the caregiving perspectives of gerontology, psychology, and education. These three chapters complement the other three chapters in two important ways. First, these three disciplines have practice capability and technical language that does not necessarily apply to or reflect the practice paradigms of the direct practice disciplines. In other words, a broader interpretation of practice and different dimensions and nuances of caregiving practice are expressed in these three chapters. Second, the caregiving science provided by this set of authors is described in ways that establish a discipline as the origin and primary home for certain key concepts in caregiver research and practice. For example, stress, strain, and coping in the caregiving experience are most often associated with psychology. Intergenerational relations is a core feature of the gerontology literature on caregiving. By recognizing the disciplinary origins of these ideas, we can begin to understand how certain concepts and constructs have enjoyed what we call a "protective status" within a discipline, even as they are embraced, applied, and measured by others engaged in collaborative work.

There are several ways to think about the assortment of chapters in these two parts. First, most of the chapters present a broad spectrum of caregiving issues as defined by a unique disciplinary focus and context. The authors provide a rich historical perspective of the discipline and of the discipline's interest in and contributions to professional caregiving issues. As you read these chapters, do think about the unique contributions of each discipline. Do these contributions stand out as adding value to current and future collaborative work? Is the potential of the discipline being fully actualized, as evidenced by the work presented in the chapter, or is there more development that needs to occur?

Second, some disciplinary contributions to caregiving have continued to mature in quality, quantity, and innovation over time while others have not. Where stasis of ideas exists, what lessons can be learned from others to keep the discipline relevant and engaged in caregiving service and/or scholarship for the near and long term?

Finally, some disciplines are clearly in caregiving leadership roles, some are followers or adopters of the work of others, and some appear largely in supporting or occasional roles? Can a discipline be a leader in all aspects of caregiving: research, education, advocacy, policy, and practice? If not, is it clear what area or areas of activity the discipline should continue to pursue and develop in the future?

In the concluding chapter we revisit these ideas and probing questions in order to offer a summary of the many contributions being made to caregiving across the professions. Embedded in this summary is a call to the professions for individual and collaborative engagement in innovative research, education, practice, advocacy, and policy development on behalf of caregiving and caregivers of the twenty-first century.

References

Administration on Aging. (n.d.). *Resources: Common caregiving terms*. http://www.aoa.gov/prof/aoaprog/caregiver/careprof/progguidance/resources/caregiving_terms.asp.

Aneshensel, C. S., Pearlin, L. I., & Schuler, R. H. (1993). Stress, role captivity, and the cessation of caregiving. *Journal of Health and Social Behavior, 34*(1), 54–70.

Antai-Otong, D. (1997). Team building in a health care setting. *American Journal of Nursing, 97*(7), 48–51.

Berg-Weger, M., Rubio, D. M., & Tebb, S. (2001). Strengths-based practice with family caregivers of the chronically Ill: Qualitative insights. *Families in Society, 82*(3), 263–272.

Gillon, S. (2004). *Boomer nation: The largest and richest generation ever and how it changed America*. New York: Free Press.

Health Plan of New York & National Alliance for Caregiving. (n.d.). *Care for the family caregiver: A place to start*. http://www.caregiving.org/pubs/brochures/CFC.pdf.

Horowitz, A. (1985). Family caregiving to the frail elderly. In C. Eisdorfer (Ed.), *Annual review of gerontology and geriatrics* (5th ed. pp. 194–246).

Macunovich, D. J. (2002). *Birth quake: The baby boom and its aftershocks*. Chicago: The University of Chicago Press.

Metlife & National Alliance for Caregiving. (2006). *2006 MetLife Foundation family caregiver awards program*. Retrieved from

Montgomery, R. J. V., Gonyea, J., & Hooyman, N. (1985). Caregiving and the experience of subjective and objective burden. *Family Relations, 34*, 19–26.

National Alliance for Caregiving & American Association of Retired Persons (NAC/AARP). (2004). *Caregiving in the U.S.* Washington: Author. http://www.caregiving.org/data/04finalreport.pdf.

National Family Caregiver Association. (n.d.). *What is family caregiving?* http://www.thefamily-caregiver.org/what/what.cfm

Robertson, D. (1992). The roles of health care teams in care of the elderly. *Family Medicine, 24*, 136–141.

Schumacher, K., Stewart, B., Archbold, P., Dood, M., & Dibble, S. (2000). Family caregiving skill: Development of the concept. *Research in Nursing & Health, 23*, 191–203.

Seltzer, M. M., & Li, L. W. (2000). The dynamics of caregiving: Transitions during a three-year prospective study. *Gerontologist, 40*(2), 165–178.

Talley, R. C., & Crews, J. E. (Eds.). (2013). *The multiple dimensions of caregiving and disability*. New York: Springer.

Travis, S. S., & Duer, B. (2000). Interdisciplinary management of the older adult with cancer. In A. Luggen & S. Meiner (Eds.), *Handbook of care of the older adult with cancer* (pp. 25–34). Pittsburg: Oncology Nursing Press.

Tuchman, L. I. (1996). The team and models of teaming. In P. Rosen, A. Whitehead, L. I. Tuchman, G. S. Jesien, A. L. Begun, & L. Irwin (Eds.), *Partnerships in family-centered care* (pp. 119–143). Baltimore: Paul Brookes Publishing.

Part II
Discipline-specific Professional Caregiving

The State of Family Caregiving: A Nursing Perspective

Katherine Morton Robinson

Family caregiving is an area that has received extensive attention in the professional and public domains. The graying of America, the looming aging and retirement of the baby-boomers, increased pressures to care for the chronically ill in their homes, and changes in health care service reimbursement systems all contribute to the generalized concerns regarding caregiving.

Nursing constitutes the largest group of all health professions (Spratley et al. 2000). Nurses practice with families of all sorts and in all settings, addressing physical, psychological, social, emotional, and spiritual needs and problems. The relationship(s) between nursing theory, nursing practice, nursing education, nursing research, and family caregiving are explored in this chapter.

Background and Current Status

Popular images of nursing include the compassionate bedside caregiver in the highly technical acute care (hospital) setting. Many do not realize that nursing is much more than caring for the acutely ill. During its early developmental years, American nursing flourished in the community. Nurses cared for both individuals and families in their homes and communities before becoming the primary bedside caregivers in hospitals (Kalisch and Kalisch 1995). Today, nursing practice includes caring for families, communities, and individuals in a variety of settings including hospitals, sub-acute and long-term care facilities, clinics, and homes. Furthermore, nurses provide services to patients and families, caregivers and care-receivers of all ages (International Council of Nurses [ICN], n. d.). Hence, it is natural for nurses, in practice and in academia, to be vitally interested in the welfare of family caregivers.

K. M. Robinson (✉)
University of North Florida, 1 UNF Drive,
Jacksonville, FL 32224, USA
e-mail: krobinso@unf.edu

R. C. Talley, S. S. Travis (eds.), *Multidisciplinary Coordinated Caregiving*,
Caregiving: Research • Practice • Policy, DOI 10.1007/978-1-4614-8973-3_2,

Theoretical Foundations of the Discipline of Nursing

The theoretical matrix for the discipline of nursing is complex. With such a wide variation in practice settings and a scope of practice involved with health promotion, disease prevention, illness and symptom management, birth and death, and work with individuals, families, communities and populations, it is extraordinarily difficult to distill the essence of nursing into one theoretical document. Not one theoretical or conceptual framework is dominant (Fawcett 2000; Meleis 1997).

In the early 1980s, the nursing industry attempted to describe its central purposes and functions in a metaparadigm of nursing (Fawcett 1984). The new paradigm, consisting of the constructs of person, environment, health and nursing, and the propositions describing their respective relationships is widely, but not universally accepted (Fawcett 2000). Other nurse theorists have suggested that the constructs of human care, environmental context and well-being (health) should be substituted for the constructs outlined above (Leininger 1995), or that the construct of caring, considered central to nursing, be added to the metaparadigm (Watson 1990). In the metaparadigm as described by Fawcett (1984), the concept of family, or one of its permutations, is included only implicitly. It is not specifically defined or mentioned.

A few nurse scientists have attempted to examine the phenomena of family caregiving within the context of one of nursing's grand theories (Andershed and Ternestedt 1999; Geden and Taylor 1999; Shyu 2000; Yamashita 1997). Many others have studied the phenomena within the context of other disciplines, such as Marxism, critical theory, feminism, and sociology (Bridges and Lynam 1993; Redding 2000; Wuest 1998).

While the grand theorists in nursing have not explicitly included the concept or construct of family in their writings, there has been theorizing about the nature of the family and its relationship to nursing through the subspecialty of Family Nursing. Three dominant models have emerged (Hanson et al. 2001; International Council of Nurses n. d.):

1. The Family Systems Stressor–Strength Model and Inventory (Hanson and Mischke 1996);
2. The Friedman Family Assessment Model (Friedman 1998);
3. The Calgary Family Assessment and Intervention models (Wright and Leahey 1984).

Each of these models describes the nature of the relationship between nurses and families, but each also draws heavily on theories from other disciplines (Hanson and Boyd 1996). As in the grand theories, none of the specific family models in nursing directly address the phenomena of family caregiving.

Theoretical Background for Family Caregiving in Nursing

As with the discipline, no single theoretical description of the relationship between nursing practice and family caregivers has emerged. Among the variety of mid-range family caregiving theories generated within the discipline, one of the most respected is Bower's Model of Intergenerational Family Caregiving (Bowers 1987). In this model, caregiving was conceptualized as anticipatory, preventive, supervisory, instrumental, or protective. Bowers was one of the earliest researchers in nursing to systematically identify caregiving functions that ranged beyond hands-on, physical (instrumental) care. Bowers' model was developed after observing adult children who were caring for frail, elderly parents. Although Bowers' model is widely cited, it has not been tested for its applicability to other family caregiving populations.

Carol Smith (1994, 1999) developed and tested a model of caregiving effectiveness, which has been refined into a midrange theory (Smith 2002). In the earlier Smith model, the variables of caregiver mutuality, preparedness, family economic stability, esteem from caregiving, and social support accounted for significant variance in the outcomes of quality caregiving (i.e., quality of life for patients and caregivers, patient's physical condition, and technological side effects). The studies from which the theory was generated included the caregivers of patients receiving lifelong mechanical ventilation, total parenteral nutrition, or continuous intravenous therapy designed to support a failing heart. Methodologies used to develop, refine, and test the theory were both qualitative and quantitative, and included the use of a number of established instruments. Sample sizes for all model testing achieved appropriate power. Smith's Caregiving Effectiveness Model is the most robust caregiving theory developed by a nurse.

In the early 1990s, Zerwekh (1991, 1992) approached the study of family caregiving from the perspective of public health nurses, resulting in The Family Caregiving Model for Public Health Nursing. Zerwekh identified three competencies for public health nurses that are considered foundational to providing family centered care: locating the family, building trust, and building strength. Different strategies used to achieve each competency were identified. The model has not been tested or modified for use in practice areas other than public health.

Other researchers have studied caregiving conceptually, but have not generated theoretical models. Schumacher et al. (Schmuacher et al. 1998, 2000) sought to review the conceptualization and measurement of five concepts related to effective family caregiving: caregiving mastery, self-efficacy, competence, preparedness, and quality. Although these concepts have not been organized into a model at this time, their definition and measurement contribute to nursing's understanding of the dynamics of family caregiving.

Numerous other studies, many of them qualitative, have endeavored to describe family caregiving in a theoretical or conceptual fashion. These young models have the potential to develop into midrange theory, but will require more testing and exploration before they can be considered at that level. A variety of types of caregivers have been studied: patients with potentially fatal illnesses (Brown and Stetz 1999), technology dependent children in socially marginalized families (Cohen 1999), care of children with serious chronic diseases (Hilbert et al. 2000; Spalding and McKeever 1998; Wilson et al. 1998), patients requiring complex care (Robinson 1999), and patients with cancer (Schumacher 1996; Steele and Fitch 1996; Stetz 1996). Numerous other conceptual descriptions exist of similar caregiving/care-receiving populations.

The Standards of Nursing Practice Related to Family Caregiving

Although family centered care is not explicitly addressed in either the metaparadigm or any of the grand theories or conceptual models of nursing, it is addressed in statements describing professional practice. Standards of practice exist both for the nursing profession in general organizations (e.g., American Nurse's Association, International Council for Nursing) and specialty organizations within the profession (e.g., American Association of Critical Care Nurses, American Rehabilitation Nurses Organization, American Association of Oncology Nurses, etc.). In each set of published standards, bylaws, or mission statements, there exists a phrase or sentence that describes the inclusion of family members in the planning and provision of nursing care (American Association of Critical Care Nurses 2004; International Council of Nurses n. d.; McCourt 1993; Oncology Nursing Society & Association of Oncology Social Work 2000). If one was to pick up any standard introductory nursing text (Delaune and Ladner 2002; Harkreader and Hogan 2004), one would also find statements, long or short, reinforcing the importance of including the family in the provision of quality care. It would appear, therefore, that there is a strong commitment at the practice level, by the profession, to provide sensitive care to families, and by extension, to family caregivers.

The State of Practice with Family Caregivers

Nurses may interact with family caregivers in a variety of settings, including hospitals, private homes, and long-term care facilities. Nursing practice with family caregivers in each of these settings will be explored.

Nurses and family caregivers in the home Most informal caregiving (87 %) is provided in private homes (National Alliance for Caregiving & AARP 2004). Family members, while they are recognized by the home health care industry as crucial contributors to patient welfare, receive only fragmented professional services. Home health care reimbursement has changed dramatically from the time of the earliest Visiting Nurse Services to the present. Third payer payments are directed towards the care of the *patient*, not the family. Home health nurses have less time to provide support for family caregivers, due to the necessary streamlining of services required by prospective payment reimbursement schemes. There is no specific allowance for care of the caregiver. Other countries, such as the UK, have mandated that the needs of family caregivers (carers) as well as their care recipients be assessed (McKenna 2003), but no such requirement or standard exists in the USA. In October 2005, on request, the Centers for Medicaid and Medicare Services (CMS) released a set of outcome measures designed to give consumers and health care providers information concerning the effectiveness of home health care programs. Notably, none of the 15 outcome measures directly address supportive or instructive care for caregivers (Health Services Advisory Group 2005; National Quality Forum 2007). A noted health care analyst and family caregiver commented on the quality of long-term home health care: "It is not cheap, but it is feasible. The lack of such relief is primarily a problem of public policy and political will" (Somers 1999, p. 1005).

There is no doubt that individual nurses and agencies work closely with family caregivers. However, the amount of care and support received by family members remains largely a function of an individual home care agency or nurse's philosophy of care. Third party payers do not financially support interventions with family caregivers.

Nurses and family caregivers in the hospital Approximately 60 % of all nurses are employed in hospitals (American Association of Colleges of Nursing 2002). This is one of the practice settings where they most frequently encounter family caregivers. Many care recipients, due to the nature of their chronic illnesses, require occasional hospitalization. The stated commitment of the profession to family centered care indicates that the care provided to family members in hospitals will be stellar, sensitive, and compassionate. Sadly, however, this is not always so. Isolated shining examples of family centered care exist in acute or chronic care settings (Ford and Turner 2001; Heermann and Wilson 2000; Hostler 1999), but family members of hospitalized patients feel these instances are few and far between.

One family caregiver describes her perceptions of nurses providing basic care during the hospitalization of her quadriplegic son:

> You usually have to tell them [hospital staff] how... but they don't ask for it. They bulldoze without knowing how, anyway. A lot of times, he [the patient] is well enough that he can say "do this, do that" and he can walk them through how to turn him or how to do certain things with him. But they tend to want to do it their way. They need to listen. (Robinson 1999, p. 115)

Other family members speak of feeling demeaned, overlooked, excluded or ignored (Dunne and Sullivan 2000; Fenwick et al. 2001; Heermann and Wilson 2000; Levine and Zuckerman 2000). In a recent interaction with a nursing student, a nurse faculty member inquired about the caregiving preparation for an 80-year-old husband who would now be providing significant care to his wife. The faculty member asked: "How is he going to handle her?" The nurse assigned to the patient responded, "I have no idea" (personal communication). One observer of the status of family centered care remarked: "Despite much rhetoric about partnership and participation, our professional language and subsequent behavior continue to reflect a hierarchical position with respect to patients and families" (Mohr 2000, p. 18).

Nurses and family caregivers in long-term care Another clinical setting where nurses have the opportunity to interact with family caregivers is in long-term care facilities. Levy-Storms and Miller-Martinez (2005) recently examined caregiver satisfaction with care during the first year of institutionalization. They found that caregivers became less satisfied with institutional care as time went on, and concluded "a meaningful caregiving role after institutionalization is not facilitated by nursing homes" (p. 160). Bauer and Nay (2003) reviewed the literature concerning family and staff partnerships in long-term care for the last 20 years. They observed that caregivers suffer considerable distress when patients are admitted to long-term care and suggested that establishing close partnerships between long-term care staff and caregivers has the potential to decrease family stress, and increase satisfaction. A group of nurse researchers from the University of Iowa has been testing a Family Involvement in Care (FIC) partnership intervention with the families of dementia patients (Jablonski et al. 2005; Maas et al. 2004; Specht et al. 2000). They concluded that the partnership intervention improves the quality of the caregiving experience for family members, and improves nursing home staff attitudes towards families (Maas et al. 2004, p. 76). Despite these findings, there continues to be relatively little family-centered care provided in long-term care facilities by nurses. As with home health care and acute care, some of the reasons for inadequate support of family caregivers relate to the practices of individual nurses and facilities. However, rather than vilifying the staff, other explanations of the paucity of professional nursing support for family caregivers in day-to-day clinical environments must be explored. There are centers of excellence where families and nurses collaborate together in mutually satisfying relationships (Archbold et al. 1995; Stewart 1995; Vander-Laan et al. 2001), but many families continue to report frustration and unhappiness with the care they receive.

Factors that Negatively Impact Nursing Practice with Caregivers

A frank discussion about family caregiving issues with practicing nurses in settings of all types would proffer many reasons for failing to include family caregivers as respected partners in the caregiving process. The first would be: "We don't have enough staff/time." Complaints about poor staffing are an almost reflexive response whenever nurses are confronted concerning quality of care issues. Although this explanation is readily and commonly offered, it should neither be ignored nor dismissed. Staffing issues are of central concern to the practices of professional nurses across all settings, throughout the United States and the rest of the world (Aiken et al. 2001; Buelow and Cruijssen 2002; Navaie-Waliser et al. 2004). CMS collates staffing data reported by nursing homes that receive Medicare and Medicaid funds. (Approximately 77 % of the reimbursement for long-term care is provided by CMS.) These data show that the average number of registered nursing (RN) hours per resident per day is only 0.64 h (Centers for Medicare and Medicaid Services 2005). These hours include the onerous record keeping responsibilities of professional nurses in long-term care. It becomes easier to understand why professional nurses are unable to provide significant support to family caregivers of residents, despite the demonstrated benefits. Hospitals have fared no better. The last 20 years have seen steady erosion in nursing full-time equivalency (FTE) positions adjusted for increased patient acuity, and inpatient and outpatient volume (Aiken et al. 1996, 2000a). As nursing departments were restructured in the 1980s and 1990s as a result of cost-saving measures, the expert nurse, the Clinical Nurse Specialist, and Nurse Educator, became increasingly rare commodities in the health care work force. Clinical specialists frequently have extensive interactions with family members. However, less than 1 % of all nurses currently employed in acute care settings in the USA are employed as Clinical Nurse Specialists, and only 4 % are employed as educators

(Spratley et al. 2001). As a result, nurses are being asked to do more for patients in less time and with less support and guidance from expert colleagues. Additionally, as the nursing work force ages, a dramatic nursing shortage has risen and is expected to persist (Kimball 2004; Levine 2001). As reimbursement has tightened, home health care nurses have been forced to complete more visits every day and prepare extensive clinical documentation, taking time away from patient and family care. In order to provide family centered care, both staffing patterns and staffing supply need to be remedied (Buelow and Cruijssen 2002).

Structural/organizational issues other than staffing also contribute to inadequate family nursing practices. In a recent study by Aiken et al. (2000a), nurse characterizations of their hospitals were reported, using a 1986 dataset and data collected in 1998. Of the 24 hospital characteristics reviewed, 18 showed declines. Nurses reported decreased satisfaction with the quality of care they were giving, as well as feeling less supported by nursing or hospital administration, less in control of their practice, and less involved in policy formation. Additionally, in 30 % of the cases, nurses reported that their Chief Nursing Executive was no longer "equal in power/authority to other top hospital officials" (p. 463). Fewer than 50 % of the nurses surveyed felt that they had enough time to get their work done. These feelings are echoed by nurses in other settings as well (Buelow and Cruijssen 2002; Navaie-Waliser et al. 2004). Other organizational barriers to the provision of family centered care were described by Rutledge et al. (2000a): lack of endorsement of a strategic philosophy of family centered care in both the service setting vision and mission, lack of materials for family education, little to no organization of outpatient services, and environmental and architectural barriers.

Caring for family caregivers, whether it is caregiver education, emotional support or needs assessment, is not valued by current reimbursement systems. In a healthcare system where productivity is of paramount importance, it is difficult to offer a service that is not valued by or compensated for by the third party payers (CMS and private health insurance). Nurses struggle to perform routine and critical assessments, administer prescribed medications and treatments, assist with diagnostic tests, evaluate patient response, and perform necessary clerical and record keeping tasks. In the rushed clinical atmosphere, family preparation for caregiving responsibility is reduced to the provision of booklets or the sharing of a video. Too often, the family is left at the bedside or in the home, anxious, full of questions, and frustrated.

Future Needs and New Directions

Professional Nursing Issues

As it has been stated, the profession is committed to family centered care as expressed in policies and standards, but not consistently carried out in practice. In many instances, work place issues such as staffing patterns and work designs do not allow for sensitive family care. These are not, however, the only explanation for inadequate family care. Nurses need to look to their own behaviors as well. In their recent analysis, Rutledge et al. (2000a) identified the following nurse/staff barriers to family centered care: nurses' lack of confidence in their communication abilities, limited follow-through on identified family problems, and lack of knowledge concerning the components of family-centered care.

Nurses struggle to attain power and control in their practice settings. They are highly knowledgeable individuals who, by tradition, law, or policy, are frequently reduced to having to request a physician's "order" for something as simple as a specialized dressing or adaptive device for a patient. By and large, nurses are educated to practice with much more autonomy than they are permitted to exercise in most health care institutions. Despite vigorous efforts by the profession, the image of nursing has been described as "powerless, dependent, unintelligent, and underpaid" (Takase et al. 2001). Sharing power with, and ceding power and knowledge to family members can be uncomfortable and threatening:

It's real intimidating to have the parents tell you, or worse yet not to ask them ahead and just do it your way and find out that is not what they had in mind. That's really threatening . . . it was intimidating to have [a parent] say "No, I don't do it this way. This is how we do it." . . . It's kind of a transfer of power. It's like abdicating my power (Heermann and Wilson 2000, p. 25).

In some practice settings, such as the critical care unit, the needs of the patient are so extensive that the family is actually viewed as interfering with patient care. When a family's needs are too overwhelming, or the nurses are too busy or tired, control may be maintained by enforcing visiting hours and asking family members to leave (Hupcey 1999).

Nurses have also been socialized by their educational processes and work environments to demonstrate knowledge, competence, and confidence in their practice. For some, it is extremely difficult to acknowledge and rely upon the expertise of a non-professional partner (family caregiver). Exhibiting expertise is part of the nursing identity.

Nursing work in acute care agencies is organized around a very task-oriented conceptualization of nursing. It is difficult for nurses to step out of the model and perform as counselors, teachers, or coaches. Some may even feel that it is "not their job." Kohnke described this issue in 1974:

> Professional nurses . . . who function according to a professional design model encounter resistance from other nurses and people in other professions . . . there are two primary reasons for resistance . . . the first derives from the poor image of nursing held by some people in other professions . . . the second is that some other professions perceive professionalism in nursing as a potential threat to their power. (p. 129)

It is no different today. In settings where nurses are harried, over-worked, under-respected, and not permitted to use all the skills and knowledge they have acquired, it is difficult to provide excellent, compassionate care to families. This is not to say that excellence in family care does not exist, but in many instances it exists not because it is supported or rewarded by the institution but in spite of the institution.

Institutional Policy and Organizational Change

What kind of organizational changes need to be made to promote professional nursing practice, including practice with family caregivers? One model, the Magnet Nursing Services Recognition Program for Excellence in Nursing Services, was originally developed for acute care settings, but has been extended to long-term care facilities and home health agencies as well. The American Nurse's Credentialing Center (ANCC), the administrator of the Magnet Nursing Service Recognition Program, states:

This program provides a framework to recognize excellence in:

1. The management philosophy and practices of nursing services;
2. Adherence to standards for improving the quality of patient care;
3. Leadership of the chief nurse executive in supporting professional practice and continued competence of nursing personnel;
4. Attention to the cultural and ethnic diversity of patients and their significant others, as well as the care providers in the system (American Nurse's Credentialing Center 2007).

Implementing organizational changes such as those recommended by ANCC does result in meaningful changes in the practice environment. Improved outcomes found in Magnet designees include (Aiken et al. 2000b; Scott et al. 1999):

1. Increased autonomy
2. Increased control over the practice setting
3. Higher RN–patient ratios
4. Increased opportunity to participate in policy decisions
5. Increased satisfaction with "having enough RNs to provide quality care"
6. Decreased nurse burn-out
7. Decreased job frustration
8. Increased job satisfaction
9. Decreased patient mortality
10. Increased patient satisfaction
11. Increased educational preparation of staff nurses.

Another group, The American Association of Colleges of Nursing (2002), issued a white paper identifying hallmarks of the professional practice environment. Early in this document, they stated: "Clinical practice refers to all direct and indirect patient care activities undertaken to provide nursing care to individuals, families, or groups" (p. 4), reaffirming nursing's commitment to family inclusion.

Although there is no direct measure of family centered care practices in the Magnet Nursing Service or AACN standards, it does seem probable that family-centered care is more likely to be practiced in a setting where a professional nursing practice model flourishes. This is an area for future study.

Nursing Education

Registered nurses are educationally prepared for practice through a variety of mechanisms. Most registered nurses today receive their initial educational preparation for nursing at either the associate degree (junior college) or baccalaureate level. There are some who receive initial preparation at the master's or doctoral level, although these are very few. In the last 5 years, 61 % of new nursing graduates received their preparation in associate degree programs, and 35 % from baccalaureate programs. The remaining 4 % were educated in hospital based diploma schools (National Council of State Boards of Nursing 2005). All students from programs preparing registered nurses write the same licensing examination following their graduation and receive the same license to practice.

In addition to the multiple points of entry for registered nurses, licensed practical or vocational nurses exist, educated in either high school or junior college programs, certified nursing assistants (prepared in on-the-job training programs), and home health aides. These multiple points of entry into the profession have created a variety of problems for nursing. There is tension between nurses prepared in different programs and confusion in the work place as to how their work-roles should be differentiated, if at all (Nichols 2001; Wisdom 2001). This multiplicity of roles also occasionally creates confusion in the minds of the public as to "who is the nurse?" In this paper, however, the discussion is limited to registered nurses.

Associate degree nurses are prepared with basic knowledge and skills that allow them to practice with individuals, families, and communities. They have minimal preparation in therapeutic communication, adult teaching and learning and case management. Baccalaureate prepared nurses, in addition to the preparation received by their associate degree nurse colleagues, receive additional education concerning family and group dynamics, leadership, research, teaching and learning, case management, and aggregate care. Some of them will also learn basic support and counseling techniques. Registered nurses with masters or doctoral degrees may be prepared to provide individual and group therapy, design and evaluate sophisticated intervention programs, conduct nursing research, or provide primary health care to patients and families.

In most health care agencies, many of the roles the nurses have been prepared for are not included in the work design, so their enactment is neither facilitated nor rewarded. With few exceptions, all nurses who function as "staff nurses" will have the same job responsibilities within an agency. A nurse with advanced degree preparation who wishes to remain "at the bedside," giving direct patient care, will be expected to perform exactly the same work as her associate degree nurse colleague. The additional skills of the nurse with the advanced degree may be lost to the patient and the family. Therefore, nursing practice is reduced to the least common denominator.

When reviewing the curricula of a basic nursing program, one will probably find a course labeled "Family Nursing." This course will include at the very least, the care of pregnant and delivering women, and infants and children. It may or may not include family theory and intervention. It is unlikely that a course relating specifically to family caregiving will be found. Family caregiving is mentioned in most textbooks, with a varying degree of emphasis. Students may graduate from a basic nursing program without receiving any formal information regarding family caregiving. They may not even work with a family caregiver during their clinical experiences. The American Association of Colleges of Nursing state in their list of essentials for baccalaureate preparation that the baccalaureate nurse will be prepared to "anticipate, plan for, and manage physical, psychological, social, and spiritual needs of the patient and family/caregiver" (American Association of Colleges of Nursing 1998, p. 13). As in the practice arena, the commitment to family caregiving is present at the level of standards, but its visibility in the classroom and clinical experiences of students is variable.

Nursing Research

Family caregiving is more visible in nursing research than either in clinical practice or education. In a recent search of the Cumulative Index to Nursing and Allied Health Literature (CINAHL), there were over 1,000 hits to a combined search of the terms "caregiver" and "nursing" in peer-reviewed journals. Of these, approximately 50 % were concerned with caregiving of the frail elderly or patients with dementia. Both Farran (2001) and Rutledge et al. (2000a, 2000b) have conducted comprehensive reviews of the caregiving research literature. The reader is referred to these analyses for a much more detailed review than is possible in this chapter.

Both Farran (2001) and Rutledge et al. (2000b) noted that the majority of nursing research that has been conducted concerning caregiving is of an exploratory, descriptive nature. Farran notes that in the 1980s, descriptive research on caregiving included a great deal of emphasis on stressors associated with caregiving and their effects on the caregivers and their social roles, as well as the resources available to caregivers. In the 1990s, studies began to focus on positive aspects of caregiving and multicultural caregiving. In the 1990s and the early part of the twenty-first century, intervention and model testing studies have become more visible but continue to represent only a small portion of the nursing research conducted on family caregiving. Craft and Willadsen (1992) identified a typology of nine categories of family-centered interventions: family support, process maintenance, integrity promotion, involvement, mobilization, therapy, caregiver support, sibling support, and parent education. The bulk of the family caregiving intervention studies that have been conducted are using psycho-educational interventions such as support groups, educational programs or strategies, and behavior management (Farran 2001; Rutledge et al. 2000b), falling under Craft and Willadsen's categories of caregiver support and parent education. The areas of family process maintenance, family mobilization, and family involvement, all cogent to caregiving, remain understudied. Of the intervention studies that have been conducted, most are small, limited to one area (not multi-center), and have not yet been replicated.

As a young academic discipline, much of the research conducted in nursing is found in master's theses and doctoral dissertations. A search of *Dissertation Abstracts International* shows that over 350 doctoral dissertations concerning family caregiving have been authored by nurses; of these, the majority are descriptive, correlational, or comparative studies. Very few manipulate an independent variable. A few test theoretical models. Not one theoretical framework, outcome, intervention, or instrument dominates.

Research gaps There are a few established programs of research that are testing models and interventions. At least two nurse scientists are involved in long-term programs of intervention research. Archbold (1991, 1995, 1999) has been studying PREP, a nursing intervention to increase preparedness, enrichment and predictability in caregiving since the early 1990s and is currently conducting a 5-year evaluation of the PREP nursing intervention funded by the National Institute of Aging, the Agency for Healthcare Research and Quality, the National Institute of Nursing Research, and National Institutes of Health. However, Archbold's work, like many others', is limited primarily to the elderly. Smith (1994, 1999) has developed and tested a model of caregiving effectiveness in patients receiving complex technologic care in the home. This body of research has resulted in the generation of a midrange theory. Smith continues to conduct intervention studies with varied groups of patients receiving technologic care in the home. Phillips (Hsueh et al. 2005; Phillips 1983, 2001; Phillips and Rempusheski 1986; Phillips et al. 1990; Phillips et al. 1995) has published extensively over the last 20 years, addressing a variety of caregiving topics, including caregiver abuse, instrument development, and transcultural aspects of caregiving. As previously noted, cursory reviews of both CINAHL and *Dissertation Abstracts International* show that the bulk of caregiving research conducted by nurses is descriptive, correlational, or comparative in nature. While there are attempts at developing and testing models of caregiving, very little research examines the effectiveness of interventions directed towards caregivers. No standard set of outcome measures has been studied.

State of the science: Informal family caregiving NINR workgroup The National Institute of Nursing Research (NINR) convened a workgroup, Research in Informal Caregiving: State of the Science, to examine the state of the science of informal caregiving research in nursing in July 2001 (NINR 2001). Three areas of research opportunities were identified: informal caregiving populations; caregiver knowledge, skills, and support; and impact on the caregiver.

The workgroup noted the paucity of population-based research of informal caregivers. Most nursing research directed towards understanding the processes of informal caregiving depends on convenience samples. Additionally, caregivers from diverse ethnic groups of all ages, both genders, and from both rural and urban populations should be included in caregiving research. The workgroup also observed that caregivers care for patients with a variety of types and severity of illnesses, and that these groups of caregivers should be studied as well.

The second area of opportunity identified was caregiver knowledge, skills, and support. In this area, the workgroup commented that it is essential to understand how caregivers best acquire their skills and how required skills and knowledge change over time. The need to develop and test research-based and caregiver-oriented interventions was emphasized. Researchers were reminded to include cultural considerations when planning caregiver research. The workgroup acknowledged that caregiving occurs over a continuum, and the needs of the caregivers are likely to change during transitions in illness. In addition to knowledge about disease management and instrumental skills, caregivers need information about available resources and need to be supported in problem solving skills and decision-making.

The third research opportunity identified by the workgroup was the impact on the caregiver. The workgroup reminded nurse researchers that although burden has been extensively studied in caregivers, not all caregivers are burdened. The variety and depth of both positive and negative aspects of the caregiving experience need to be considered. Other areas that need to be studied include strategies employed by caregivers for personal health maintenance, impact of caregiving on other members of the caregiving family, and strategies that can be implemented to ameliorate negative responses and reinforce positive responses to the act of caregiving.

Extramural funding for family caregiving research has been limited. During the first 14 years of NINR funding, only 114 grants were awarded to study family caregiving. The NINR emphasized the importance of studying family (informal) caregiving by convening the workgroup in 2001, issuing the first R0-1 call for papers in 2001, and identifying informal caregiving as a research priority in 2002. Since 2001, an additional 157 grants have been awarded by the NINR. It is more difficult to quantify numbers of funded studies awarded to nurse researchers who are examining aspects of family caregiving, but other institutes in the National Institutes of Health, private foundations, and intramural funding sources have awarded such grants. The increased availability of NINR funding and its emphasis on family caregiving should result in a whole new generation of intervention and outcome studies related to family caregiving and nursing.

Summary and Conclusions

As a discipline, nursing has the potential to contribute extensively and meaningfully to the health and well being of both caregivers and care-receivers. To offer its best, however, significant professional and policy changes must be made.

One of the first changes required does not necessitate effort by any policymaking body external to the discipline. The culture within which nurses practice, whether it be their academic culture or their work culture, needs to be reconstructed in such a way as to see families and their needs as central, not peripheral to nursing practice. Family care can no longer be a "nice extra" or a luxury; it must become a core component of what nurses do. The groundwork for this cultural change has been laid in the standards of the profession; the enactment is left to the practicing nurse and to the profession's leaders.

Support for family caregivers cannot be consistently rendered if it continues to be an undervalued, non-reimbursed service. Hospitals and other health care agencies should be reimbursed adequately to allow them to provide this necessary service.

Professional environments must be created that allow nurses to practice using all the skills and knowledge they have acquired in their education and during their careers. If professionals do not feel respected, valued, and satisfied, it is difficult for them to provide creative, compassionate, and individualized care to families. The time has come for health care agencies to understand that nurses of varying levels of education bring different skills to the clinical work place, and assignments and workloads should be modified accordingly. Nurses can no longer be treated as interchangeable cogs on a wheel.

Family caregiving needs to be more specifically and critically addressed in nursing curricula and textbooks. The stated commitment of the profession to family centered care needs to be operationalized in every course and every clinical experience. Nurses who have been out of the formal educational setting for sometime should be offered the opportunity to learn about family caregiving.

Nurses must also have the tools to provide care to family caregivers. Quality assessment guides, educational and support programs, and evaluation tools, all derived from excellent research, need to be available to the practicing nurse. The wealth of knowledge about caregiving must be distilled into useable forms.

References

Aiken, L., Sochalski, J., & Anderson, G. (1996). Downsizing the hospital nursing workforce. *Health Affairs, 15*(4), 88–92.

Aiken, L., Clarke, S., &, Sloane, D. (2000a, Oct). Hospital restructuring: Does it adversely affect care and outcomes? *Journal of Nursing Administration, 30*(10), 457–465.

Aiken, L., Havens, D., & Sloane, D. (2000b). The magnet nursing services recognition program: A comparison of two groups of magnet hospitals. *American Journal of Nursing, 100*(3), 26–36.

Aiken, L., Clarke, S., Sloane, D., Sochalski, J., Busse, R., Clarke, H., et al. (2001). Nurses' reports on hospital care in five countries: The ways in which nurses' work is structured have left nurses among the least satisfied workers, and the problem is getting worse. *Health Affairs, 20*(3), 43–53.

American Association of Colleges of Nursing. (1998). *The essentials of baccalaureate education or professional nursing practice*. Washington: Author.

American Association of Colleges of Nursing. (2002). *Your nursing career: A look at the facts.* http://www.aacn.nche.edu/education/Career.htm. Accessed 18 Mar 2007.

American Association of Critical Care Nurses. (2004, March). *Standards for acute and critical care nursing practice.* http://www.aacn.org/AACN/practice.nsf/ad0ca3b3bdb4f33288256981006fa692/5e3c9805e57b3b0888256a6b00791f35?OpenDocument. Accessed 18 Mar 2007.

American Nurses' Credentialing Center. (2007). *Magnet nursing services recognition program.* http://www.nursingworld.org/ancc/magnet/index.html. Accessed 23 Mar 2007.

Andershed, B., & Ternestedt, B. (1999). Involvement of relatives in care of the dying in different care cultures: Development of a theoretical understanding. *Nursing Science Quarterly, 12*(1), 45–51.

Archbold, P. (1991). An interdisciplinary approach to family caregiving research. *Communicating Nursing Research, 24,* 27–42.

Archbold, P. (1999). Grant number 5R01AG17909–02 [Grant Abstract]. Washington: National Institute of Nursing Research. (Principal Investigator)

Archbold, P., Stewart, B., Miller, L., Harvath, T., Greenlick, M., Van-Buren, L., et al. (1995). The PREP system of nursing interventions: A pilot test with families caring for older members: Preparedness (PR), enrichment (E), and predictability (P). *Research in Nursing and Health, 18*(1), 3–16.

Bauer, M., & Nay, R. (2003). Family and staff partnerships in long-term care: A review of the literature. *Journal of Gerontological Nursing, 29*(10), 46–53.

Bowers, B. (1987). Intergenerational caregiving: Adult caregivers and their aging parents. *Advances in Nursing Science, 9*(2), 20–31.

Bridges, J., & Lynam, M. (1993). Informal carers: A Marxist analysis of social, political, and economic forces underpinning the role. *Advances in Nursing Science, 15*(3), 33–48.

Brown, M., & Stetz, K. (1999). The labor of caregiving: A theoretical model of caregiving during potentially fatal illness. *Qualitative Health Research, 9*(2), 182–197.

Buelow, J., & Cruijssen, M. (2002). Long-term care nurses speak out: Midwest nurses speak freely about their likes and dislikes in long-term care. *Nursing Homes, 51*(3),50, 52–54, 69–70.

Centers for Medicare and Medicaid Services. (2005). *Nursing home compare: About the nursing home staff.* http://www.medicare.gov/NHCompare/Include/DataSection/Questions/SearchCriteria.asp?version=default&browser=IE%7C6%7CWinXP&language=English&defaultstatus=0&pagelist=Home&CookiesEnabledStatus=True. Accessed 25 Feb 2007.

Cohen, M. (1999). The technology-dependent child and the socially marginalized family: A provisional framework. *Qualitative Health Research, 9*(5), 654–668.

Craft, M., & Willadsen, J. (1992). Interventions related to family nursing. *Nursing Clinics of North America, 27,* 517–540.

Delaune, S., & Ladner, P. (2002). *Fundamentals of nursing: Standards and practice.* Clifton Park: Delmar.

Dunne, K., & Sullivan, K. (2000). Family experiences of palliative care in the acute hospital setting. *International Journal of Palliative Nursing, 6*(4), 170–174.

Farran, C. (2001). Family caregiver intervention research: Where have we been? Where are we going? *Journal of Gerontological Nursing, 27*(7), 38–46.

Fawcett, J. (1984). The metaparadigm of nursing: Current status and future refinements. *Image: Journal of Nursing Scholarship, 16,* 84–87.

Fawcett, J. (2000). *Analysis and evaluation of contemporary nursing knowledge: Nursing models and theories.* Philadelphia: F.A. Davis.

Fenwick, J., Barclay, L., & Schmied, V. (2001). Struggling to mother: A consequence of inhibitive nursing interactions in the neonatal nursery. *Journal of Perintatal and Neonatal Nursing, 15*(2), 49–64.

Ford, K., & Turner, D. (2001). Stories seldom told: Pediatric nurses' experiences of caring for hospitalized children with special needs and their families. *Journal of Advanced Nursing, 33*(3), 288–295.

Friedman, M. (1998). Family nursing: Focus, evolution, and goals. In M. Friedman (Ed.), *Family nursing: Research, theory and practice* (pp. 31–48). Stamford: Appleton and Lange.

Geden, E., & Taylor, S. (1999). Theoretical and empirical description of adult couples' collaborative self-care systems. *Nursing Science Quarterly, 12*(4), 329–334.

Hanson, S., & Boyd, S. (1996). *Family health care nursing: Theory, practice and research.* Philadelphia: F.A. Davis.

Hanson, S., & Mischke, K. (1996). Family health assessment and intervention. In P. Bomar (Ed.), *Nurses and family health promotion* (2nd ed, pp. 165–202). Philadelphia: Saunders.

Hanson, S. M., Gedaly-Duff, V., & Kaakinen, J. R. (2001). *Family health care nursing* (3rd ed.). Philadelphia: F.A. Davis.

Harkreader, H., & Hogan, M. (2004). *Fundamentals of nursing: Caring and clinical judgment.* Philadelphia: Saunders.

Health Services Advisory Group. (2005, July). *National quality forum: National voluntary consensus standards for home health care.* http://hhqi.hsag.com/poa/NQF_Endorsed_Measures.pdf. Accessed 1 Mar 2007.

Heermann, J., & Wilson, M. (2000). Nurses' experiences working with families in an NICU during implementation of family-focused developmental care. *Neonatal Network, 19*(4), 23–29.
Hilbert, G. A., Walker, M., & Rinehart, J. (2000). "In it for the long haul:" Responses of parents caring for children with Sturge-Weber syndrome. *Journal of Family Nursing, 6*(2), 157–159.
Hostler, S. (1999). Pediatric family-centered rehabilitation. *Journal of Head Trauma Rehabilitation, 14*(4), 384–393.
Hsueh, K., Phillips, L., Cheng, W., & Picot, S. (2005). Assessing cross-cultural equivalence through confirmatory factor analysis. *Western Journal of Nursing Research, 27*(6), 755–771.
Hupcey, J. (1999). Looking out for the patient and ourselves—the process of family integration into the ICU. *Journal of Clinical Nursing, 8*(3), 253–262.
International Council of Nurses. (n. d.). *The ICN definition of nursing*. http://www.icn.ch/definition.htm. Accessed 1 Mar 2007.
Jablonski, R., Reed, D., & Maas, M. (2005). Care intervention for older adults with Alzheimer's disease and related dementias: Effect of family involvement on cognitive and functional outcomes in nursing homes. *Journal of Gerontological Nursing, 31*(6), 38–48.
Kalisch, P., & Kalisch, B. (1995). *The advance of American nursing*. Philadelphia: J. B. Lippincott.
Kimball, B. (2004, May). Health care's human crisis: Rx for an evolving profession. *Journal of Issues in Nursing, 9*(2). http://nursingworld.org/ojin/topic24/tpc24_1.htm. Accessed 11 Mar 2007.
Kohnke, M. (1974). *The case for consultation in nursing: Designs for professional practice*. New York: Wiley.
Leininger, M. M. (1995). *Transcultural nursing: Concepts, theories, research and practice*. New York: McGraw Hill.
Levine, L. (2001). *A shortage of registered nurses: Is it on the horizon or already here?* Washington: Congressional Research Service.
Levine, C., & Zuckerman, C. (2000). Hands on/hands off: Why health care professionals depend on families but keep them at arm's length. *Journal of Law Medicine and Ethics, 28*(1), 5–18.
Levy-Storms, L., & Miller-Martinez, D. (2005). Family caregiver involvement and satisfaction with institutional care during the 1st year after admission. *Journal of Applied Gerontology, 24*, 160–174.
Maas, M., Reed, D., Park, M., Specht, J., Schutte, D., Kelley, L., et al (2004). Outcomes of family involvement in care intervention for caregivers of individuals with dementia. *Nursing Research, 53*(2), 76–86.
McCourt, A. (1993). *The specialty practice of rehabilitation nursing: A core curriculum*. Skokie: Rehabilitation Nursing Foundation.
McKenna, H. (2003). Discussion: Comments on "home care versus institutionalization: Family caregiving and senile brain disease.". *International Journal of Nursing Studies, 40*, 471–472.
Meleis, A. (1997). *Theoretical nursing: Development and progress* (3rd ed.). Philadelphia: Lippincott.
Mohr, W. (2000). Partnering with families. *Journal of Psychosocial and Mental Health Nursing Services, 38*(1), 15–22, 38–39.
National Alliance for Caregiving & AARP. (2004). *Caregiving in the U.S.* Washington: Authors.
National Council of State Boards of Nursing. (2005). *2004 Annual Report*. Washington: Author.
National Institutes of Health. (2005). *CRISP: Computer retrieval of information on scientific projects*. http://crisp.cit.nih.gov/. Accessed 27 Feb 2007.
National Institute of Nursing Research. (2001, July). *Executive summary*. http://ninr.nih.gov/ninr/research/dea/workgroup.pdf. Accessed 1 June 2007.
National Quality Forum. (2007). *National Quality Forum announces publication of new report on home health care performance measures: Additional priority areas, 2005–2007*. http://www.qualityforum.org/pdf/news/pr3HospReportAvail7–14-06.pdf. Accessed 25 Mar 2007.
Navaie-Waliser, M., Karuturi, L., & Reisch, K. (2004). Increasing job satisfaction, quality care, and coordination in home health. *Journal of Nursing Administration, 34*(2), 88–82.
Nichols, E. (2001). Educational patterns in nursing. In K. Chitty (Ed.), *Professional nursing: Concepts and challenges* (3rd ed, pp. 33–53). Philadelphia: Saunders.

Oncology Nursing Society, & Association of Oncology Social Work. (2000). *Joint position on end-of-life care*. http://www.ons.org/publications/positions/EndOfLifeCare.shtml. Accessed 14 Mar 2007.

Phillips, L. (1983). Abuse and neglect of the frail elderly at home: An exploration of theoretical relationships. *Journal of Advanced Nursing, 8*(5), 379–392.

Phillips, L. (2001, April). *Community-based intervention research: Lessons learned and thoughts on the state of the science*. Paper presented at the annual meeting of the Communicating Nursing Research Conference, Seattle, WA Communicating Nursing Research, 34(29), 45–53.

Phillips, L., & Rempusheski, V. (1986). Caring for the frail elderly at home: Toward a theoretical explanation of the dynamics of poor quality family caregiving. *Advances in Nursing Science, 8*(4), 62–84.

Phillips, L., Morrison, E., & Chae, Y. (1990). The QUALCARE scale: Developing an instrument to measure quality of home care: Family caregiving. *International Journal of Nursing Studies, 27*(1), 61–75.

Phillips, L., Morrison, E., Steffl, B., Chae, Y., Cromwell, S., & Russell, C. (1995). Effects of the situational context and interactional process on the quality of family caregiving. *Research in Nursing & Health, 18*(3), 205–216.

Redding, S. (2000). Hospice forum. Control theory in dying: What do we know? *American Journal of Hospice and Palliative Care, 17*(3), 204–208.

Robinson, K. (1999). Family caregiving of patients requiring complex care: Doing what you gotta do (Doctoral dissertation, University of Florida, 1999). Dissertation Abstracts International, 60, 4523.

Rutledge, D., Donaldson, N., & Pravikoff, D. (2000a). Caring for families of patients in acute or chronic health care settings: Part I—Principles. *Online Journal of Clinical Innovations, 3*(2), 1–26.

Rutledge, D., Donaldson, N., & Pravikoff, D. (2000b). Caring for families of patients in acute or chronic health care settings: Part II—Interventions. *Online Journal of Clinical Innovations, 3*(3), 1–52.

Schumacher, K. (1996). Reconceptualizing family caregiving: Family-based illness care during chemotherapy. *Research in Nursing & Health, 19*(4), 261–271.

Schumacher, K., Stewart, B., & Archbold, P. (1998). Theory. Conceptualization and measurement of doing family caregiving well. *Image: Journal of Nursing Scholarship, 30*(1), 63–69.

Schumacher, K., Stewart, B., Archbold, P., Dodd, M., & Dibble, S. (2000). Family caregiving skill: Development of the concept. *Research in Nursing & Health, 23*(3), 191–203.

Scott, J., Sochalski, J., & Aiken, L. (1999). Review of magnet hospital research: Findings and implications for professional nursing practice. *Journal of Nursing Administration, 29*(1), 9–19.

Shyu, Y. I. L. (2000). Role tuning between caregiver and care receiver during discharge transition: An illustration of role function mode in Roy's Adaptation Theory. *Nursing Science Quarterly, 13*(4), 323–331.

Smith, C. (1994). A model of caregiving effectiveness for technologically dependent adults residing at home. *Advances in Nursing Science, 17*(2), 27–40.

Smith, C. (1999). Caregiving effectiveness in families managing complex technology at home: Replication of a model. *Nursing Research, 48*(3), 120–128.

Smith, C. (2002). Caregiving effectiveness model evolution to a midrange theory of home care: A process for critique and replication. *Advances in Nursing Science, 25*(1), 50–64.

Somers, A. (1999). Long term care at home. *New England Journal of Medicine, 341*(13), 1005.

Spalding, K., & McKeever, P. (1998). Mother's experiences caring for children with disabilities who require a gastrostomy tube. *Journal of Pediatric Nursing, 13*(4), 234–242.

Specht, J., Kelley, L., Manion, P., Maas, M., Reed, D., & Rantz, M. (2000). Who's the boss? Family/staff partnership in care of persons with dementia. *Nursing Administration Quarterly, 24*(3), 64–77.

Spratley, E., Johnson, A., Sochalski, J., Fritz, M., & Spencer, W. (2000). *The registered nurse population: Findings from the National Sample Survey of Registered Nurses: March 2000*. U.S. Department of Health and Human Services, Health Resources and Service Administration, Bureau of Health Professions, Division of Nursing. http://bhpr.hrsa.gov/healthworkforce/reports/rnsurvey/rnss1.htm. Accessed 14 Mar 2007.

Steele, R., & Fitch, M. (1996). Coping strategies of family caregivers of home hospice patients with cancer. *Oncology Nursing Forum, 23*(6), 955–960.

Stetz, K. (1996). Needs and experiences of family caregivers during marrow transplantation. *Oncology Nursing Forum, 23*(9), 1422–1427.

Stewart, E. (1995). Family matters. Family-centered care for the bereaved. *Pediatric Nursing, 21*(2), 181–184.

Takase, M., Kershaw, E., & Burt, L. (2001). Nurse-environment misfit and nursing practice. *Journal of Advanced Nursing, 35*(6), 819–826.

Vander-Laan, R., Brandys, C., Sullivan, I., & Lemsky, C. (2001). Integration through a city-wide brain injury network and best practices project. *NeuroRehabilitation, 16*(1), 17–26.

Watson, J. (1990). Caring knowledge and informed moral passion. *Advances in Nursing Science, 13*(1), 15–24.

Wilson, S., Morse, J., & Penrod, J. (1998). Absolute involvement: The experience of mothers of ventilator-dependent children. *Health and Social Care in the Community, 6*(4), 224–233.

Wisdom, K. (2001). Nursing roles in the health care delivery system. In K. Chitty (Ed.), *Professional nursing: Concepts and challenges* (3rd ed, pp. 335–359). Philadelphia: Saunders.

Wright, L., & Leahey, M. (1984). *Nurses and families: A guide to family assessment and intervention*. Philadelphia: F.A. Davis.

Wuest, J. (1998). Setting boundaries: A strategy for precarious ordering of women's caring demands. *Research in Nursing and Health, 21,* 39–49.

Yamashita, M. (1997). Family caregiving: Application of Newman's and Peplau's theories. *Journal of Psychiatric and Mental Health Nursing, 4*(6), 401–405.

Zerwekh, J. (1991). A family caregiving model for public health nursing. *Nursing Outlook, 39*(5), 213–217.

Zerwekh, J. (1992). Laying the groundwork for family self-help: Locating families, building trust, and building strength. *Public Health Nursing, 9*(1), 15–21.

Professional Gerontology and Caregiving

Miae Chun, Lewina O. Lee and Bob G. Knight

Professional Gerontology and Caregiving

Gerontology and professional gerontologists have been involved with research on caregiving and with services to caregivers since caregiving emerged as a focus of policy and program development in the USA. In this chapter, we focus primarily on family caregiving, with secondary attention to the role of gerontology in preparing, planning, and managing professional caregiving services for the frail elderly. Given the nature of the field of gerontology, our focus is almost entirely on the care of frail older adults. We believe that many, and probably most, caregiving issues are more determined by the nature of the chronic illness or functional impairment that necessitates the caregiving than by age as such, at least for adult care recipients. In the following sections, we discuss demographic changes that will shape the nature of caregiving, the history of gerontology as it relates to the relationship between gerontology and caregiving, thoughts on the strengths that gerontologists can bring to work with caregivers, and finally, examples of the ways in which gerontologists provide services to the frail elderly and to family caregivers.

M. Chun (✉)
Department of Social Work, Chongshin University,
31–3 Sadang 3-dong, Dongjak-gu, Seoul 156–763, South Korea
e-mail: miaechun@hotmail.com

L. O. Lee
Department of Epidemiology, Boston University School of Public Health
VA Boston Healthcare System 150 South Huntington Avenue Boston, MA 02130, USA
e-mail: lol@bu.edu

Department of Veterans Affairs Boston Healthcare System, Boston, MA, USA

B. G. Knight
University of Southern California, 3715 McClintock Avenue,
Los Angeles, CA 90089–0191, USA
e-mail: bknight@usc.edu

R. C. Talley, S. S. Travis (eds.), *Multidisciplinary Coordinated Caregiving*,
Caregiving: Research • Practice • Policy, DOI 10.1007/978-1-4614-8973-3_3,

Background and Current Status

Demographic Trends that Affect Caregiving

There are several population trends that have profound implications for elders, family caregivers, and professional gerontology. First, demographic trends in the USA show and project an increase in the absolute number and the relative percentage of the older population (65+ years old). The older population grew from 25.7 million persons in 1980 to 40.3 million persons in 2010. The proportion of the total population that was aged 65 and over increased from 11.3 % in 1980 to 12.4 % in 2000 and 13.0 % in 2010 (Siegel 1999; U.S. Census Bureau 2011a). Among those aged 65 and older in 2010, the fastest rate of population growth between 2000 and 2010 was observed in the age 65–69 cohort. As the first Baby Boomers turned 65 in 2011, we expect to see a rapid expansion of the elderly population in the coming decade. Projections based on Census 2010 data indicate that the older adult population will reach 54.8 million (16.1 % of the total population) in 2020, 72.1 million (19.3 %) by 2030, and 88.5 million (20.2 %) by 2050 (U.S. Census Bureau 2008a, b).

Despite recent evidence suggesting a gradually increasing male to female ratio among the older population, the sex ratio continues to be lower in older age groups and this pattern is projected to hold in 2050. In 2010, the male to female ratio was 76:100 for the 65+ age group and 48:100 for the 85+ age group. The proportion of men aged 65+ grew from 41.2 % in 2000 to 43.1 % in 2010, and was predicted to reach 45.1 % in 2050 (U.S. Bureau of the Census 2008b, 2011b).

Second, the prevalence of disabilities, chronic conditions (e.g., diabetes, hypertension), and dementia are higher among individuals in older age groups (Brault 2012; Karel et al. 2012; Taylor and Lynch 2011). In 1999, the Centers for Disease Control and Prevention reported that among persons aged 65 and over, 50 % (16.3 million) reported having a disability. Across all age groups, older adults had the highest prevalence rate for disability in functional activities (such as seeing words or letters in newsprint, hearing normal conversation, having one's speech understood, lifting or carrying 10lbs, climbing a flight of stairs or walking three city blocks), activities of daily living (ADLs), and instrumental activities of daily living (IADLs). Older adults were also reported to have higher rates of chronic diseases. Projections also indicate that the number of disabled individuals in the community and long-term care will increase from nearly 6 million in 1980 to approximately 20 million in 2060 (Dwyer 1996). Since the burden of providing personal care to frail older adults already falls on families, these trends and estimates suggest that greater numbers of families will be affected by the demands of caring for a physically ill or demented relative.

Third, while women had steadily increased their participation in the labor force across the twentieth century (Dwyer 1996), they also tend to take on the role of caregiver for elderly relatives and friends. Between 1970 and 2009, women's participation in the labor force increased from 43.3 to 59.2 % (U.S. Department of Labor, Bureau of Labor Statistics 2010). In a national longitudinal survey of caregivers in the USA, 67 % of unpaid caregivers to individuals aged 50+ and 68 % of care recipients were female (National Alliance for Caregiving and American Association of Retired Persons 2009a, b). Findings from the 2004 data collection wave indicate that although female caregivers were slightly less likely to be working when compared with their male counterparts, on average, female caregivers provided more hours and higher levels of care than male caregivers. Additionally, more women than men (42 vs. 34 %) felt that they did not have a choice in taking on the caregiving role (NAC and AARP 2004). At the time of the 2009 survey, almost three-quarters (74 %) of caregivers were employed at some point since they began providing care (NAC and AARP 2009b), suggesting that caregivers are often juggling multiple responsibilities. As daughters are the main source of care for impaired older adults who do not have a spouse, the conflict between meeting work and caregiving responsibilities is likely to be a source of stress for these women. Consequently, there will be an increased demand for community-based services that can supplement care responsibilities of working women. Regardless of gender differences, it is important to note the high levels of caregiving stress: About one in six caregivers rated their health as fair or poor, over half (54 %) rated the emotional stress of caregiving as at least moderately stressful, and nearly a quarter (23 %) of caregivers reported having at least moderate levels of financial hardship due to caregiving (NAC and AARP 2009b).

Fourth, the elderly population is becoming more diverse. The number of elders among various minority races is growing much more rapidly than the number of non-Hispanic White elders and is expected to continue to rise over the next half century (Siegel 1999). Comparing Census data from 2000 and 2009, Hispanic and Asian elders showed the highest population growth across all ethnicity at 59.2 and 64.4 % respectively. The size of the elderly population was estimated at 2.8 million for Hispanics and 1.3 million for Asians in 2009 (U.S. Census Bureau 2010). Consequently, there will be a greater need for an understanding and integration of cultural diversity issues in the applied work of professional gerontologists. Reviews of ethnic caregiving research (e.g., Aranda and Knight 1997; Connell and Gibson 1997; Janevic and Connell 2001; Knight and Sayegh 2010) have contributed to an increased interest in racial, ethnic, and cultural differences in the dementia caregiving experience.

Fifth, the higher rate of divorce and remarriages since the 1970s (e.g., Graphic Sociology 2009) suggest that the Boomer cohort, at least, will be facing the challenges of assigning caregiving responsibilities in divorced and blended families. Will male care recipients be cared for by ex-wives or by daughters for whom they were the noncustodial parent? Will daughters be willing to care for step-parents? The ratio of dependent elders to potential caregivers, already higher due to declining birth rates, becomes even higher if step-parents are added to the picture.

In sum, the aging of our population suggests that there will be an increased need for professionals who are knowledgeable of aging and caregiving issues to work with ethnically diverse older adults and their families and with new and evolving family structures.

Short History of Gerontology

To better understand the various aspects of the field of gerontology, we will look briefly at the history of its development. Before World War II, aging research was conducted mostly in biology, followed by psychology and sociology; however, in those years, aging research was primarily focused within each discipline. There was limited sharing of research findings through research conferences because researchers were identified only by their discipline of origin.

Historical events facilitated the creation of professional gerontology (Peterson 1987). After the Great Depression of the 1930s, new programs were initiated in many areas. One of these new programs, the Social Security Act, was passed in 1935 as an income maintenance program for the elderly. This program was initially administered by social workers who did not necessarily have an understanding of aging. The Medicare and Medicaid programs of 1965 have been major sources of health care support for older adults and for the poor (overlapping categories of program participants). Through these programs, nursing homes, hospitals, and home care services are offered to older people. Another important legislation for the older population is the Older Americans Act of 1965, which created the National Aging Network (57 state and territorial Agencies on Aging, and 666 Area Agencies on Aging). The Aging Network has played a major role in facilitating and operating a variety of programs, such as meals on wheels, ombudsman and legal service programs, transportation services, senior centers, day care programs, and respite services. All these services and programs created job opportunities in order to serve older adults. Moreover, it was necessary to create training programs for currently employed professionals, so that they could learn the background on the processes of aging and/or the current conditions of older people. For this reason, new courses dealing with life span development and aging were developed in various educational settings including college and universities. Also, the Older American Act made funds available to college and universities for career and short-term training starting in 1966 (Peterson 1987). As the field develops, a growing number of professionals are making long-term commitments to gerontology.

Another significant marker of the development of gerontology is the history of the Gerontological Society of America (GSA). It grew out of the Club for Research on Ageing organized in 1939 (Achenbaum 1987). In order to encourage, legitimize, and disseminate research in aging, the Club members decided to establish a journal (currently called *The Journal of Gerontology*) and other organizational supports. The 1945 charter of the Gerontological Society, Inc. stated their organizational objectives:

> to promote the scientific study of aging; to foster the growth and diffusion of knowledge relating to the problems of aging; to afford a common meeting ground for representation of the various scientific fields; all without profit to the corporation or its members. (*Journal of Gerontology* 1946, p. 134).

This new Society contributed to gerontology because it promoted multidisciplinary research in a variety of established fields of inquiry that utilized both theory and empirical data, such as biology, clinical medicine, behavioral and social sciences, and social research, policy, and practice (Achenbaum 1987). In addition, the Society translated research into practice in order to disseminate findings to the professional community and help them deal with the problems of aging. The GSA newsletter became *The Gerontologist*, which was designed to appeal to a more diverse reading audience, and later became oriented to professionals working with older adults. *The Journal of Gerontology* and *The Gerontologist* are the two major journals in gerontology today. *The Gerontologist* has been the leading outlet for research and model practice papers on caregiving.

The creation of the National Institute on Aging (NIA) in 1975 became a major funding source for both biomedical and social/psychological studies of aging (Peterson 1987). NIA focuses on research, research training, and faculty career development. Major diseases of older persons (such as Alzheimer's disease, stroke, Parkinson's disease, etc.) and major social problems (such as caregiving) are investigated through its funding. Funds support master's degree, predoctoral, postdoctoral, and faculty development training at a number of colleges and universities and have been instrumental in expanding gerontological instruction within several related professions. The NIA, and to some extent the National Institute of Mental Health (NIMH) and the National Institute of Nursing Research (NINR), and the Alzheimer's Association have been the leading funding agencies for research on caregiving and for the evaluation of interventions designed to assist family caregivers.

The development of master's level professional gerontology and caregiving The history of the University of South Florida (USF), Department of Gerontology, the first degree-awarding program in Gerontology, and the Department of Applied Gerontology at the University of North Texas (formerly known as the Center for Studies in Aging) illustrate the emergence of federal funding for training programs for aging. The USF was chartered in 1956 and an Institute on Aging was created in 1965 in response to the large and growing numbers of retirees relocating to Florida. With a grant from the Administration on Aging (AoA) in 1967, the Institute on Aging became a Master's in Aging Studies program. USF started with the master's program because of the available market of students. Historically, a principal focus of the USF program has been the training of gerontological professionals to manage long-term care facilities and other programs for the care of frail older adults (S. Reynolds, personal communication, March 6, 2002).

The Department of Applied Gerontology at the University of North Texas, one of the nation's oldest career training programs in gerontology, was established in 1967 also through a grant from the U.S. Administration on Aging (D. A. Peterson, personal communication, May 15, 2002). The Department offers master's degrees and a graduate-level specialist certificate (University of North Texas 2002). The master's degree program has three majors: administration of long-term care and retirement facilities, administration of aging organizations, and applied gerontology. This program prepares students to become administrators of skilled nursing facilities, continuing care retirement communities, assisted living facilities, home health care agencies, advocacy groups for older adults, government offices on aging at all levels, senior centers, and others. This program more clearly focused on services for older adults and trains gerontologists as practitioners.

In 1975, the Leonard Davis School of Gerontology at the University of Southern California (USC) was established based on a gift provided by Leonard Davis. The USC School of Gerontology was the first professional school (i.e., an independent unit reporting directly to central university administration dedicated to training gerontologists) in the world. Both undergraduate and master's degree programs were offered, with a focus on professional services in gerontology, including direct service delivery, administration, and policy development and evaluation. The focus on professional training and education led to successful application for Administration on Aging funding for a service learning program then called the Andrus Older Adult Center in the late 1970s, a multipurpose senior services program that developed quickly into a counseling center for older adults. Under Steven Zarit's leadership, this service learning center provided support groups and counseling for caregivers, with an active research program on caregiver burden and interventions to assist caregivers. The intertwined nature of gerontology training, research, and caregiving is very clearly illustrated in this sequence of events.

Oregon State University, University of Massachusetts in Boston, and Baylor University in Texas established master's programs in gerontology in 1970s, followed by the Sagmond University in southern Illinois, University of Akron in Akron, OH., Ohio University in Oxford, OH., University of Florida, and Florida State University in 1980s (D. A. Peterson, personal communication, May 15, 2002). As of 2012, GradSchools.com listed 108 master's programs in gerontology in the US, with 25 being distance learning programs and the remainder on campus or mixed. This spread of master's programs in gerontology illustrates the recognition of and response to increasing elderly population.

PhD programs in the 1990s The next phase of the development of gerontology as a discipline in its own right occurred with the emergence of Ph.D. programs in gerontology (or aging studies) in the 1990s. For the first time, doctoral level researchers and professors are being trained in gerontology per se, rather than being trained in a constituent discipline and then specializing in aging. For example, the USC School of Gerontology established the first doctoral program in gerontology in 1989, quickly followed by the University of Massachusetts at Boston. The curriculum of the gerontology Ph.D. program at USC includes content courses in psychology, sociology, physiology, social policy, theories of aging, research methods, and a distinguished lecture series that exposes the students to the leading researchers in aging. Graduates have taken positions in academic, public sector, and private sector settings. Several students have pursued research projects on caregiving with particular attention to cross cultural and cross national studies of caregiving to frail older adults, again illustrating the close relationship between the development of gerontology and caregiving studies.

Subsequently, during 1995–1997, three more PhD programs—the University of South Florida, the University of Kansas, and the University of Kentucky—were established focusing on interdisciplinary research training in gerontology. The University of Maryland, Baltimore (UMB) and the University of Maryland Baltimore County (UMBC) jointly offered a Ph.D. program in gerontology in the Fall of 2001.

As of 2012, GradSchools.com listed 28 PhD programs in gerontology in the USA, six were online programs and the remainder were on campus or hybrid. Currently, a total of six Ph.D. programs are available nationwide. Among these programs, University of Kansas has a research project for targeting support services in caregiver careers supported by the Alzheimer's Association (University of Kansas 2002), and USC has a research project on ethnic comparison studies on caregivers' emotional and physical distress outcomes, and coping strategies. In addition, Alzheimer's Disease Research Center (ADRC)s are placed under gerontology programs in the University of Kentucky (University of Kentucky 2002) and USC. ADRC provides education and information about all aspects of Alzheimer's disease (AD) for health care professionals, families, and communities.

Potential Strengths of Gerontologists for Serving Caregivers

According to Peterson (1987), gerontology has two orientations: *discipline* and *practice*. Gerontology as a *discipline* devotes itself to the study of the processes of aging. Gerontologists have tried to promote the acquisition of new knowledge or greater insight into the meaning of aging. On the other hand, gerontology is a field of *practice* in which professionals and paraprofessionals plan, provide, and administer a variety of services to aging individuals.

Gerontologists are trained in both discipline and practice. A gerontologist can practice as a service provider, but can also understand what aging entails, from biological experiments on life span extension to difficult choices regarding allocation of health care resources (e.g., Moody 2000). Understanding the processes involved in aging as well as the social issues confronting the elderly population is a great advantage of gerontologists. In this section, the potential strengths of gerontologists will be discussed in four parts: interdisciplinary background, skilled interdisciplinary communication/collaboration, research grounded in gerontology, and caregiving relevant roles of gerontologists.

Interdisciplinary Background: Biology, Psychology, Sociology

Gerontology is typically defined as the study of the processes of aging. Aging affects multiple aspects of the person: biological, psychological, and social. Therefore, gerontology is an interdisciplinary discipline. In order to understand the processes of aging, we have to study biological, psychological, and sociological aspects as well as those multiple and interrelated changes that affect the biological behavior and social aspects of our lives. A number of fields, each with its own body of knowledge and methods of research, contribute to the knowledge about the process of aging or older adult lives.

In gerontology training, students are exposed to the physiology of human development, growth, and aging with a major emphasis on the physiology of the later years and implications for health maintenance. Theories of the biology of aging and the effects of age on functional integrity of our body are also taught in gerontology programs. In addition, students learn the major components of psychology such as perception, cognitive processes, personality, sexuality, and lifestyles. Social gerontology includes the life course perspective on the sociological theories of marriage and the family, intergenerational relationships, work and retirement, and other forms of social organization. As a result of exposure to a broad knowledge base, gerontologists are well trained in interdisciplinary issues of aging.

Skilled in Interdisciplinary Communication/Collaboration

Gerontology training is provided under the instruction of multidisciplinary faculty. Faculty members themselves are either trained in an interdisciplinary area of gerontology, or in one specific field of study such as sociology, psychology, or something else. Regardless of their training, faculty members have been working together for their research in gerontology and sharing their ideas within a multidisciplinary gerontology community. Therefore, communication or collaboration between faculty members who have different backgrounds is an essential aspect of the gerontology field. Usually, those faculty members understand the broader context of aging processes, and share their research experiences or ideas with other faculty or students. Gerontology training also brings outside practitioners or public policy makers in the gerontology field so that students learn about the field as well as develop communication skills with them. By the very nature of the multidisciplinary training experience, gerontologists are well prepared for working in interdisciplinary teams and programs. This multidisciplinary preparation is frequently lacking in single discipline training that often focuses on developing a disciplinary identity. Unfortunately, this narrow focus can lapse into disciplinary chauvinism, which can later interfere with cross discipline communication.

Grounded in Gerontology Research

Gerontology training is rooted in research on aging and on current cohorts of older adults. A well-trained gerontologist will have a broad, research-based comprehension of older adults, the context in which they live, and ways to address the problems of aging, including caregiving issues. Many professionals trained in other disciplines will have solid training and knowledge related to their professional discipline, but may have little knowledge about older adults that is based in scientific gerontology. When individuals are not well grounded in scientific knowledge about older adults, they may well draw upon common conventional wisdom or folklore about older adults. Thus, even highly trained professionals may remain uninformed about the problems of frail older adults and their caregivers. In such instances, even well meaning professionals may inadvertently do things to older adults and their families rather than for them, because they lack the accurate knowledge base upon which high quality professional service depends.

Caregiving Relevant Roles of Gerontologists

As a result of their multidisciplinary background, gerontologists are in a good position to be members of teams assisting caregivers of older adults. Gerontologists can take on several roles relevant to caregiving by providing: (1) health education, (2) case management, (3) support groups, (4) counseling, (5) community-based care management, (6) long-term care management, and (7) policy analysis and development.

Health education As a result of their exposure to a broad and interdisciplinary training, gerontologists can provide education about: (1) the aging process, (2) the nature and expected course of the care recipient's illness (i.e., Alzheimer's disease), (3) related health, financial, housing, and legal issues; and (4) access to formal services. This information can be disseminated when gerontologists act as case managers, support group leaders, counselors, or care managers.

Case management Case management is a widely used service involving assessment, information, and referral data and coordination of services (Olshevski et al. 1999). Case management is intended to help access available services for elders and their families (Toseland et al. 1995). In the case of caregiving, caregivers most often seek help for their relative. Morrow-Howell (1992) described the core functions of case management with frail older adults as casefinding, assessment, care planning, follow-up, and reassessment. Casefinding entails conducting community outreach, determining eligibility of older adults for services, and completing intakes. Gerontologists can begin to help caregiving families by assessing the physical, psychological, and social functioning of the care recipient, followed by the caregiver, and other family members. Gerontologists' understanding of the physical (e.g., chronic illnesses), psychological (e.g., dementia, depression, grief), and social (e.g., isolation) problems which are common in later life can guide this assessment process. Administration of screening instruments such as the Mini Mental State Examination, the Geriatric Depression Scale, and assessment of ADLs/IADLs can inform gerontologists of the need to refer the older adult for a neuropsychological evaluation, psychological treatment, and/or homemaker services. At the care planning stage, gerontologists evaluate what support is provided by the older adult's informal network, and what form of help the informal network is willing to provide because the effectiveness of community-based services is likely to depend on how they interface with the family (Noelker and Bass 1989). A comprehensive assessment enables gerontologists to develop a care plan to support the frail older adult and the caregiver, and to involve other family members and agencies in specific roles. Once the care plan has been formulated, gerontologists play an important role in contracting with the caregiver, other family members, and other providers to carry out the plan, implement it, and monitor its progress (Toseland et al. 1995). Gerontologists' knowledge of information required by specific mental health programs and agencies serving older clients can help determine an older adult's eligibility for these services. Gerontologists' understanding of community services catering to the elderly and their fluidity of their roles as case managers enable them to address gaps in the service network within a community via different pathways, such as by acting as advocates for older adults' needs and coordinating services among several different agencies, or developing resources for caregivers through church or civil groups.

Support groups Support groups can offer information, emotional support, and the exchange of ideas on how to manage difficulties to caregivers of demented or frail older adults. Knight (2004) described the spectrum of support group formats which ranged from informational groups with drop-in membership to groups with consistent membership and groups likened to psychotherapy groups. Although outcome studies of support groups has generally reported evidence for null or very small effects on changing burden or emotional distress (Knight et al. 1993; Sorensen et al. 2002), Knight (2004) suggested that such results could be inconclusive for reasons such as caregivers having derived maximum benefit from attending support groups before studies began. On the positive side, attending support groups may provide caregivers with the sense that they are not alone with their problems, normalize the feelings and experiences associated with caregiving, and allow caregivers to share their experience and specific advice about problems. In other instances, support groups may enhance stress for some caregivers, for example, when an early-stage caregiver hears about the problems of later-stage dementia, or when members of a support group suffer from serious mental disorders or personality disorders.

As a result of their multidisciplinary background, gerontologists are in a good position to act as support group leaders to: (1) disseminate health education (see previous section for more detailed information); (2) develop support within the group; (3) examine how to cope with the emotional aspects of caregiving; (4) teach caregivers how to care for themselves; (5) explore how to improve relationships with the care recipient and other family members; (6) provide access to formal services; (7) explain and validate sources of potential differences between caregivers (e.g., nature of care recipients' disease, relationships with care recipients, gender differences); and (8) help group members understand how caregiving experiences and approaches to problems may vary due to these individual differences.

Counseling Gerontologists can carry out individual or family counseling sessions to ease caregiving burden. Individual counseling can help decrease caregiving burden, identify positive steps to be taken, and facilitate deriving meaning and growth from stressful encounters (Olshevski et al. 1999). Family meetings can address the tensions and imbalances in the family system created by the care recipient's disabilities (Zarit et al. 1985), and also address the issue of providing more support to the primary caregiver. Thus, gerontologists are in the position of helping individuals and families solve a situational problem and offer information to family members to increase their control over the situation (Olshevski et al. 1999).

Community-based care management Community-based services assist families by relieving them of some care responsibilities while allowing them to keep the care recipient in the home. Types of services available to caregivers include in-home respite, homemaker and home health aide services, home-delivered meals, transportation and escort services, friendly visitor programs, senior centers, adult day care programs, overnight out-of-home respite programs, and short-term and overnight respite in a facility.

Gerontologists are knowledgeable of activities appropriate for older clients with diverse interests and levels of functioning, and of compensatory techniques and environmental adaptations that can help impaired older adults function most effectively. Consequently, gerontologists can play an important role in the planning, implementation, and evaluation of therapeutic and recreational activities for older adults in community-based agencies (i.e., senior centers, day care facilities, nursing homes). In addition, gerontologists can act as case managers in these agencies or manage the programs available in these agencies.

Manage long-term care Long-term care is a wide range of health and health-related support services for people who cannot take care of themselves over an extended period of time regardless of physical or mental problems. Since the early 1970s, expansions in Medicare and Medicaid as well as expanded coverage by private insurance policies prompted a dramatic increase in the use of professional home care services for the chronically impaired. In the past several years, there have been increased investments on a wider range of long term care services, including assisted living facilities, congregate housing, adult foster care, and board and care homes (McCall 2001). Since long-term care is an umbrella term which covers a wide range of services, its goals are often broad, complex, and call for an integrated approach to health-care delivery. It often requires the collaboration of a team of specialists that can cater to patients' medical, social, and personal needs. Consider the two major age-related disabling conditions, namely stroke and dementia. In the former, care recipients may require rehabilitative services to restore their former level of functioning. Conversely, among demented patients who will not see a recovery of functioning, service may require medical treatment to prevent deterioration combined with counseling to assist patients in socially and emotionally adjusting to stages of their decline (Organization for Economic Co-operation and Development (OECD), 2005. In the above instances and many others, the goal of long-term care is to maximize their independence, not to cure (Evashwick 1996). Most long-term care is provided by friends and family (Doty 1986) in their own communities. However, as elderly persons' functions deteriorate, it may reach the point that friends or family members are no longer able to take care of elderly patients. For this reason, it is necessary to have nursing facilities. Currently, about 5 % of the elderly population lives in long-term care facilities. However, when the term "long-term care management" is used, it usually means skilled and/or intermediate nursing facilities. Here, we are broadening the term to include all 24-hour care facilities for older adults.

There are challenges for administrators of long-term care systems. Thinking of ways to improve the continuum of care through various measures, successful examples include multidisciplinary care assessment teams, which assist informal caregivers with available care alternatives and what might be the best choice for the care recipients. Alternatively, establishment of quality assessment and monitoring of outcomes in long-term care settings can allow for better regulation of long-term care services. Drawing from their practical training on service provision and delivery, and their knowledge in the biological and psychological aspects of aging, gerontologists are particularly apt for the tasks of assessing the quality of long-term care and identifying its deficits.

Other challenges for gerontologists in the long-term care domain include balancing the desire to meet patients' and staff's needs with the funding limits imposed by tight Medicaid reimbursement and stringent federal and state regulations (Evashwick and Langdon 1996). Without appropriate training and sufficient experience, these challenges may remain unsolved. Although balancing these competing demands is not an easy task, gerontologists may be the best professionals for this complex job.

In fact, long-term care administration courses are offered in gerontology programs (USC, USF, and others). Also, graduates of gerontology programs get administration positions in various long-term care facilities. Since they understand the various aspects of elderly persons as individuals and as a population, gerontologists are a good fit for the position. Gerontologists usually get training on biological, psychological, and social aspects of elderly persons as well as current trends and policies. They understand how the long-term care system works and also learn how to work with families of older adults.

Policy analysis and development The graduates of gerontology programs are well equipped to analyze policies and develop programs not only for elderly persons but also for their caregivers as gerontologists understand the various issues and policy alternatives with regard to caregiving as well as to elderly persons. During the course of education, students of gerontology not only learn the policies for the elderly and their caregivers but also practice and sharpen their skills to analyze the policies to help improve the condition of services for the elderly and/or caregivers. In addition, because of their deep understanding of the characteristics and the needs of elderly persons, gerontologists could be the best persons to develop programs and policies for the elderly persons and caregivers. Therefore, gerontologists are in a good position to serve as a policy analyst and program developers for elderly persons and caregivers.

Future Needs and New Directions

With an understanding of the history of gerontology, the nature of gerontological training programs, and the skills of professional gerontologists, we can turn to the question of the contributions that gerontologists can make in services for caregivers.

In this section, we discuss the roles that gerontologists can play in interdisciplinary teams working with caregivers, the role that gerontologists can play in bring life span models of understanding adult development and aging to the understanding of caregiving, and what gerontologists have to offer in understanding likely future directions in caregiving services.

Interdisciplinary Team Practice

As we argued earlier, gerontologists can play an important role in interdisciplinary services for caregivers, especially the caregivers of older adults, and also caregivers of adults who are either physically or cognitively frail. Gerontologists are specifically trained to work with older adults, and a sizable portion of the gerontology knowledge base is research on caregiving, especially caring for persons with acquired cognitive impairment and persons with chronic physical disabilities. The range of skills, as noted above, includes case management which was formally recognized in 1992 with the creation of geriatric case management certifications (Commission for Case Manager Certification 2002) and the inclusion of gerontologists along with social workers and nurses in this certification process (National Academy of Certified Care Managers 2002). Other skills include health education, counseling, leading support groups, and managing programs in both community-based and institutional long-term care. Although these roles can be filled by persons from various disciplines, the gerontologist would bring a specialization in knowledge about older adults and a higher degree of experience and comfort in thinking and working across the typical disciplinary boundaries that divide health care, mental health care, and social services as developed using younger adult models of service delivery.

The interdisciplinary background should also be helpful in enabling the gerontologist to facilitate communication among interdisciplinary team members. The world views and communication styles of persons trained in specific traditional disciplines differ in ways that make planning services for caregivers and care receivers difficult for everyone. Each traditional discipline approaches the tasks of assessment and intervention with distinct assumptions concerning the logic of assessment, the appropriate focus of professional efforts, the locus of responsibility, and the pace of action in gerontological interventions (Qualls and Czirr 1988). For example, in medicine, the focus is on ruling out problems by systematically eliminating hypotheses until a single problem solution is identified. In psychosocial professions (psychology, social work), the emphasis is on encompassing a broader view of the problem, factors contributing to it, and interacting elements that may affect the outcome of assessment and intervention (Smyer and Qualls 1999). The gerontologist, who has had to master communicating with persons of different disciplines since the beginning of his/her training, can help translate among the other team members.

Education of Gerontologists

In principle, gerontologists are trained to think in terms of life span development, covering the adult life span and later life. The classic picture of caregiving for frail elderly has been that of the middle-aged daughter caring for elderly parents (Brody et al. 1989). However, the most likely person to assume caregiving responsibility is the wife or husband of a disabled elder (Soldo and Myllyuoma 1983; Stone et al. 1987). Since spouses are the first in line for caregiving duties, the caregiver and care receiver are often of approximately the same age. With the rapidly increasing proportion of persons living into the old-old years, it is more and more common to see young-old children (e.g., recently retired couples who had planned on leisure time and travel) caring for old-old parents. There is increasing attention as well to other types of caregiving: growing numbers of elderly parents caring for middle aged or young-old children with psychosis or developmental disabilities (e.g., St. Onge and Lavoie 1997; Kropf 1997), and grandparents caring for their grandchildren (Burton 1992). Census data in 2009 indicated that the number of American children living in a household maintained by a grandparent increased by 64 % over the past two decades: 7.8 million children lived with at least one of their grandparents, up from 4.7 million in 1991 (Jayson 2011). In other words, approximately 4.97 million American children were identified as the grandchild of a householder, among which 2.03 million were headed by grandmothers (U.S. Census Bureau 2011b). Grandmothers in this family type were also more likely than grandparents in other family types to face economic hardship. They also reported more personal distress and parenting stress than mothers (Musil et al. 2002). Multigenerational homes present another form of caregiving with increasing prevalence in recent years, especially among families of color or families of recent immigrants (Musil et al. 2005). Various circumstances such as teenage pregnancy, substance use and abuse, marital disruptions can contribute towards the phenomenon. Multigenerational living arrangements are often found in such instances, such as grandparents caring for children while parents work, or adult children moving back to grandparents' home after divorce.

Given the diverse patterns in which caregiving can occur in the family context, Musil et al. (2005) suggested that ethnic heritage could serve as a way to strengthen intergenerational relationships within families and thereby illuminate professionals and families in caring for frail elderly members. They explained that younger generations can increase the self-esteem of older generation and provide the latter with an exchange resource by displaying an interest in their ethnic history and heritage. Equipped with knowledge about different ethnicities, gerontologists can help strengthen family ties by helping young family members understand that older people may recount their past as a way of providing coherence and meaning to their lives, and to encourage young adults engage in life review projects with elder family members. Sharing of ethnic heritage can also reinforce continuity with the past. For instance, creating a cookbook of ethnic recipes can encourage sharing between generations. Chapters in national ethnic organizations (e.g., Jewish Council for the Aging, National Association for Hispanic Elderly) exist in many communities and provide information to families in drawing on their ethnic heritage as caregiving resources. When caregiving is viewed as broader than simply caring for the frail elderly, caregiving moves into a life span context and the focus can change from the frail elderly as the presumed recipients of care to the nature of caregiving itself, including the observation that older adults provide care as well as receive it. When families are viewed in a life span context (e.g., Knight and McCallum 1998), we become aware that all families have aging members, middle aged members, young adult members, and children. These changes in perspective can avoid polarizing public debates into battles between services for young and old and remind us that we are all related (Binstock 1992).

Life span developmental psychology also focuses our attention on explanations for age differences other than the developmental processes roughly indexed by chronological age. Other major influences on observed differences between age groups at any given point in time include cohort effects and time effects. Cohort effects are differences between successive generations, what makes Boomers different from the World War II generation. Time effects are changes in society that affect everyone (i.e., all cohorts) at about the same time. For example, the increasing emphasis on home care over institutional care in recent decades changes family caregiving for everyone. An awareness of these other influences on age differences can provide a different viewpoint on how to think about adapting services for older adults (e.g., Knight 2004).

Cohort differences, for example, suggest that we need to constantly revise services for older adults because the nature of the older population changes as each new cohort becomes old. An advantage of this type of thinking is that we could, in principle, plan ahead and devise service programs and policies for the next generation of older adults by looking at what is happening with today's middle-aged cohorts. A shift to this kind of future-oriented planning would help to avoid the structural lag described by Riley (Riley et al. 1995) in which programs and policies stay a generation or two behind the needs of the current cohort, because of the time it takes policy and programs to get implemented. That is, a need is identified based on those who are elderly today. It takes a decade or two for the laws to get passed, regulations to get written, and programs to be implemented and disseminated nationwide. By that time, the cohort whose needs the programs were to meet has passed away and a different cohort is elderly.

Education of Family Caregivers

What are the likely future needs of caregivers in the early twenty-first century? There will likely be greater numbers of older adults with dementia, simply because there will be greater numbers of older adults. It is possible that vascular dementias may decline, since there is some evidence that cardiovascular health has improved for the Boomer generation (see Knight and Maines 2001). As noted earlier in the section on demographic changes, older adults will be more likely to have divorced, women are more likely to have careers, children are more likely to be step-children or to have a noncustodial parent who now needs care. These changes in family structure and duties all have implications for caregiving and may eliminate traditional potential caregivers just at a time when the largest cohort becomes elderly. It would seem wise to start planning for these changes soon, and to rethink the reliance on traditional family caregiving as the traditional family becomes scarce.

For the post-Boomer generation or Generation X, declining fertility rates during the last three decades of the twentieth century will severely limit the number of adult children available to provide care or assistance to older parents (Crimmins and Ingegneri 1990). This trend is especially true of the more educated and affluent (Wolf 1994). Post-boomers are more likely to be single parents (p. 211) and more likely have higher education (p. 84), women are more likely to have a career (p. 297) and are less likely to have children (p. 115) (Mitchell 2000). As younger generations of women pursue higher education, they are more likely to delay birth of child, and this leads to increase in the possibility of having fewer children. Having fewer children increases the probability that an elder parent will have no proximate adult children while proximity plays an important role in caregiving and co-residency. Moves by the elderly nearer their children are frequently made with retirement, widowhood, divorce, illness, or frailty (Wolf 1994; Crimmins and Ingegneri 1990). Still, without available children, the elderly must look to siblings and other kin or obtain paid services or housing. It is clear that we need preparation for future care for the elderly.

Policy Analysis and Development

Old-age policies and programs constituted over one-third of the federal budget in the 1990s (Stechenrider and Parrott 1998). Aging policy encompasses the innumerable programs directed toward senior citizens and toward an aging population such as Medicare, Social Security, the Older Americans Act, home-delivered meals, subsidized housing, legal assistance, and transportation services.

Since gerontologists are trained in research and understand aging individuals and trends, gerontologists are in a good position to analyze or develop policies for elderly persons. For example, let us say, policy makers developed a day program for elderly persons in rural area. If they do not understand the physical limitations of the elderly persons in that rural area and have not included a transportation component along with the day program, the newly provided program would be useless. Therefore, an understanding of elderly individuals and the aging population is important in policy development.

Conclusions

In this chapter, we have explored the contributions of gerontology as a discipline and as a profession to caregiving. The interdisciplinary nature of gerontology, its use of the life span perspective, and the substantive focus on caregiving as a content area within gerontology all create the potential for important contributions of gerontologists to improving programs and policies intended to support and assist caregivers as they support the frail members of our society.

References

Achenbaum, A. (1987). Reconstructing GSA's history. *Gerontologist, 27*(1), 21–29.

Aranda, M. P., & Knight, B. G. (1997). The influence of ethnicity and culture on the caregiver stress and coping process: A sociocultural review and analysis. *Gerontologist, 37,* 342–354.

Binstock, R. H. (1992). Aging, disability, and long-term care: The politics of common ground. *Generations, 16*(1), 83–88.

Brault, M. W. (2012). Americans with disabilities: 2010. Current population reports. www.census.gov/prod/2012pubs/p70–131.pdf. Accessed 25 July 2012.

Brody, E. M., Hoffman, C., Kleban, M. H., & Schoonover, C. B. (1989). Caregiving daughters and their local siblings: Perceptions, strains, and interactions. *Gerontologist, 29*(4), 529–538.

Burton, L. M. (1992). Black grandparents rearing children of drug-addicted parents: Stressors, outcomes, and social service needs. *Gerontologist, 32*(6), 744–751.

Centers for Disease Control and Prevention (1999). Prevalence of disabilities and associated health conditions among adults—United States. mortality and morbidity weekly report, 50(7). http://www.cdc.gov/mmwr/preview/mmwrhtml/mm5007a3.htm. Accessed 13 March 2007.

Center for Medicare and Medicaid Services. (2007). Nursing home compare, Baltimore. Retrieved 22 March 2007. www.medicare.gov/NHcompare/Home.asp.

Commission for Case Manager Certification. (2002). *The evolution of CCMC.* Rolling Meadows: Author.

Connell, C. M., & Gibson, G. D. (1997). Racial, ethnic, and cultural differences in dementia caregiving: Review and analysis. *Gerontologist, 37,* 355–364.

Crimmins, E. M., & Ingegneri, D. G. (1990). Interaction and living arrangements of older parents and their children: Past trends, present determinants, future implications. *Research on Aging, 12*(1), 3–35.

Doty, p. (1986). Family care of the elderly: The role of public policy. *Milbank Quarterly, 64*(1), 34–75.

Dwyer, J. W. (1996). The effects of illness on the family. In R. Blieszner & V. Hilkevitch Bedford (Eds.), *Aging and the family: Theory and research* (pp. 401–421). Westport: Praeger.

Evashwick, C. J. (1996). Definition of the continuum of care. In C. J. Evashwick (Ed.), *The continuum of long-term care: An integrated systems approach* (pp. 1–14). San Francisco: Delmar Publishers.

Evashwick, C., & Langdon, B. (1996). *The continuum of long-term care: An integrated systems approach.* San Francisco: Delmar Publishers.

Graphic Sociology. (December 2009). Figure 5. http://thesocietypages.org/graphicsociology/2009/12/. Accessed 27 July 2012.

Janevic, M. R., & Connell, C. M. (2001). Racial, ethnic, and cultural differences in the dementia caregiving experience: Recent findings. *Gerontologist, 41,* 334–347.

Jayson, S. (2011 June 29). Census: More kids live with a grandparent in the house. USA Today. http://www.usatoday.com/news/health/wellness/story/2011/06/More-kids-live-with-a-grandparent-in-the-house-Census-says/48965076/1. Accessed 20 July 2012.

Journal of Gerontology. (1946). Certificate of incorporation of the Gerontological Society Inc. *Journal of Gerontology, 1*(1), 134–137.

Karel, M. J., Gatz, M., & Smyer, M. A. (2012). Aging and mental health in the decade ahead: What psychologists need to know. *American Psychologist, 67,* 184–198.

Knight, B. G. (2004). *Psychotherapy with older adults* (3rd ed.). Thousand Oaks: Sage Publications.

Knight, B. G., & Maines, M. (2001). Mental disorders and mental health services in late life: Issues for public health and public policy. In G. Lesnoff-Caravaglia (Ed.), *Aging and public health: Technology and demography—Parallel evolutions* (pp. 69–92). Springfield: C. C. Thomas.

Knight, B. G., & McCallum, T. J. (1998). Adapting psychotherapeutic practice for older clients: Implications of the contextual, cohort-based, maturity, specific challenge model. *Professional Psychology: Research and Practice, 29*(1), 15–22.

Knight, B. G., & Sayegh, p. (2010). Cultural values and caregiving: The updated sociocultural stress and coping model. *Journals of Gerontology: Psychological Sciences, 65B,* 5–13.

Knight, B. G., Lutsky, S. M., & Macofsky-Urban, F. (1993). A meta-analytic review of interventions for caregiver distress: Recommendations for future research. *Gerontologist, 33,* 240–249.

Kropf, N. P. (1997). Older parents of adults with developmental disabilities: Practice issues and service needs. *Journal of Family Psychotherapy, 8*(2), 37–54.

McCall, N. (2001). Long term care: Definition, demand, cost, and financing. In N. McCall (Ed.), *Who will pay for long term care? Insights from the partnership program* (pp. 3–31). Chicago: Health Administration Press.

Mitchell, S. (2000). *American generations: Who they are, how they live, what they think.* Ithaca: New Strategist Publications.

Moody, H. R. (2000). *Aging: Concepts and controversies*. Thousand Oaks: Pine Forge Press.

Morrow-Howell, N. (1992). Clinical case management: The hallmark of gerontological social work. *Journal of Gerontological Social Work Special Issue: Geriatric Social Work Education, 18*(3–4), 119–131.

Musil, C., Youngblut, J., Ahn, S., & Curry, V. (2002). Parenting stress: A comparison of grandmother caretakers and mothers. *Journal of Mental Health and Aging, 8*(3), 197–210.

Musil, C. M., Warner, C. B., Stoller, E. P., & Andersson, T. E. (2005). Women and intergenerational caregiving in families: Structure, ethnicity, and building family ties. In M. L. Wykle, P. J. Whitehouse, & D. L. Morris (Eds.), *Successful aging through the life span* (pp. 143–158). New York: Springer.

National Academy of Certified Care Managers. (2002). Eligibility criteria. http://www.NACCM.net. Accessed 8 Mar 2007.

National Alliance for Caregiving and American Association for Retired Persons. (April 2004). Caregiving in the U.S. http://assets.aarp.org/rgcenter/il/us_caregiving.pdf. Accessed 9 Mar 2007.

National Alliance for Caregiving & American Association for Retired Persons. (2009a). Caregiving in the U.S. 2009. http://www.caregiving.org/data/Caregiving_in_the_US_2009_full_report.pdf. Accessed 25 July 2012.

National Alliance for Caregiving and American Association for Retired Persons. (2009b). Caregiving in the U.S. 2009: A focused look at those caring for someone age 50 or Older. assets.aarp.org/rgcenter/il/caregiving_09.pdf. Accessed 25 July 2012.

Noelker, L. S., & Bass, D. M. (1989). Home care for elderly persons: Linkages between formal and informal caregivers. *Journal of Gerontology, 44,* 563–570.

Olshevski, J. L., Katz, A. D., & Knight, B. G. (1999). The context of stress reduction: Community services and resources for caregivers. In J. Olshevski, A. Katz, & B. Knight (Eds.), *Stress reduction for caregivers* (pp. 117–135). Ann Arbor: Brunner/Mazel.

Peterson, D. A. (1987). *Career paths in the field of aging: Professional gerontology*. Lexington: Lexington Books.

Qualls, S. H., & Czirr, R. (1988). Geriatric health teams: Classifying models of professional and team functioning. *Gerontologist, 28,* 372–376.

Riley M. W., Kahn R. W., & Foner A. (Eds.). (1995). *Age and structural lag: Society's failure to provide meaningful opportunities in work, family, and leisure*. New York: Wiley.
Siegel, J. S. (1999). Demographic introduction to racial/Hispanic elderly populations. In T. Miles (Ed.), *Full-color aging: Facts, goals, and recommendations for America's diverse elders* (pp. 1–19). Washington, DC: Gerontological Society of America.
Smyer, M. A., & Qualls, S. H. (1999). The context and pragmatics of practice. In M. Smyer & S. Qualls (Eds.), *Aging and mental health* (pp. 257–283). Malden: Blackwell.
Soldo, B. J., & Myllyuoma, J. (1983). Caregivers who live with dependent elderly. *Gerontologist, 23,* 605–611.
Sorensen, S., Pinquart, M., & Duberstein, p. (2002). How effective are interventions with caregivers? An updated meta-analysis. *Gerontologist, 42,* 356–372.
Stechenrider, J. S., & Parrott, T. M. (1998). Introduction: The political environment and the new face of aging policy. In J. S. Steckenrider & T. M. Parrott (Eds.), *New directions in old-age policies (1–12).* Albany: State University of New York Press.
St. Onge, M., & Lavoie, F. (1997). The experience of caregiving among mothers of adults suffering from psychotic disorders: Factors associated with their psychological distress. *American Journal of Community Psychology, 25*(1), 73–94.
Stone, R., Cafferata, G. L., & Sangl, J. (1987). Caregivers of the frail elderly: A national profile. *Gerontologist, 27,* 616–626.
Taylor, M. G., & Lynch, S. M. (2011). Cohort differences and chronic diseases profiles of differential disability trajectories. *The Journals of Gerontology, Series B: Psychological Sciences and Social Sciences, 66,* 729–738.
Toseland, R. W., Smith, G. C., & McCallion, p. (1995). Supporting the family in elder care. In G. Smith, S. Tobin, E. Robertson-Tchabo, & p. Power (Eds.), *Strengthening aging families* (pp. 3–24). Thousand Oaks: Sage.
University of Kansas. (2002). 1999: A report on sponsored research the University of Kansas. http://www.kstate.edu/research/awards/archives/ awards99.pdf. Accessed 9 Mar 2007.
University of Kentucky. (2002). Sanders-Brown Alzheimer's Disease Research Center (ADRC): Overview. http://www.mc.uky.edu/coa/ADRC/adrc.htm. Accessed 8 Mar 2007.
University of North Texas. (2002). Applied gerontology: Opportunities for graduate students: Master's program. http://www.unt.edu/pais/grad/gager.htm. Accessed 9 Mar 2007.
U.S. Census Bureau. (August 2008a). Table 2. Projections of the population by selected age groups and sex for the United States: 2010 to 2050 (NP2008-T2). http://www.census.gov/population/www/projections/summarytables.html. Accessed 26 July 2012.
U.S. Census Bureau. (August 2008b). Table 3. Percent distribution of the projected population by selected age groups and sex for the United States: 2010 to 2050 (NP2008-T3). Accessed 25 July 2012.
U.S. Census Bureau (June 2010). Table 10. Resident population by race, Hispanic origin, and age: 2000 and 2009. www.census.gov/compendia/statab/2012/tables/12s0010.pdf. Accessed 25 July 2012.
U.S. Census Bureau (2011a). The Older Population: 2010. http://2010.census.gov/2010census/data/. Accessed 25 July 2011.
U.S. Census Bureau (2011b). Current Population Survey, 2011 Annual Social and Economic Supplement. http://www.census.gov/hhes/families/data/cps2011.html. Accessed 20 July 2012.
U.S. Department of Labor, Bureau of Labor Statistics. (December 2010). Women in the labor force: A databook. www.bls.gov/cps/wlf-databook2011.htm. Accessed 25 July 2012.
Wolf, D. A. (1994). The elderly and their kin: Patterns of availability and access. In L. G. Martin & S. H. Preston (Eds.), *Demography of aging* (pp. 165–194). Washington, DC: National Academy Press.
Zarit, S., Orr, N., & Zarit, J. (1985). *The hidden victims of Alzheimer's disease: Families under stress.* New York: New York University Press.

Social Work, Direct Care Workers, and Family Care Provider Challenges: Crisis in Care

Nancy R. Hooyman

Social workers, direct care workers, and family caregivers are critical in ensuring health and well-being for older adults. With an aging population and an ongoing shortage of professionals focused on care of older adults, society and the caregiving community face unprecedented challenges in meeting the growing demand for high-quality care.

This chapter addresses a crisis in care for older adults that cuts across three different levels of caregivers: professional health care providers, with a focus on geriatric social workers; underpaid direct care or frontline workers (case aides, home health and home care aides, personal care workers, homemaker or chore workers); and unpaid informal family caregivers, typically women in families. Such interconnections among caregivers are emphasized; the author argues that sexism, racism, and ageism underlie all three levels of care. Women, the primary providers of care across these levels and the highest number of adults in poverty, frequently face negative economic consequences in old age because of their multiple caregiving roles across the life course. In addition, the low value placed by our society on caregiving work creates many of the challenges faced by unpaid and underpaid caregivers of older relatives. These challenges, particularly the gendered nature of care, must be addressed from practice, education, research, and policy perspectives in order to promote is to promote effective care to rapidly growing population age 85 years and over who are most in need of long-term assistance.

Although social workers, direct care workers, and family members provide care to persons of any age with chronic health or mental disabilities, this chapter focuses on caring for older adults. The rationale for this is that gerontological social work has, until recently, been a low priority for the social work profession, while the demand for caregiving of elders is growing dramatically. In addition, the author suggests that the dynamics of the gendered nature and low status of caregiving for persons with chronic disabilities are relatively similar across vulnerable populations.

N. R. Hooyman (✉)
CSWE National Center on Gerontological Social Work Education,
School of Social Work, University of Washington, Campus Box 354900,
4101 15th Avenue, NE, Seattle, WA 98105–6299, USA
e-mail: hooy@u.washington.edu

R. C. Talley, S. S. Travis (eds.), *Multidisciplinary Coordinated Caregiving*,
Caregiving: Research • Practice • Policy, DOI 10.1007/978-1-4614-8973-3_4,

Background and Current Status

Crisis in Care in Social Work

By 2010, it is estimated that most health care workers will spend at least 50 % of their time with older adults, and the demands on all three levels of care are increasing dramatically (Bureau of Labor Statistics 2004). Nursing and medicine, similar to social work, are not yet preparing enough graduates to meet the needs of the rapidly growing older population (Blanchette and Flynn 2001) or work effectively with older adults (Division of Nursing, Bureau of Health Professions 2001; Government Accounting Office 2001; Fulmer et al. 2001; Kimball and O'Neill 2001; University of Illinois Nursing Institute 2001). Although the crisis in care affects numerous health care providers, this chapter focuses upon the social work profession.

Among health and mental health providers, social work is distinguished by addressing the social, environmental, and ethical aspects of aging in addition to the physical and psychological considerations (Scharlach et al. (2000). Social work emphasizes the interaction of the person with the environment and interventions focused on individual, family/group, community, and organizational change. The person-in-environment perspective has multiple implications for changing systemic factors to reduce the stress facing older adults and families (e.g., removing barriers to enhance access to services) as well as modifying individual and family capacities to deal with environmental demands.

The values that underlie social work's person-in-environment perspective create a distinctive professional ethic. These values include respect for the dignity, worth, and uniqueness of each human being, the right to self-determination, and the right of individuals to have access to the basic resources of our society. Committed to social justice, social work aims to address inequities across the life course and foster the empowerment of historically disadvantaged persons by increasing their capabilities and opportunities to achieve health and well-being (Damron-Rodriguez 2005).

Social work practitioners bring skills of biopsychosocial assessment, diagnosis, and coordination of resources, and evidence-based interventions with both older adults and their family members. Through information, coordination of resources, education, individual and family counseling, group work, advocacy, and community and organizational change, social workers assist individuals, families, and communities to develop solutions to problems facing them. Evidence-based interventions to enhance older adults' problem-solving capacities and resilience are one of the most basic and critical components of gerontological social work. In addition, social workers understand the organization of service systems, how to access them and influence them to be more responsive to older adults' needs (e.g., advocacy and policymaking), and how to develop, monitor, and evaluate resources. Such micro and macro knowledge, skills, and values are at the core of social work education. Accordingly, the perspective of social work case managers/service providers is generally broader, encompassing more psychosocial, environmental, and ethical considerations than other professions.

The need for gerontological social workers is well documented (Berkman et al. 2000; Rosen and Persky 1997; Scharlach et al. 2000). According to the National Institute of Aging (1997), 60,000–70,000 geriatric social workers will be needed by 2020, yet less than 10 % of that projected need is currently available. The Bureau of Labor Statistics (2004) predicts that the demand for geriatric social workers will increase by over 30 % in large part because of the aging baby boom cohort. In addition, US News and World Report ranks geriatric social work as one of the top 20 careers in terms of growth potential. In fact, it can be argued that virtually all social workers will work in some capacity with older adults and their families. A huge gap exists between the opportunities for and genuine need for gerontological social workers and their professional preparation. This gap is due in part to inadequate gerontological content in social work curriculum, limited gerontological expertise among social work faculty, and lack of student interest in working with the growing aging population (Scharlach et al. 2000).

Education and Training

Professional preparation of gerontological social workers has markedly changed over the past 40 years. In the 1970s and early 1980s, social work programs seeking to prepare their graduates with gerontological competencies care typically developed aging specializations or concentrations. In fact, nearly 50 % of Master of Social Work (MSW) programs offered a specialization in aging in 1984 (Nelson and Schneider 1984). Students were often recruited to these specializations because of the availability of Administration on Aging training grants and stipends to academic institutions. Many students who insisted "I don't want to work with old people" were otherwise convinced by a paid placement in a long-term setting with excellent field supervisors. In numerous instances, once students entered the aging field, they were surprised by how much they learned from and enjoyed working with older adults, and some became employed by their field agency after graduation.

In the early 1980s, the Council on Social Work Education sponsored the development of model specialized gerontological social work course syllabi (Schneider 1984; Schneider et al. 1984a, b). These were not widely adopted for a variety of reasons, including limited funding, competing interests, and lack of faculty "buy in" to the need for specialized gerontological content (Rosen et al. 2000). In 1981, a group of approximately 12 social work faculty members formed the Association for Gerontology in Social Work Education (AGE-SW) and agreed to do "whatever it takes to promote gerontology at our programs" (Schneider 2001). Despite their commitment, interest in aging care declined dramatically in the next 20 years with (a) the cutbacks in Title IVE funding under the Administration on Aging and in most other public sources of support for training gerontological social workers, and (b) the national—and necessary—emphases on the needs of and funding for low-income children and families in the late 1980s and early 1990s. During that time, well-established aging concentrations were often eliminated due to lack of student interest and demand, or alternatively, lack of faculty expertise in gerontology; this decline is captured by the fact that 34 % of programs had an aging concentration in 1992, and only 27 % in 2002 (Cummings and DeCoster 2003).

Because of the past lack of gerontology content throughout social work curricula, few social work students have received the knowledge or skills to work with an aging population unless they specialized in gerontological practice, either through an advanced practice concentration or a certificate program. However, interest in aging specializations continued to decline in the 1990s, when only 2 % of students identified aging as their concentration in 1992, compared with 6 % in 1983 (Damron-Rodriguez et al. 1997; Petersen 1987). Moreover, less than 5 % of students took any advanced aging courses in the past. In the 1990s, nearly 75 % of social work programs did not have faculty with the focused expertise to teach geriatric social work, about 60 % did not offer a specialization in aging, and relatively few students chose to take gerontology courses (CSWE SAGE-SW 2001; Damron-Rodriguez et al. 1997; Gibelman and Schervish 1997; Gleason Wynn 1995; Kropf et al. 1993; Lubben et al. 1992; Rosen et al. 2002; Scharlach et al. 2002; Takamura 2001).

Given this trend, it is not surprising that approximately 16 % of baccalaureate and 4 % of master's graduates work in services to older adults (Gibelman and Schervish 1997; Teare and Sheafor 1995). A major reason for these low percentages of trained and employed gerontological social workers has been the lack of aging-enriched learning opportunities in required foundation social work courses and field practica (first year MSW or junior/senior year of the BSW; Damron-Rodriguez 2005). Fortunately, this pattern is changing as a result of nearly $ 49 million invested by the John A. Hartford Foundation in the Geriatric Social Work Initiative (GSWI), which is described more fully under the section on "Practice and Education."

Although the Hartford Foundation's investments have resulted in dramatic progress, a gap persists between practice needs and professional preparation. For example, in a national survey of a sample of licensed social workers, conducted in 2005 by the National Association of Social Workers, 75 % of respondents reported that they work in some capacity with older adults but are not adequately prepared to do so. To illustrate, child welfare or school social workers increasingly deal with grandparents who are the primary caregivers for grandchildren, but lack the knowledge and skills to assist them with the economic, legal, and health care issues faced. Child welfare practitioners committed to kinship care typically lack the competencies to work with older kin. In fact, given the current and projected rapid increase in the older population, it can be argued that few health and social service settings do and will not involve social workers' interacting with older people and/or their families (Berkman et al. 1996; Scharlach et al. 2000). Given these patterns, all social work graduates, not just those who choose specialized aging courses or concentrations, need foundation competencies to work with older adults and their families.

Two primary factors underlie the shortage of social workers prepared to work effectively with older adults and their families: limited faculty and demand. Given our culture's focus on youth and the perceived low status of older adults, both faculty and students often hold ageist attitudes and fear aging, whether for themselves or their family members. These negative attitudes partially explain how often students will say "I don't want to work with older people," or "nursing homes are just places to die," and how faculty members will question the need for and relevance of infusing aging content in their courses. In contrast, students in the 1980s and 1990s were largely interested with populations that have the "potential to change" or "to contribute to society," which translated into a focus on children and youth, particularly those historically disadvantaged by racism or poverty. This pattern can be explained in part by the association of death with old age and students' infrequent contact with older persons (Damron-Rodriguez et al. 1997). Accordingly, students have generally been unaware of the diversity and richness of the aging population, the complexity of effective multimodal interventions, and the range of community-based gerontological practice settings available. The wide availability of Title IVE child welfare funding for social work student stipends compared to the absence of federal training funds in aging has also intensified students' gravitation toward working with younger generations.

Sexism may underlie the challenges of recruiting faculty, students, and practitioners to address age-related issues. Women form the majority of older adults, formal and informal caregivers of elders, and gerontological social workers. Further, the median salary of social workers in aging is less than any other practice area (NASW 2005). The gendered nature of social work and of caregiving becomes interrelated with the low status of women and older adults in our society, making older women one of the "least attractive" practice populations for young social work students. Until social work educators confront both ageist and sexist attitudes, recruiting students in the absence of financial incentives is likely to remain difficult.

Another barrier is that both students and faculty often fail to see the interconnections of aging with and across different substantive areas. For example, students who intend to work with families may not recognize that every family includes older members, resulting in complex multigenerational family dynamics. As another illustration, students who are committed to feminist practice may be unaware that the majority of older adults are women, many of whom often live in poverty. Aging issues also cross cut the domains of health, mental health, substance abuse, interpersonal violence, and multicultural practice. When faculty members fail to articulate these interconnections to students, aging content tends to be viewed as an "add onto the last class session"; older adults are seen as a separate population.

A primary reason for this "add on" or compensatory curricular approach is that the Council on Social Work Education, the profession's accrediting body, requires extensive foundation content, including content on numerous "at-risk" populations (CSWE 2001). The Educational Policy and Accreditation Standards provide clear guidance about curriculum content for baccalaureate (BSW) generalist education and foundation curriculum for the first year of the MSW. As a result, many social work faculty members feel that too many content demands are placed on an already crowded curriculum and that the curriculum bucket is "too full." When that is the case, they may make minimal efforts to include content on older adults in foundation courses. If that is the case, they attempt to meet accreditation expectations at a minimum. Fox example, they may invite an older person as a guest speaker in a foundation cultural diversity course or address illness, death, and dying rather than the elders' strengths in the last class session in the Human Behavior and Social

Environment course—a point when student engagement in the course is typically low. As another example, foundation social policy courses usually include a review of Social Security and Medicare, yet may not explicitly relate these policies to older adults and changing economic, health care, and demographic needs. At the undergraduate level, aging may be included in contemporary social problems courses, therefore focusing on the negative conditions that face some older people and overlooking their strengths, resilience, and contributions to society. When aging is treated in separate curricular units, it remains somewhat invisible, secondary and peripheral to the curriculum as a whole. As a result, the pedagogy, structure or objectives of courses are not fundamentally changed to ensure that aging is among the organizing curricular themes and embedded throughout the curriculum. Of even greater concern is that these "add on" approaches are unlikely to change students' largely negative attitudes toward aging, excite them about their potential contributions in working with older people, or recruit them to the field.

In summary, the historical pattern of too few faculty prepared to teach gerontological social work content, too few students interested in gerontological careers, and too little outcomes-based gerontological research is well documented (CSWE SAGE-SW 2001). At this point in the development of gerontological social work education, more identification of the need is not required. Instead, what is necessary is the best and most creative thinking about how to break this historical pattern. One way to alter this pattern is through structural changes in social work curricula and new models for transforming gerontological social work education. These directions will be discussed later in the chapter under "Future Needs/Directions in Education and Training."

Crisis in Care Among Direct Care Workers: The Underpaid Caregivers

Ageist and sexist attitudes along with gender-based patterns of care, which underlie the low status of geriatric social work, also influence the conditions faced by frontline workers who comprise the majority of paid (underpaid) caregivers within long-term care settings. They are the "eyes and the ears" of the long-term care system, providing "high touch" intimate, personal, and physically/emotionally challenging care. Yet, these frontline workers generally do not feel prepared, respected, or valued. The typical direct care worker or aide is a middle aged, single mother, with minimal education and living in poverty. Racial inequities in terms of education and employment opportunities partially explain the predominance of African American, Asian, and Latina women, many of whom are immigrants, among such hands-on care providers. Language or cultural differences in communication may interfere with meeting older patients' needs. Our society's lack of public recognition of the hard, socially and economically important work of caregiving is, in turn, reflected in difficult working conditions. These include low pay, limited training, and low status of such direct care workers. Within the long-term care system, paraprofessionals are typically paid $ 7–9 an hour, without benefits. Not surprisingly, the turnover rate is high, with 90 % of direct care staff replaced annually (DSHS 2003; Olson 2003; Wichterich 2000).

Little other compensation exists for such hard, underpaid work. The heavy workload is often a repetition of single tasks, and the risk of personal injury from physical work is high. Older patients who may hold racist attitudes may be disrespectful or even verbally or physically abusive toward workers of color. Because of fiscal pressures and continuous turnover, training is typically limited and supervision inadequate. As a result, most direct care workers lack basic competencies essential to quality care, particularly effective interpersonal communication skills (Levy-Storms 2005). In addition, there are few incentives for direct care workers to obtain more training or education.

The low societal value placed on caregiving within the long-term care system can create problems not only for the workers, but also for older adults, family members, and formal providers of care. Long-term care settings face difficulties recruiting direct care staff: morale among workers is low, turnover is high, and labor shortages and diminished quality of care plague the long-term care system. In fact, at least 40 states currently face shortages of such direct care staff (HHS 2003). Public policy also creates inadequate staffing levels in long-term care settings. Managed care, early discharges, and increased care at home have intensified the demand for intensive, complex long-term direct care. However, fiscal pressures to reduce costs threaten the quality of care. By keeping reimbursement rates low, the federal government sets the near-poverty level wages and undervalues the career paths of direct care staff in long-term care that may negatively affect the physical and mental health and well-being of frail elders. As the predominant long-term care recipients, older women, who are frequently poor, are most often negatively impacted by the adverse work environments faced by their low-income female caregivers.

The policy and educational implications for change are discussed later in the chapter under "Future Needs/Directions."

Crisis in Care Among Families: The Unpaid Caregivers

Over 70 % of older adults receive long-term care in their own homes or other community-based settings. As a result, families are the primary providers of care, comprising 70–80 % of informal providers (HHS 2003; Doty et al. 2001; National Academy on an Aging Society 2000; Spillman and Pezzin 2000). In fact, parent care has become a predictable and nearly universal experience across the life course, yet most adults are inadequately prepared for this role and responsibility.

In addition, the demands on family caregivers to provide long-term care will grow commensurately with the aging of the population, particularly the rapid growth of those over age 85 who are most likely to have chronic illnesses. These expectations on families to provide "high tech" in addition to "high touch" care are intensified by (1) older adults and families' preferences for home care; (2) federal and state policies that provide incentives to discharge patients quickly from hospitals, thus leading to medically oriented acute care, postacute and rehabilitative care (e.g., intravenous drug therapy, ventilator assistance, and wound care) being provided in home care and community-based settings; and (3) pressures to reduce health care costs generally. The estimated costs for home care, which the government would need to absorb if family care were not available, would be nearly $ 94 million a year (AOA 2003; LaPlante et al. 2002).

Sexist attitudes toward women's roles and responsibilities and the low value placed on the importance of caregiving also underlie the gendered nature of unpaid family care, which is socially invisible and undervalued work. Socialized to assume care roles, women form over 70 % of family caregivers (National Association of State Units on Aging 2003). Women who are caregivers to older parents spend an average of 22 h a week providing care (National Academy on an Aging Society 2000). Many of these women juggle multiple roles and responsibilities of wife, daughter, granddaughter, employee, and parent to dependent children, although the greatest conflicts tend to be between informal care responsibilities and employment (Brody 2004; Spillman and Pezzin 2000). Among all types of caregivers (primary and secondary), 36 % are wives, 29 % are daughters, 8 % are sons, 20 % are other female relatives (nieces, granddaughters, etc.), and the remainder is male relatives. Among primary caregivers (e.g., one family member assumes most of the responsibility), 48 % are spouses/partners, and 74 % are women, with very few sons or other male relatives as primary caregivers (National Association of State Units on Aging 2003; Matthews and Heidon 1998; Seltzer and Li 2000; Spillman and Pezzin 2000; Stone 2000; Tennstedt 1999).

Types of care also vary by gender and family relationship. Spouses perform 80 % of caregiving tasks, especially household chores and personal care that consume 40–60 h per week. Male caregivers are typically husbands/partners. Among adult children, daughters are more likely than sons to be involved in caring for (e.g., help with daily tasks such as bathing, dressing, and eating) as well as caring about (e.g., relational aspect of care involves trust, rapport, compassion, comfort, communication, sense of psychological responsibility). In general, sons tend to focus on more circumscribed and sporadic tasks (house and yard maintenance, financial management, occasional shopping trip) than on personal, hands-on care (Sanders and MacFarland 2002). In addition, sons generally place more importance on completing care goals and less on emotional well-being. Given this gender-based division of caregiving tasks, daughters tend to experience more stress than sons, even when they both are performing similar tasks across similar time periods (Dautzenberg et al. 1999; Gerstel 2001; Martin 2000). Accordingly, sons and husbands are more likely to utilize formal services than are daughters or wives (Hughes et al. 1999; Seltzer and Li 2000). These gender-based patterns tend to persist across cultures, with women of color even less likely than their Caucasian counterparts to utilize formal services to reduce their care demands (Aranda and Knight 1997; Navaie et al. 2001).

In the past decade, gerontological social work scholarship has been part of the extensive caregiving research that has identified the needs and burdens of caregiving. Rather than more documentation of caregivers' needs, evidence-based interventions and policy changes, which value and support the societally important work of caring for older adults, are critical to preventing caregiving stress across the life span.

Future Needs/Directions Across the Three Levels of Caregivers

Practice and Education

The demand for more gerontological social workers cannot readily be separated from the need for geriatric social work education. The social work profession is both challenged and well suited to address the aging of our society. It is challenged because of the inadequate preparation of social workers to meet the care demands inherent in the growing aging population. Yet, it is well suited by its distinctive psychosocial and person-in-environment perspective relevant to enhancing the well-being of older adults and their families.

The need to expand the number of gerontological social work specialists is even more acute among populations of color, since the number of minority elders will grow faster than majority older populations between now and 2030 (US Administration on Aging 2002). In addition, all social workers, regardless of their primary field of practice, need to have at least a basic level of competence in working with older adults. Such an approach is congruent with the advanced generalist model of social work education and with the profession's accrediting standards.

Multifaceted approaches are essential to increase the number of gerontological social workers: faculty and programmatic development, student recruitment and support, curriculum and organizational change, and increase in practicum placements in agencies serving older adults. Central to all these initiatives is to engage key stakeholders at various levels: deans/directors, faculty, students, field instructors, practitioners, and older adult consumers. In addition, preparation to be culturally competent caregivers cross cuts all initiatives. Since the majority of social work graduates will work in some capacity with older adults and their families, as indicated by the 2005 NASW data, gerontological knowledge, skills, and values must be embedded within required foundation courses rather than relying upon specializations or concentrations which reach only a small percentage of students. Curricular initiatives must therefore address both content and process in changing social work to include aging-enriched learning opportunities for all students.

For over two decades, the John A. Hartford Foundation has addressed the shortage of geriatric physicians and nurses. Since 1998, the foundation has also provided critical leadership in preparing gerontological social work practitioners, scholars, and educators. These Geriatric Social Work Initiatives include programs for faculty scholars, doctoral dissertation support, practicum placements using a rotational model, faculty and programmatic development, and curriculum enrichment. The recognition of the need for structural, curricular, and organizational changes to infuse gerontological competencies throughout the curriculum to reach the majority of students was central to the faculty development (CSWE Strengthening Aging and

Gerontological Education in Social Work or SAGE-SW) and the curriculum change projects (Geriatric Enrichment in Social Work Education or GeroRich) funded from 1999–2004. The two projects complemented each other, with SAGE-SW focusing on faculty development and course content, and Geriatric Enrichment funding 67 undergraduate and graduate programs nationwide to transform their curricula and organizational culture and create long-term sustainable change. The CSWE National Center for Gerontological Social Work Education (Gero-Ed) builds upon these curricular accomplishments by fostering a model of curriculum infusion and transformation among social work programs nationally. Restructuring curriculum through infusion—permeating foundation curriculum with aging content taken by all students—was a strategy to ensure that all social workers who work with older adults have basic knowledge and skill competencies. As a result of the Hartford initiatives, the interest in and enthusiasm for gerontological social work among key stakeholders are dramatically increasing. Ongoing outcomes-based research will determine the impact of these curriculum initiatives on students, faculty, practitioners, and educators as well as their long-term sustainability after funding has ended.

The need to improve the recruitment and preparation of direct care workers is acute, but seldom recognized by both public and private funders. The nature of the long-term care work environment is one of the most important predictors of job satisfaction and turnover among hands-on caregiving workers. This is shaped primarily by the management style and quality of supervision. The job satisfaction of direct care workers is likely to be enhanced by changes in the organizational environment that support worker autonomy and a sense of personal responsibility for one's work (e.g., involvement in care planning meetings) and provide training and feedback from supervisors (Olson 2003). Improved working conditions must also include increases in wages and benefits, which are discussed under the section on Future Policy Directions.

The need for family caregiver education and training is extensively documented in the caregiving research. Most families, despite good intentions, rarely prepare in advance for taking care of an older relative. Fear of such responsibilities and denial that "this won't happen to me" underlie inadequate preparation. In fact, a crisis, such as a broken hip, a diagnosis of Alzheimer's disease, or an imminent hospital discharge, is typically when families first confront their care responsibilities. During such dramatic changes, families often lack the time or energy to turn to the growing educational resources provided by corporations, employee assistance programs, religious institutions, hospitals, long-term care facilities, the self-help sections of bookstores, or the media. An obstacle to such planning is that most families do not define themselves as "caregivers" until the level and intensity of care increases (Montgomery and Kosloski 2001). While education and training are increasingly available to family caregivers, an ongoing challenge is how to provide information to families and their older relatives to foster open discussion and planning before intensive caregiving is needed. In other words, educational interventions for the general public should focus on planning for care responsibilities and preventing caregiving stress, rather than providing information to ameliorate it after the fact.

Families enmeshed in caregiving are eager for education. A danger, however, is that some educational approaches inadvertently imply that families can reduce their stress by becoming more efficient and faster at their tasks. In many instances, training that is a one-way transmittal of information cannot alleviate the stress of continuous daily care. The goal of educational programs should not be increased efficiency or cost savings, but caregiver resilience and well-being. Instead, educational programs must offer opportunities for caregivers to provide input and to experience a sense of mastery and empowerment rather than be blamed or undervalued (Stone 2000). The strengths perspective of social work is conducive to caregiver empowerment. Social workers are well positioned to work with families to locate needed resources and services for both themselves and their older relatives. In fact, it is social work's emphasis on how the environment, including structural factors such as discrimination, health disparities, and service barriers, affects caregiver burden that distinguishes it from other professions that may interact with family members. With its systems perspective, social workers recognize that the client system includes family caregivers, not just the care recipient.

Research

The need for research includes both formal and informal levels of care. With the growth of the oldest-old, more ways must be found to provide cost-effective quality services, without placing disproportionate burdens upon families as a low-cost alternative to formal care. The need for outcomes-based research to guide service expenditures is intensifying with current fiscal constraints and cutbacks. Quality assurance is even more critical, given the trend toward less centralized, often privatized services, and more "outsourced" contracts. Social workers—as with all health care professionals—are increasingly expected to demonstrate professional competence, cost-effectiveness, and accountability.

Little attention has been given to developing empirical evidence regarding the added value of gerontological social work in health and long-term settings, evidence essential to funding both services and educational initiatives. Well-designed studies are needed to document the distinctive contributions of gerontological social work and "best practices" for improving the health and well-being outcomes of older adults and their family caregivers. Continuous quality improvement evaluation and data collection of program innovations and increased practice accountability are also essential (Scarlet et al. 2000). As one example of the type of research needed, the Geriatric Social Work Initiative at Boston University, funded by Atlantic Philanthropies, is conducting a randomized clinical trial to investigate whether specific geriatric social work interventions are cost-effective and lead to improved health and social outcomes for older persons and their families.

A predominant theme in social work is the integration of research and practice. While the quality and significance of social work research is growing rapidly, research findings are often not utilized by practitioners faced with heavy workloads and limited time. In addition, practitioners may not see the relevance of research to their practice, even though social work education programs prepare all graduates to utilize empirical evidence. Ways to translate research to practice and to disseminate findings widely are ongoing challenges for the profession. Fortunately, the Society for Social Work and Research (SSWR) is providing national leadership regarding evidence-based practice, and the National Association of Social Workers is committed to providing their membership with useful research findings. The Institute for the Advancement of Social Work Research (IASWR) provides leadership for the development, dissemination, and utilization of scientific knowledge in social work. In addition, the Campbell Collaboration and the Practice Guidelines Coalition are working to identify effective interventions and translate research findings into implications and guidelines for practice, but these groups have not yet addressed interventions for older adults.

Policy

The lack of societal recognition for the benefits of social work with older adults, as well as the gendered nature of social work practice partially underlies the inadequate salaries for gerontological social workers. As noted earlier, gerontological social work is the lowest paying field in social work practice (NASW 2005). The prevalence of small, private nonprofit agencies with constrained budgets delivering services also influences the low salaries in aging. In addition, qualifications for employment in many aging settings are often less rigorous than in mental health, health, or child welfare, where employees are typically required to have advanced training and/or a clinical license. Questions need to be raised whether the low status of older adults, oftentimes viewed as "unproductive" and resistant to change, or the predominance of women in geriatric social work, underlies these salary and qualification differences in qualification requirements. Less rigorous employment qualifications stem, in part, from the lack of standards for educational credentials in gerontology, in general, and in social work practice with older adults, in particular (Austin 2005; Berkman et al. 1996; Scharlach et al. 2000). The 2005 White House Mini-Conference on Aging on Geriatric Healthcare Workforce Issues recommended more federal funding for the education and reimbursement of health care providers, including geriatric social workers. In addition, the 2005 Social Work Congress identified ten imperatives for the future of the profession, including assure excellence in aging knowledge, skills, and competencies at all levels of social work education, practice, and research. Although substantial change in the geriatric workforce is unlikely in the short run, awareness of the documented need for gerontologically competent social workers has been raised.

Not surprisingly, both low wages and inadequate benefits (e.g., health care, sick leave, bonuses, dependent care assistance, child care, and transportation) are critical factors in the recruitment and retention of direct care workers. Women of color predominate among underpaid caregivers, suggesting that ageist, sexist, and racist attitudes may play out in these economic disparities. The federal government, through

Medicaid, determines wage levels, although some states have implemented "pass throughs" based on a set dollar amount for workers per hour or patient day, or as a percentage of the increased reimbursement rate. The recruitment and retention of direct care workers qualified to provide patient-centered care was another recommendation from the 2005 White House Mini-Conference on Geriatric Workforce Issues. With cuts in Medicare and Medicaid, substantial improvement in the wages of direct care workers will not occur in the foreseeable future. Initiatives that substantially increase labor costs in health and long-term care are unlikely to be supported by the government or by individual recipients who share the costs of care. The extent to which caregiving is viewed as "women's work" or not socially valued as hard, essential, and productive work may also influence policymakers' resistance to increasing wage levels and benefits for direct care workers.

Drawing upon the classic concept of H. G. Mills (1959), gender inequities in family caregiving are a social problem, not a "private trouble." Thus, Mills argues that care of older adults is socially important and hard work that must be supported with public resources and shared by both men and women. Ultimately, caregiving values of collectivity and community must provide a counterbalance to our societal values of individualism, family privacy, and residual public policy. Caregiving values must become public values, rather than divided along economic, racial, and gender lines.

Current social policies tend to view families as a low-cost way to provide long-term care rather than essential care providers to be supported through education and policy. Policies to support family caregivers should take account of the diversity of family structures (e.g., families of color, gay/lesbian/bisexual/transgender families, and kinship care) and needs, and strive for gender equity in both the home and societal institutions. In other words, public/private, political/personal, formal/informal, work/home spheres of responsibility cannot be separated from one another. Changes to support family caregivers are needed in societal values, public policy, the workplace, educational and religious institutions, and the private sphere of home and family.

One way to support family caregivers is through economic supports. Caregiver or attendant allowances, common in other industrialized nations, or cash and counseling programs that define the consumer as the caregiver, would be the first step in legitimizing and making more visible the important work of caregiving. Cash and counseling programs recognize the replacement costs (e.g., what society would have to spend if families were not providing care) high and families' economic contribution to society. Not surprisingly, consumers who are disabled or older prefer to pay a family member as their caregiver rather than a stranger (Simon-Rusinowitz et al. 2005). Economic supports could be used to help pay for services for the care receiver or supports for the family unit. Such supports would also recognize the economic costs of caregiving for older women, who have moved in and out of the labor force across the life span as they cared for young children or parents, grandparents, adult children, siblings, and husbands. Attaching a market value to the socially necessary work of caring could also provide both women and men with more choice about assuming a caregiving role or working outside the home. Accordingly, modifications in Social Security and other pension systems could be made to recognize the years spent out of the labor force by many women caregivers, yet such changes are unlikely with the increased focus on privatization (Gonyea and Hooyman 2005). Adequately compensating family caregivers, regardless of gender, provides societal recognition that the work of caring for older relatives is a service to society that is just as important as the manufacture of airplanes or the development of software. In doing so, the affective or emotional ties of caregiving are unlikely to be diminished, given the strength and predominance of these ties.

Economic supports cannot alleviate the emotional and physical stress of care. Services to support family caregivers that take account of the wide range of needs and family structures are essential, whether they are flexible, accessible respite care, or educational and support groups tailored to caregivers' needs. A family-centered approach to service delivery would provide resource choices for caregivers across the life span, including them in care planning and benefiting both the care provider and the care receiver. Estes et al. (1993) recommend community gerontology teams encompassing both formal and informal caregivers, including representatives from senior, children's, and other social action groups, to bring an intergenerational comprehensive approach to empower both older adults and their caregivers. Pilot projects funded by the Kellogg Foundation provide a single access point through one phone call, and multiple options based on consumer's values and circumstances. Nontraditional settings, such as religious institutions, community centers, local businesses, and other community sites, can enhance caregivers' access to services. Neighborhood-based Gatekeeper Outreach models (e.g., utility meter readers, customer service representatives, bank tellers, apartment managers, bartenders, and postal carriers) can identify vulnerable older adults and their caregivers and connect them with services through information and referral. In the long run, our society must move beyond defining issues related to long-term care as an individual or family problem to that of a societal need requiring a comprehensive universal long-term policy.

Summary

An underlying assumption of this chapter is that the gender inequities and low status of both formal (e.g., direct care workers, professional social workers) and informal (e.g., family members) care providers need to be addressed by professional organizations, unions, advocates for older care recipients, educational institutions, and federal policymakers. Without improved recruitment, education/training, and retention of both informal and formal care providers, the well-being of frail older adults is at risk. Strategies for mobilizing family caregivers for change in existing long-term care and health policies and formulating new legislation and practices are essential to creating more choices for men and women caregivers and recipients. In doing so, we need to rethink how problems facing caregivers are defined and how solutions are formulated so that we may contemplate alternatives today's accepted wisdom (Dalley 1988).

This analysis of the gendered nature and structure of care in our society is intended to raise questions and suggest long-range changes in economic and social policies and practices related to the important work of caregiving. Long-term directions have been suggested, while recognizing that incremental change, although limited, is essential to a vision for the future: "The vision of a world as we would like it to be is essential to progress toward that world" (Miller 1994, p. 30). The directions of gender justice and a model of comprehensive, accessible social care are not yet feasible. Nevertheless, the very act of questioning and challenging the assumptions underlying the basis of daily living and care within and outside the home can have profound repercussions over time on our values, attitudes, and polices toward professional, direct care and family caregivers. Social change typically occurs in a series of short-run increments in which agendas are partially and unevenly implemented. It is the author's belief that in the long run, both male and female professional and family caregivers within the field of social work could benefit from implementation of a model of care that bridges home and work along with informal and formal spheres and that ensures a choice, increased economic supports, and public respect within both domains.

References

American Association of Colleges of Nursing. (2001). *2000–2001 Enrollment and graduations in baccalaureate and graduate programs in nursing*. Washington, DC: Author.

Aranda, M., & Knight, B. C. (1997). The influence of ethnicity and culture on the caregiver stress and coping process: A sociocultural review and analysis. *Gerontologist, 37,* 342–354.

Austin, C. (2005). The future of social work with older adults. *Families in Society* (Special Issue), *86*(3).

Blanchette, P., & Flynn, B. (2001). Geriatric medicine: An approaching crisis. *Generations, 25*(1), 80–85.

Berkman, B., Damron-Rodriguez, J., Dobrof, R., & Harry, L. (1996). Social work. In S. M. Klein (Ed.), *A national agenda for geriatric education: White papers* (pp. 53–85). New York: Springer.

Berkman, B., Silverstone, B., Simmons, W. J., Volland, P. J., & Howe, J. L. (2000). Social work gerontological practice: The need for faculty development in the new millennium. *Journal of Gerontological Social Work, 34,* 5–23.

Brody, E. (2004). *Women in the middle: Their parent care years* (2nd ed.). New York: Springer.

Bureau of Labor Statistics. (1999). *Occupational employment projections to 2008*. Washington, DC: Author.

Bureau of Labor Statistics. (2004). *Social workers*. http://stats.bls.gov/oco/ocos060.htm. Accessed 2 Jan 2007.

Carmel, S., & Cwikel, J. (1992). Changes in knowledge, attitudes and work preferences following courses in gerontology among medical, nursing, and social work students. *Educational Gerontology, 18,* 329–342.

Council on Social Work Education (CSWE). (2001). *Educational policy and accreditation standards*. Alexandria: Author.

Council on Social Work Education Strengthening Aging & Gerontological Education in Social Work. (CSWE SAGE-SW). (2001). *Strengthening the impact of social work to improve the quality of life for older adults & their families: A blueprint for the new millennium*. Alexandria: Author.

Cummings, S. M., & DeCoster, V. A. (2003). The status of specialized gerontological training in graduate social work education. *Educational Gerontology, 29,* 235–250.

Dalley, G. (1988). *Ideologies of caring: Rethinking community and collectivism*. London: McMillan.

Damron-Rodriguez, J. (2005). *Reality check: Social work*. (2005, July 16). Presented at the Min-Conference on Geriatric Healthcare Workforce Issues, the White House Conference on Aging, Washington, DC.

Damron-Rodriguez, J., & Lubben, J. E. (1994). Multidisciplinary factors in gerontological curriculum adoption in schools of social work. *Gerontology and Geriatrics Education, 14*(4), 39–52.

Damron-Rodriguez, J., Villa, V., Tseng, H. F., & Lubben, J. E. (1997). Demographic and organizational influences on the development of gerontological social work curriculum. *Gerontology and Geriatrics Education, 17*(3), 3–18.

Dautzenberg, G. H., Diederiks, J., Philipsen, H., & Tan, F. (1999). Multigenerational caregiving and well-being: Distress of middle aged daughters providing assistance to elderly parents. *Women and Health, 29*(4), 57–74.

Division of Nursing, Bureau of Health Professions. (2001). The national sample survey of registered nurses March 2000: Preliminary findings. Washington, DC: Author.

Doty, P. J., Stone, R. I., Jackson, M. E., & Drabek, J. L (2001). Informal caregiving. In C. J. Evashwick (Ed.), *The continuum of long-term care* (2nd ed., pp. 132–154). Albany: Delmar.

Estes, C., Swan, J., Bergthold, L., Binney, E., Carrell, D., Casper, M. et al. (1993). *The long-term care crisis*. Newbury Park: Sage.

Federation of Nursing & Health Professionals. (2001). *The nurse shortage: Perspectives from current direct care nurses and former direct care nurses*. Washington, DC: Author.

Fulmer, T., Flaherty, E., & Medley, L. (2001). Geriatric nurse practitioners: Vital to the future of healthcare for elders. *Generations, 25*(1), 72–75.

Gerstel, N. (2001). Men's caregiving: Gender and the contingent character of care. *Gender and Society, 15*(2), 197–217.

Gibelman, M., & Schervish, P. H. (1995). Pay equity in social work—not. *Social Work, 40*(5), 622–629.

Gibelman, M., & Schervish, P. H. (1997). *Who we are: A second look*. Washington, DC: National Association of Social Workers.

Gleason Wynn, P. E. (1995). Addressing the educational needs of nursing home social workers. *Gerontology and Geriatrics Education, 16*(2), 31–36.

Gonyea, J., & Hooyman, N. (2005). Reducing poverty among older women: Social Security reform and gender equity. *Families in Society, 86*(3), 338–346.

Government Accounting Office. (2001). *Nursing workforce: Emerging nurse shortages due to multiple factors* (GAO-91–944). Washington, DC: Author.

Hayslip, B., Shore, R. J., Henderson, C., & Lambert, P. (1998). Custodial grandparenting and grandchildren with problems: Their impact on role satisfaction and role meaning. *Journal of Gerontology: Social Sciences, 53B*, S164–S174.

Hughes, S. L., Giobbie-Hurder, A., Weaver, F. M., Kubal, J. D., & Henderson, W. (1999). Relationship between caregiver burden and health-related quality of life. *Gerontologist, 39*, 534–535.

Institute of Medicine. (1994). *Training physicians to care for older Americans: Progress, obstacles and future directions*. Washington, DC: National Academies Press.

Kimball, B., & O'Neill, E. (2001). *Health care, human crisis: The American nursing shortage*. Princeton: Robert Wood Johnson Foundation.

Kropf, N. P., Schneider, R. L., & Stahlman, S. D. (1993). Status of gerontology in baccalaureate social work education. *Educational Gerontology, 19*(7), 623–634.

LaPlante, M. P., Harrington, C., & Kang, T. (2002). Estimated paid and unpaid hours of personal assistance services in activities of daily living provided to adults living at home. *Health Services Research, 37*, 397–415.

Lubben, J., Damron-Rodriguez, J., & Beck, J. (1992). A national survey of aging curriculum in schools of social work. *Journal of Gerontological Social Work, 42*, 61–75.

Martin, C. (2000). More than the work: Race and gender differences in caregiving burden. *Journal of Family Issues, 21*(8), 986–1005.

Matthews, S. H., & Heidon, J. (1998). Meeting filial responsibilities in brothers-only sibling groups. *Journals of Gerontology, 50B*, S278–S286.

Miller, D. (1994). What is needed for true equality: An overview of policy issues for women. In L. Davis (Ed.), *Building on women's strengths* (pp. 27–56). New York: Haworth.

Mills, C. W. (1959). *The sociological imagination*. New York: Oxford University Press.

Montgomery, R., & Kosloski, K. (2001). *Change, continuity and diversity among caregivers. Caregiving resources for the aging network*. Washington, DC: Administration on Aging.

National Academy on an Aging Society. (2000, May). *Helping the elderly with activity limitations* (Caregiving #7). Washington, DC: Author.

National Association of Social Workers (NASW) Center for Workforce Studies. (2005). *Assuring the sufficiency of a frontline workforce: A national study of licensed social workers. Preliminary report*. Washington, DC: Author.

National Association of State Units on Aging (NASUA). (2003). *The aging network implements the National Family Caregiver Support Program*. Washington, DC: Administration on Aging.

National Institute on Aging. (1984). Report on education and training in geriatrics and gerontology. Bethesda: Department of Health and Human Services.

National Institute on Aging (1997). Personnel for health needs of the elderly through the year 2020. Bethesda: Department of Health and Human Services.

Navaie, W. M., Feldman, P. H., Gould, D. A., Levine, C., Kuerbis, A. N., & Donelan, K. (2001). The experiences and challenges of informal caregivers: Common themes and differences among White caregivers and Hispanics. *Gerontologist, 41*(6), 733–741.

Neal, M. B., Ingersoll-Dayton, B., & Starrels, M. E. (1997). Gender and relationship differences in caregiving patterns and consequences among employed caregivers. *Gerontologist, 37*, 804–816.

Nelson, G., & Schneider, R. L. (1984). The current status of gerontology in graduate social work education. Washington, DC: CSWE: Series in Gerontology.

Olson, L. K. (2003). *The not-so golden years: Caregiving, the frail elderly and the long-term care establishment*. New York: Rowman & Littlefield.

Peterson, D. A., & Wendt, P. F. (1990). Employment in the field of social work: Implications for educating professionals. *Social Work, 35*(5), 412–415.

Rosen, A., & Persky, T. (1997). Meeting the mental health needs of older people: Policy and practice issues for social work. In C. Saltz (Ed.), *Social work responses to the 1995 White House Conference on Aging: From issues to actions* (pp. 45–54). New York: Haworth Press.

Rosen, A., & Zlotnik, J. L. (2001a). Demographics and reality: The "disconnect" in social work education. *Journal of Gerontological Social Work, 36*(3/4), 81–97.

Rosen, A., & Zlotnik, J. L. (2001b). Social work's response to a growing older population. *Generations, 25*(1), 69–71.

Rosen, A., Zlotnik, J. L., Curl, A., & Green, R. (2000). *CSWE SAGE-SW National Competencies survey and report*. Alexandria: Council on Social Work Education.

Rosen, A., Zlotnik, J. L., & Singer, T. (2002). Basic gerontological competence for all social workers: The need to "gerontologize" social work education. *Journal of Gerontological Social Work, 399*(1/2), 25–36.

Sanders, S., & McFarland, P. (2002). Perceptions of caregiving role by son's caring for a parent with Alzheimer's disease. *Journal of Gerontological social Work, 37*, 61–75.

Scharlach, A., Damron-Rodriguez, J., Robinson, B., & Feldman, R. (2000). Educating social workers for an aging society: A vision for the 21st century. *Journal of Social Work Education, 36*(3), 521–538.

Scharlach, A., Simon, J., & Dal Santo, T. (2002). Who is providing social services to today's older adults? Implications of a survey of aging services personnel. *Journal of Gerontological Social Work, 38*(4), 5–17.

Schneider, R. (Ed.) (1984). *Gerontology in social work education: Faculty development and continuing education*. Alexandria: Council on Social Work Education.

Schneider, R. (2001, Spring). A 20 year retro-history of AGE-SW. *AGE-SW Newsletter, 1*, p. 4. http://www.agesocialwork.org/spring2001feature.html. Accessed 26 Jan 2007.
Schneider, R., Decker, T., Freeman, J., & Syran, C. (1984a). *A curriculum concentration in gerontology for graduate social work education.* Washington, DC: Council on Social Work Education.
Schneider, R., Decker, T., Freeman, J., & Syran, C. (1984b). *The integration of gerontology into social work educational curricula.* Washington, DC: Council on Social Work Education.
Seltzer, M., & Li, L. W. (2000). The dynamics of caregiving: Transitions during a three-year prospective study. *Gerontologist, 36,* 165–178.
Simon-Rusinowitz, L., Mahoney, K. J., Loughlin, D. M., & Sadler, M. D. (2005). Paying family caregivers: An effective policy option in the Arkansas Cash and Counseling Demonstration and Evaluation. In R. Caputo (Ed.). *Challenges of aging on U.S. families: Policy and practice implications* (pp. 83–106). Binghamton: The Haworth Press.
Spillman, B. C., & Pezzin, L. E. (2000). Potential and active family caregivers: Changing networks and the "sandwich generation." *Milbank Quarterly, 78,* 347–374.
Stone, R. (2000). *Long-term care for the elderly with disabilities: Current policy, emerging trends and implications for the 21st century.* New York: The Milbank Memorial Fund.
Takamura, J. C. (2001). Towards a new era in aging and social work. *Journal of Gerontological Social Work, 36*(3/4), 1–11.
Teare, R., & Sheafor, B. (1995). *Practice-sensitive social work education.* Alexandria: Council on Social Work Education.
Tennstedt, S. (1999). *Family caregiving in an aging society. Symposium on an Aging Society.* Washington, DC: Administration on Aging.
University of Illinois Nursing Institute (2001). Who will care for each of us? America's coming health care crisis. Chicago: University of Illinois Nursing Institute.
U.S. Administration on Aging. (2002). *A profile of older Americans.* Washington, DC: Author.
Wichterich, C. (2000). *The globalized woman: Reports from a future of inequality.* New York: St. Martens Press.

Psychological Aspects of Caregiving

Laura M. Arnstein and Ronald T. Brown

Psychological Aspects of Caregiving

Over the past decade, an extensive literature has emerged within psychology related to the caregiving of disabled family members. A search of the major database of psychological research, PsychINFO, revealed over 12,000 articles, books, or chapters related to caregiving. To date, a majority of the psychological literature has focused on caregiving for older adults, including geriatric issues, with less literature devoted to pediatric populations.

Significant and dramatic changes in the delivery of health care within this country have, in part, fueled interest in this area. First, with advanced technologies in medical care, individuals are surviving previously unsurvivable illnesses, thereby resulting in an increase in the need for caregiving by family members. Second, increased costs of health care in this country have resulted in a movement toward home-based care of individuals who in previous years may have been hospitalized or treated in a residential or rehabilitation care facility. As a result of these two factors, record numbers of adults are providing care for disabled parents, spouses, and children.

This chapter focuses on current and future contributions of psychology as a discipline and psychologists as health service providers to caregivers. We also focus on psychological caregiving science and its implications for caregiver practice.

L. M. Arnstein (✉)
College of Medicine, Genetics & Developmental Pediatrics,
Medical University of South Carolina, Rutledge Tower,
135 Rutledge Ave., RT 396, Charleston, SC 29403, USA
e-mail: carpentl@musc.edu

R. T. Brown
University of North Texas at Dallas, Office of the President,
7300 University Hills Bouleverd,
Dallas, TX 75241 USA

R. C. Talley, S. S. Travis (eds.), *Multidisciplinary Coordinated Caregiving*,
Caregiving: Research • Practice • Policy, DOI 10.1007/978-1-4614-8973-3_5,

Current Status

The process of caregiving may be conceptualized as a developmental process affected by multiple variables. A review of the literature reveals that caregivers frequently evidence difficulties with overall adjustment, and are at-risk for the development of depression, anxiety, and somatic symptoms that require intervention. Given that caregivers are at increased risk for serious psychological and physical difficulties, psychologists have specifically focused their efforts on improving the quality of life of caregivers through practice, education/training, research, and policy/advocacy.

Psychological Practice

The literature suggests that caregiving impacts both physical and mental health. Caregiving has been clearly linked with physical morbidity in studies using a variety of methodologies, including self-report ratings of physical health, health care utilization, and direct measurement of immune function (Shulz et al. 1990). Haug et al. (1999), in a longitudinal 2-year investigation of elderly caregivers, found significant decreases in physical and mental health during this period.

Similarly, Grant et al. (2002a, b) followed a sample of 119 caregivers for 18 months. They found that caregivers had higher systolic blood pressure at rest than did noncaregivers, and the caregivers whose spouses were residentially placed or deceased showed improvement in physical symptoms, while caregivers who continued to provide care showed no change in physical symptoms.

The psychological literature suggests that caregiving is associated with diminished health status, which is related to difficulties in adhering to self-care regimens, including medication adherence, attending appointments with health care providers, and exercising routine health behaviors that are compatible with good health care (e.g., diet, exercise, and sleep; Connell and Gallant 1999).

The physically deleterious impact of caregiving has been addressed by Schulz and Beach (1999), who studied 400 elderly spousal caregivers ranging in age from 66 to 96 years. Findings revealed that even after controlling for demographic factors, illnesses, and subclinical cardiovascular disease, spouses who provided care and simultaneously reported perceived emotional and mental strain had higher frequencies of mortality than did noncaregiving comparison controls. These data suggest that caregiving is an independent risk factor that compromises health and is also associated with mortality.

Caregiver Variables

Specific caregiver characteristics play an important role in predicting the physical and psychological well-being of caregivers. These characteristics identified in the literature include ethnicity, gender, social support, stress appraisal, and coping style.

Ethnicity The majority of studies examining ethnicity have focused on the differences between African-American and Caucasian caregivers (for review see, Dilworth-Anderson et al. 2002). In general, findings reveal that, relative to their majority Caucasian counterparts, minority caregivers report greater social supports from informal social networks. In addition, some investigations have demonstrated fewer depressive symptoms among African-American caregivers relative to other groups, although other studies have revealed few differences (Dilworth-Anderson et al. 2002). Differences in coping strategies among African-American caregivers (Differences in coping strategies used by African-American, as opposed to those used by Caucasians) have been found in some studies. For example, African-American caregivers evidence greater use of prayer and religion as a means of coping, relative to their Caucasian counterparts. Clearly, there is a dearth of literature related to cultural and ethnic variance in adaptation to the caregiving experience. The field is ripe for additional studies in this area, particularly research focusing on specific cultures and ethnic groups other than African-American and Caucasian individuals (e.g., Asian-Americans, Hispanics).

Gender In the majority of studies reviewed, female caregivers have reported more psychiatric symptoms than their male counterparts (Yee and Schulz 2000). Bookwala and Schulz (2000), in an investigation of approximately 300 elderly spousal caregivers, provided important data indicating that women experience greater stressors and depressive symptoms associated with the caregiving experience than do their male counterparts. Further, some experts have suggested that women respond differently to the role demands associated with caregiving than men (Yee and Schulz 2000). However, females were found to be personally engaged in a greater number of caregiving behaviors, while men were more apt to obtain informal assistance with caregiving tasks. In addition, males and females have been found to employ differential coping strategies. For example, in a longitudinal investigation of parents of adult children with mental retardation (Essex et al. 1999), mothers were found to use more problem-focused coping strategies relative to fathers. No differences were found for emotion-focused coping strategies. In addition, less use of emotion-focused coping strategies relative to problem-focused coping styles buffered the impact of caregiving for mothers, yet not for fathers.

Social Support Social support is often operationally defined as the number of individuals who the caregiver may turn to for utilitarian support, social and activity support, and refers to the caregiver's satisfaction with perceived support. Caregivers who have a strong social network with which they are satisfied are more likely to have a positive caregiving experience than those with a perceived weaker social support network (Dunkin and Anderson-Hanley 1998). Specifically, caregivers who report greater satisfaction with their social support network reveal less depressive symptoms, greater life satisfaction, and fewer health problems. In fact, the issue of social support is a robust predictor of caregiver outcome and a viable predictor of outcome in caregivers of patients with stroke (Grant et al. 2000), cancer (Gilbar 2001), and dementia (Pot et al. 2000), as well as for children with chronic health conditions (Horton and Wallander 2001).

Appraisal of Stress Some experts have suggested that an individual's response to stress is contingent upon the appraisal of a stressor's significance (Lazarus and Folkman 1984). Some investigators have applied this model to the caregiving literature and, not surprisingly, found a general consensus that caregivers who appraise their experiences as more stressful generally evidence poorer outcomes. For example, Harvey et al. (2001) investigated 154 caregivers and found that negative appraisal strongly predicted psychological distress (Harvey et al. 2001).

Coping Coping strategies, such as problem solving skills, may be the most important predictor of adjustment among caregivers (Chwalisz 1996). Social problem solving involves effective coping responses to everyday problems. A study of caregivers of stroke victims found that social problem-solving abilities were related to caregiver depressive behavior and health (Grant et al. 2001). In a study examining stress in parents of children with autism, distancing (acting as if nothing is wrong) and escape-avoidance coping styles led to increased depression (Dunn et al. 2001). Failure to use coping styles such as positive reappraisal (being inspired, finding faith) and confrontive coping (expressing anger) were associated with poorer outcomes. In a study of the families of 174 children with traumatic brain injuries or orthopedic injuries, acceptance of the disability was associated with lower burden, while denial was associated with greater distress (Wade et al. 2001).

Some researchers have hypothesized that specific coping strategies are more effective in certain situations (goodness-of-fit; Lazarus and Folkman 1984). For example, problem-focused efforts may be more effective in controllable situations while emotion-focused strategies may be more effective in uncontrollable situations. Park et al. (2001) tested this hypothesis using a group of 305 gay men (244 caregivers for HIV positive partners and 61 noncaregivers). They concluded that goodness-of-fit was very important for problem-focused coping and somewhat important for emotion-focused coping.

Schulz et al. (1997) examined the health effects of caregiving in over 500 elderly married couples in which the spouse's affliction with an illness resulted in health problems as well as problems associated with alterations in mental status. Findings revealed that over one-half of the caregivers were found to have adverse mental or physical sequelae related to the caregiving experience. Specifically, caregivers participating in this investigation relative to comparison controls were found to have higher rates of depressive and anxiety related symptoms. These caregivers evidenced poor self-care behaviors, including inadequate rest and exercise. In addition, they received less medical care and a higher frequency of prescriptive medications than their counterparts who were not involved in the caregiving experience. Lack of time and energy for self-care has been implicated as a causal factor in caregivers' distress.

Depression In terms of the psychological adjustment of caregivers, the presence of depressive symptoms is the most frequently cited condition. Grant et al. (2000) examined self-reports of psychological adjustment among caregivers of stroke survivors. Findings revealed significant depressive symptoms among caregivers that were best predicted by levels of social support and physical functioning.

Schulz et al. (1995) provided a careful review of studies of caregivers of patients with dementia. Findings revealed a high prevalence of depressive symptomatology among caregivers. More importantly, those investigations that employed structured diagnostic interviews revealed high rates of clinical depression and anxiety. Similarly, in a review of studies regarding the impact of stroke on caregivers, Low et al. (1999) found a pattern of increased strain, depression, and anxiety in caregivers of stroke survivors.

Schulz et al. (1990), in reviewing the literature regarding the psychiatric effects of caregiving, concluded that most studies reveal elevations in depressive symptoms among caregivers when compared to noncaregiving comparison controls. Some caregivers were also at increased risk for psychiatric illness. Although many of the participants in the various studies met specific criteria for a psychiatric disorder, it is difficult to differentiate true psychiatric pathology from typical reactions to those stressors associated with the caregiving experience.

Marks et al. (2002) presented data from a very large study employing over 8,000 participants. Findings revealed important information to suggest that prior to the caregiving experience, adjustment problems were essentially nonexistent. However, with the commencement of the caregiving experience, depressive symptomology among caregivers showed a marked increase. Interestingly, in some cases, although the transition was associated with more depressive symptoms, some caregivers also reported increases in life purpose.

Perhaps not surprisingly, given the data regarding the prevalence of psychiatric distress among caregivers, several studies have found that caregivers are more likely to be using psychotropic medications (Schulz et al. 1995) than those who are not providing care for the disabled. The aforementioned studies are important as the data suggest significant health and mental health risk associated with the caregiving experience.

However, findings have revealed marked variability in overall adjustment associated with the caregiving experience. As noted previously, one-half of the samples in the Schulz et al. (1997) investigation demonstrated adequate adaptation, while the remainder evinced significant adjustment difficulties, including mental and physical strains. We review interventions that show particular promise.

Education and Training by and for Psychologists

Another body of literature has focused on the efficacy of psychoeducational approaches in assisting caregivers. In their review of the literature, Sinnakaruppan and Williams (2001) conclude in support of the importance of education for caregivers that the pervasive need among caregivers of the head injured is information. Specifically, caregivers wanted honest information about the behavioral sequelae of head injury and strategies for managing behavioral changes (e.g., agitation and emotional liability) in the person needing care. Group interventions often focus on both education and social support. Educational interventions are typically provided in a package of several techniques and strategies designed to assist caregivers in their efforts. However, patient education is significantly under-administered, and when such programs are implemented, the patient as well as the caregiver frequently misses or does not attend to much of the information provided. According to Toseland and Rossiter (1989), the typical group intervention provides education and knowledge about the patient's condition, encourages self-care behaviors for the caregiver, and focuses on the importance of social support for the caregiver. Studies that have examined attendance, requests for additional groups by caregivers, and subjective reports from both the participant and the provider, have generally reported positive effects. However, when outcomes are measured using standardized instruments in well-designed clinical trials, significant group effects are generally lacking (Toseland and Rossiter 1989).

Promotion of Health Behaviors

Given the rather guarded prognosis for caregiver health (including cardiovascular risk factors), predisposing these individuals to cardiac problems and even mortality, many of the intervention packages have included positive health behaviors as part of their core ingredients. Unfortunately, with the exception of exercise programs, these health-promoting components have rarely been independently evaluated.

King et al. (2002) conducted a randomized controlled trial of a home-based exercise program for 100 female caregivers. The experimental group received 15–20 min phone calls 1–2 times per month to monitor exercise progress and to provide feedback to the caregivers. The control group received phone calls that only included nutritional advice. Both the control and experimental arms demonstrated improvements in measures of psychological distress. In addition, and most importantly, the exercise group demonstrated reductions in stress-induced cardiovascular reactivity and improvements in quality of sleep.

Social Problem Solving Therapy

One of the most promising caregiver interventions is social problem-solving therapy. This treatment teaches caregivers to use problem-solving skills to address specific caregiving issues (e.g., transportation, medical crises situations, and loneliness) and to manage negative responses (i.e., difficulties in patient management, feelings of guilt, and sexual problems) to caregiving. In a review of the literature regarding psychosocial interventions for caregivers of individuals with dementia, Pusey and Richards (2001) conclude that those interventions employing a problem-solving and behavioral approach were generally effective in enhancing psychological well-being, with results affecting coping, stress, and decreasing depression.

Grant et al. (2002a, b) examined a 13-week telephone problem-solving intervention study for caregivers of recent stroke survivors. This well-designed study included a control group and an attention control group. Findings revealed positive outcomes for the problem-solving arm, including enhanced problem-solving skills, better physical and mental health, and better caregiver preparedness relative to the control groups.

Research

The methodological rigor across psychological studies on caregiving has been somewhat variable, although there has been some excellent research characterized by well-controlled study designs, extremely large cohorts of participants, and measures with sound psychometric properties. Although the majority of studies have been disease-specific (e.g., focusing on patients with closed head injury and dementia), some research suggests that response to caregiving is not disease specific; rather, the adjustment of the caregiver, in part, is due to individual characteristics of the caregiver rather than patient characteristics.

The literature regarding intervention programs for caregivers has improved greatly in the past decade. Early investigations focusing on intervention programs for caregivers were typically weaker than more recent studies, and the earlier studies often failed to incorporate the gold standard measurement and clinical controls typically employed in controlled clinical trials. The initial studies were often not experimental in design; specifically, they did not employ random assignment to treatment groups, nor did they include control groups. Further, they often failed to employ standardized instruments and instead relied extensively on the use of clinical impressions of health care providers and on self-reports of satisfaction from the caregivers. The majority of these investigations focused on social support, psychoeducational approaches, self-help groups, respite care, and behavioral approaches.

The corpus of literature suggests that some caregivers demonstrate better adaptation to the caregiver role than others. Interestingly, we have reviewed evidence to suggest that males from minority populations may cope better than their majority White female counterparts. In addition, evidence suggests that those individuals who have better established social support networks, those who appraise the task as less stressful, and those who evidence more adaptive coping skills tend to fare better in the caregiving role.

Despite lacking empirical rigor, the findings of earlier studies generally yielded positive results, suggesting that caregivers were satisfied with the treatment programs provided and endorsed benefits from them. Unfortunately, more recent studies, which employ better experimental methodology and standardized outcome measures, have produced less favorable results and have called into question previous assumptions about the efficacy of many caregiver interventions. Thus, the more rigorous the design of these intervention trials, the weaker are the findings to support their efficacy. Cooke et al. (2001) reached a similar conclusion after reviewing 40 studies that examined the effect of psychosocial interventions for caregivers. These authors reported that two-thirds of the intervention studies did not demonstrate improvement on any outcome measure. Those studies that did yield some positive effects include respite care, education, exercise programs, and social problem-solving therapy.

Respite Care

Respite interventions typically provide services such as daycare, home respite care, and institutional respite care. A meta-analysis of eight respite/care planning studies revealed a small to moderate effect of this type of intervention on caregiver distress (Knight et al. 1993). Results of such studies often show that the caregivers want continued respite care and report positive outcomes on nonstandardized measures, such as a reduction in feelings of isolation and increased self-esteem. However, group differences have typically not been demonstrated on well-standardized and psychometrically sound instruments, including caregiver burden, stress, or mood disturbance (Bourgeois et al. 1996). Interestingly, several authors have noted that families are reluctant to use respite services; these opportunities are often underutilized. Given the findings that respite care has shown some benefit for patients, including fewer hospitalizations and greater community involvement, additional efforts are needed in support of caregivers' use of respite interventions, especially at earlier points in the caregiving process.

Social Support

Given that social support has been demonstrated to predict good adjustment and adaptation during the caregiving process, numerous intervention efforts have focused on evaluating the efficacy of social support clinical interventions. Interventions with a social component typically involve support groups, social skills training, scheduled social activities, and interventions that aim to teach the caregiver to recruit social support from existing social networks.

The majority of studies that have demonstrated a positive effect of social support have used social support in combination with other interventions, such as education. Pillemer and Suitor (2002) conducted a study to examine the independent effect of social support enhancement on 115 caregivers of individuals with Alzheimer's disease. The investigation employed an intervention that included peer volunteers who also had a family member with Alzheimer's. These volunteers were trained to provide social support to the targeted caregivers and to avoid advice giving or problem-solving. Each volunteer was individually matched to a treatment group participant and visited the participant over an 8-week period. Findings revealed no treatment effect on either caregiver depression or self-esteem, despite very positive evaluations of the program by treatment participants. These results suggest that social support alone is unlikely to have a dramatic effect on the domains assessed. However, future research may demonstrate the efficacy of social support interventions that aim to influence participants' recruitment of social support networks from their environments.

Policy and Advocacy

For this reason, we conclude with recommendations for future programmatic and research efforts that psychology and psychologists can contribute to the science and practice of family caregiving.

Determinants of Outcome for Caregivers

Our review of the literature suggests that there are specific variables that mediate and moderate the overall adjustment and adaptation of the caregiver. Both patient variables and caregiver variables are associated with the general outcome of caregivers in response to the caregiving experience.

Patient Variables

Patient variables such as diagnosis, patient age, and types of behaviors have been evaluated as possible mediator or moderator variables between caregiving and distress. Interestingly, most evaluated patient variables are not strongly related to caregiver distress. In general, most studies have not found positive associations with variables such as functional impairment, cognitive impairment, and specific diagnosis of the patient; patient variables that have been associated with caregiver distress in the research literature include patient problem behaviors and the patient's overall level of impairment.

In a review of the literature related to dementia caregiving, Dunkin and Anderson-Hanley (1998) found that behavior problems among patients, including agitation, argumentativeness, and combativeness, present a greater burden to caregivers than do actual functional impairments (e.g. difficulties with daily living skills) or psychiatric impairments (e.g., delusions and hallucinations). For example, Anderson et al. (2002) examined behavior problems in individuals with severe traumatic brain injury. Findings revealed that high levels of behavior problems affecting management significantly influenced familial problems and, as a result, increased psychological distress among caregivers.

Further, in addition to behavior and management problems associated with the care of a disabled patient, the overall level of impairment has shown to be an important factor in caregiver distress. For example, Schulz et al. (1990) reviewed the literature regarding the psychiatric effects of caregiving on the caregiver and found that caregivers of patients with greater impairments exhibited more depressive symptomology. In a review of studies focusing on burden among caregivers of the mentally ill, all studies revealed positive associations between depressive symptomology among caregivers and amount of care and burden. Thus, the greater care provided, the greater the psychological burden. However, the specific diagnosis of the patient was not associated with reported burden in caregiving (Baronet 1999). The general corpus of findings suggests that patients who evidence greater physical and emotional impairments have caregivers who exhibit and report greater distress. Specifically, the data suggest that the presence of behavior and management problems among patients is associated with the greatest levels of distress among caregivers. However, an interesting finding is that regardless of the level of impairment, caregivers who have a close relationship with the patient are less distressed than are those who do not have this type of relationship (Dunkin and Anderson-Hanley 1998).

In summary, patient variables are generally less salient than caregiver variables in predicting caregiver adaptation. The most important patient variables include the patient's problem behaviors and overall level of impairment, and caregiver variables such as caregiver demographics, social support, and coping responses play important roles in predicting outcome. Recently, several researchers have recognized the need to synthesize this information to create a comprehensive model of caregiving. The dominant models of caregiving are stress process models. Several related stress process models based on Lazarus and Folkman's stress-appraisal-coping paradigm have been proposed (1984). In its simplest form, this model states that an individual's response to a stressor depends on the individual's appraisal of the significance of that stressor. Szmukler et al. (1996) applied this model to caregiving and suggested that the caregivers' response (e.g. adaptive coping, depression, etc.) to stressors such as caregiving demands depends on the judgment of the significance of the demand. This model, known as the stress-coping model of caregiving has been supported by research showing that caregivers who make negative appraisals of caregiving exhibit more psychological distress (Harvey et al. 2001). The stress process model of caregiving proposed by Haley et al. is also an adaptation of the stress-appraisal-coping paradigm. It suggests that a variety of factors, including stress appraisal, social support, and coping responses, mediate the relationship between caregiving stress and caregiver well-being (Goode et al. 1998). The stress process models play an important role in guiding our understanding of those factors that mediate the physical and psychological impact of caregiving and of those interventions that are most likely to be effective.

Education and Training by and for Psychologists

Our review of this growing psychological caregiving literature suggests that more research needs to be conducted to evaluate the efficacy of packaged interventions involving education, social support, and exercise. Promising interventions include cognitive behavioral approaches that aim to teach problem solving and other coping skills. Further, research that focuses on positive adaptation versus inadequate adaptation will be important in both predicting psychological and physical risk factors as well as identifying essential ingredients for programs of psychological intervention.

Research

Current research falls short in the identification of a specific mechanism underlying health and mental health adaptation to the caregiving experience. Studies focusing on mediating and moderating variables (e.g., immune response and self-care behaviors) represent a first step in the identification of mechanisms underlying both positive and poor outcomes.

Clearly lacking in this area are sound, controlled clinical trials designed to evaluate treatment outcome. Frequently, the available literature has revealed studies with less adequate control groups, and when there are control groups, there is a failure to randomly assign individuals to groups. In addition, many of the studies are characterized by dependent measures that are not gold standard, and raters that are not blind to treatment conditions. When studies in this area have been more methodologically rigorous, treatment effects have frequently been small or even nonexistent.

Additional studies characterized by methodologically sound research designs are sorely needed in this area. In particular, longitudinal studies are needed, as they will examine adaptation over time and capture the developmental changes inherent in the caregiving experience, functions in which crosssectional studies are limited. Given the compelling data with regard to individual differences and the prediction of outcome, future studies will need to capture the heterogeneity of caregiver populations to determine the specific variables that predict adjustment to the caregiving experience. For example, studies of ethnicity have been primarily devoted to African-American caregivers, while there is little research focused specifically on caregivers who are Hispanic and Asian-American. As noted previously, other methodological problems in this area have included poor control groups, small sample sizes that limit generalizability, and dependent measures of questionable reliability and validity.

With respect to treatment studies, problems characteristic to this research area include dependent measures and unrealistic end points given the short time period of intervention. Within this very complex area of intervention, it is necessary to have treatment studies that either follow caregivers over a lengthy time period to permit an adequate assessment of the intensity of the intervention, or to have outcome variables specific to the skills being taught in the intervention program. Further, as with many treatment outcome studies, samples have been primarily those of convenience, with all participants selected on the basis of seeking services. This entire program of research has been difficult to interpret due to ambiguity in operational definitions, which are necessary to programmatic research. For example, the literature has been less than clear with regard to the operational definition of "caregiver," with definitions ranging from an individual in the home where the caregiver is the only caregiver, to an individual providing occasional support, to a relative residing in the community.

Many critical questions remain to be addressed. First, it is recommended that future studies examine caregiver characteristics and then match them to specific interventions that might prove efficacious. For example, one might predict that those individuals who experience significant isolation as a result of the caregiving experience may in fact benefit from social support interventions, while those caregivers with individual skill deficits might benefit from a coping skills training program. In addition, many of the available treatment programs have been characterized by multi-push efforts whereby several interventions are provided (e.g., information giving and social support and skills training). For those programs that have proved to be effective, research that attempts to dismantle the essential ingredients of these programs will prove fruitful. Also, there is a need for greater theoretical focus on research in caregiving. This includes identifying underlying mechanisms for relationships and interventions that rely on specific models demonstrated in correlational studies. In particular, stress process models have shown promise for guiding research efforts with caregivers. Finally, the development of a psychometrically reliable and valid instrument for identifying the needs, symptoms, and critical competence of caregivers represents a future important goal in this area.

Policy and Advocacy

In this chapter, we anticipate that significant policy implications will emerge from a program of psychological research. In particular, we hope that a standard of care will be developed for caregivers based on empirical evidence. Further, policy recommendations need to develop strategies to identify caregivers in the community (e.g., the use of outreach coordinators and the use of care coordinators in primary care settings) and provide empirically supported intervention programs ideally matched to the caregivers' specific needs. Finally, it has been our clinical experience that many caregivers perform exceptionally well in the face of significant demands and adversities. Systematically studying these individuals who evidence good adaptation to the caregiving experience will be a productive task. Hopefully, we can focus on the identification of the resources and beliefs that they bring to the caregiving experience. It is hoped that by this type of systematic investigation, we can effect positive change and improve the quality of life for both patients and their caregivers.

Conclusions

Caregiving is affected by the caregiver's physical and mental health. A growing psychological literature suggests that caregivers are at risk for a number of psychiatric disorders, including depression, anxiety, and other adjustment difficulties.

The caregiving experience places individuals at risk for general health problems, including serious chronic diseases. Compromised caregiver health has been attributed to poor immune responses associated with stress, coupled with poor self-care behaviors, such as lack of sleep, poor nutrition, lack of exercise, and the failure to comply with prescribed treatment procedures and protocols.

We are only beginning to understand the deleterious effects caregiving can exert on emotional adjustment and adaptation. Fortunately, variables that are likely to be associated with positive adaptation to the caregiving role are emerging from caregiving research. Nonetheless, this literature is only in its beginning stage, and given the increasing strides in medical technologies and health care, more individuals will likely survive catastrophic illnesses and disabilities, and will need caregivers.

References

Anderson, M. L., Parmenter, T. R., & Mok, M. (2002). The relationship between neurobehavioral problems of severe traumatic brain injury (TBI), family functioning and the psychological well-being of the spouse/caregiver: Path model analysis. *Brain Injury, 16,* 743–757.

Baronet, A. (1999). Factors associated with caregiver burden in mental illness: A critical review of the research literature. *Clinical Psychology Review, 19,* 819–841.

Bookwala, J., & Schulz, R. (2000). A comparison of primary stressors, secondary stressors, and depressive symptoms between elderly caregiving husbands and wives: The caregiver health effects study. *Psychology and Aging, 15,* 607–615.

Bourgeois, M. S., Schulz, R., & Burgio, L. (1996). Interventions for caregivers of patients with Alzheimer's disease: A review and analysis of content, process, and outcomes. *International Journal of Aging and Human Development, 43,* 35–92.

Chwalisz, K. (1996). The perceived stress model of caregiver burden: Evidence from the spouses of persons with brain injuries. *Rehabilitation Psychology, 41,* 91–114.

Connell, C. M., & Gallant, M. P. (1999). Caregiver health behavior: Review, analysis, and recommendations for research. *Activities. Adaptation, and Aging, 24,* 1–16.

Cooke, D. D., McNally, L., Mulligan, K. T., Harrison, M. J. G., & Newman, S. P. (2001). Psychosocial interventions for caregivers of people with dementia: A systematic review. *Aging & Mental Health, 5,* 120–135.

Dilworth-Anderson, P., Williams, I. C., & Gibson, B. E. (2002). Issues of race, ethnicity, and culture in caregiving research: A 20-year review (1980–2000). *Gerontologist, 42,* 237–272.

Dunkin, J. J., & Anderson-Hanley, C. (1998). Dementia caregiving burden: A review of the literature and guidelines for assessment and intervention. Neurology, *51*, S53–60.

Dunn, M. E., Burbine, T., Bowers, C. A., & Tantleff-Dunn, S. (2001). Moderators of stress in parents of children with autism. *Community Mental Health Journal, 37,* 39–52.

Essex, E. L., Seltzer, M. M., & Krauss, M. W. (1999). Differences in coping effectiveness and well-being among aging mothers and fathers of adults with mental retardation. *American Journal on Mental Retardation, 104,* 545–563.

Gilbar, O. (2001). Parent caregiver adjustment to cancer of an adult child. *Journal of Psychosomatic Research, 52,* 295–302.

Goode, K. T., Haley, W., Roth, D. L., & Ford, G. R. (1998). Predicting longitudinal changes in caregiver physical and mental health: A stress process model. *Health Psychology, 17,* 190–198.

Grant, J. S., Bartolucci, A. A., Elliot, T. R., & Giger, J. N. (2000). Sociodemographic, physical, and psychosocial characteristics of depressed and non-depressed family caregivers of stroke survivors. *Brain Injury, 14,* 1089–1100.

Grant, J. S., Elliot, T. R., Giger, J. N., & Barolucci, A. A. (2001). Social problem-solving abilities, social support, and adjustment among family caregivers of individuals with a stroke. *Rehabilitation Psychology, 46,* 44–57.

Grant, I., Adler, K. A., Patterson, T. L., Dimsdale, J. E., Ziegler, M. G., & Irwin, M. R. (2002a). Health consequences of Alzheimer's caregiving transitions: Effects of placement and bereavement. *Psychosomatic Medicine, 64,* 477–486.

Grant, J. S., Elliot, T. R., Weaver, M., Barolucci, A. A., & Giger, J. N. (2002b). A telephone intervention with family caregivers of stroke survivors after hospital discharge. *Stroke, 33,* 278–290.

Harvey, K., Burns, T., Fahy, T., Manley, C., & Tattan, T. (2001). Relatives of patients with severe psychotic illness: Factors that influence appraisal of caregiving and psychological distress. *Social Psychiatry and Psychiatric Epidemiology, 36,* 456–461.

Haug, M. R., Ford, A. B., Strange, K. C., Noelker, L. S., & Gaines, A. D. (1999). Effect of giving care on caregivers' health. *Research on Aging, 21,* 515–538.

Horton, T. V., & Wallander, J. L. (2001). Hope and social support as resilience factors against psychological distress of mothers who care for children with chronic physical conditions. *Rehabilitation Psychology, 46,* 382–399.

King, A. C., Baumann, K., O'Sullivan, P., Wicox, S., & Castro, C. (2002). Effects of moderate intensity exercise on physiological, behavioral, and emotional responses to family caregiving: A randomized controlled trial. *Journal of Gerontology, 57A*, M26–36.

Knight, B. G., Lutsky, S. M., & Macofsky-Urban, F. (1993). A meta-analytic review of interventions for caregiver distress: Recommendations for future research. *Gerontologist, 33,* 240–248.

Lazarus, R. S., & Folkman, S. (1984). *Stress, appraisal, and coping*. New York: Springer.

Low, J. T., Payne, S., & Roderick, P. (1999). The impact of stroke on informal carers: A literature review. *Social Science & Medicine, 49,* 711–725.

Marks, N. F., Lambert, J. D., & Choi, H. (2002). Transitions to caregiving, gender and psychological well-being: A prospective US national study. *Journal of Marriage and Family, 64,* 657–667.

Park, C. L., Folkman, S., & Bostrom, A. (2001). Appraisals of controllability and coping in caregivers and HIV+men: Testing the goodness of fit hypothesis. *Journal of Consulting and Clinical Psychology, 69,* 481–488.

Pillemer, K., & Suitor, J. J. (2002). Peer support for Alzheimer's caregivers. Is it enough to make a difference? *Research on Aging, 24,* 171–192.

Pot, A. M., Deeg, D. J. H., van Dyck, R., & Jonker, C. (2000). Psychological distress of caregivers: The mediator effect of caregiving appraisal. *Patient Education and Counseling, 34,* 43–51.

Pusey, H., & Richards, D. (2001). A systematic review of the effectiveness of psychosocial interventions for carers of people with dementia. *Aging & Mental Health, 5,* 107–119.

Schulz, R., & Beach, S. (1999). Caregiving as a risk factor for mortality. *Journal of the American Medical Association, 23,* 2215–2219.

Schulz, R., Visintainer, P., & Williamson, G. M. (1990). Psychiatric and physical morbidity effects of caregiving. *Journal of Gerontology, 45,* 181–191.

Schulz, R., O'Brien, A. T., Bookwala, J., & Fleissner, K. (1995). Psychiatric and physical morbidity effects of dementia caregiving: Prevalence, correlates, and causes. *Gerontologist, 35,* 771–791.

Schulz, R., Newsom, J., Mittelmark, M., Burton, L., Hirsch, C., & Jackson, S. (1997). Health effects of caregiving: The caregiver health effects study: An ancillary study of the cardiovascular health study. *Annals of Behavioral Medicine, 19,* 110–116.

Sinnakaruppan, I., & Williams, D. M. (2001). Family carers and the adult head injured: A critical review of carers' needs. *Brain Injury, 15,* 653–672.

Szmukler, G. I., Burgess, P., Herman, H., Benson, A., Colusa. S., & Bloch, S. (1996). Caring for relatives with serious mental illness: The development of the Experience of Caregiving Inventory. *Social Psychiatry and Psychiatric Epidemiology, 31,* 137–148.

Toseland, R. W., & Rossiter, C. M. (1989). Group interventions to support family caregivers: A review and analysis. *Gerontologist, 29,* 438–448.

Wade, S. L., Borawski, E. A., Taylor, G., Drotar, D., Yeates, K. O., & Stancin, T. (2001). The relationship of caregiver coping to family outcomes during the initial year following pediatric traumatic injury. *Journal of Consulting and Clinical Psychology, 69,* 406–415.

Yee, J. L., & Schulz, R. (2000). Gender differences in psychiatric morbidity among family caregivers: A review and analysis. *Gerontologist, 40,* 147–164.

Occupational Therapy Perspectives of Caregiving

Janet L. Valluzzi

Occupational therapy (OT) skilled services focus on assisting all persons, groups, organizations, or populations to engage in everyday life activities, broadly described as "occupation." OT skilled services are designed to help recipients perform to the best of their ability, using their environment to be able to do the things they need and want to do. With the occupational therapy practitioner's help, the person in therapy identifies desired performance changes to support health, well-being, life satisfaction, and full participation in society (Fleming-Cottrell 2005; Law et al. 2001). Services typically include customized treatment programs to improve one's ability to perform daily activities; comprehensive home and job site evaluations with adaptation recommendations; sensory, cognitive, motor, or social performance skills assessments and treatment; adaptive equipment recommendations and training in use; and guidance to family and other informal caregivers (AOTA 2006c). Many of these services are designed to help a person learn to self-manage his or her health condition or disability with support from informal and formal caregivers.

Informal or family caregivers are generally considered to be those who provide care without pay and who share personal ties with the care recipient (HHS 2004a). In 2004, there were an estimated 44.4 million informal caregivers, aged 18 and older, who provided unpaid care to an adult aged 18 or older (National Alliance for Family Caregiving and AARP 2004). This estimate would be expected to increase if it included informal caregivers less than age 18 and informal caregivers of care recipients younger than age 18.

Occupational therapy practitioners recognize that partnering with family members and other informal caregivers can be a powerful way to facilitate better outcomes for clients. As a result, OT practitioners increasingly value the family or informal caregiver role for the provision of OT services to the caregiver, the care recipient, or to the caregiver and care recipient dyad (Wilkens Blank and Finlayson 2007). The role of the caregiver may be enhanced by an OT assessment of family or informal caregiver need for emotional support, as well as their need for knowledge and skills

J. L. Valluzzi (✉)
2151 Jamison Avenue #609, Alexandria, VA 22314, USA
e-mail: Janet.Valluzzizilla@cms.hhs.gov

R. C. Talley, S. S. Travis (eds.), *Multidisciplinary Coordinated Caregiving*,
Caregiving: Research • Practice • Policy, DOI 10.1007/978-1-4614-8973-3_6,

to safely provide care in home settings (Brachtesende 2004). Dr. Shirley Behr chaired a 2005 committee that reported to the AOTA Board of Directors on the role of OT for families and caregiving across the life span (Behr et al. 2005). The committee produced a report, *Families and Caregivers across the Lifespan,* which notes that OT practitioners are uniquely qualified to evaluate both the care recipient and the family or informal caregiver to promote the care recipient's highest level of function and full participation in society (Behr et al. 2005).

Occupational therapy services to family or informal caregiver client may be exemplified by describing the scenario of Jackie, a busy mid-career executive who is leading an active professional, social, and home life. So far, her aging parents have been relatively self-sufficient in their own home. Her father assists her mother, who had a heart attack several years ago, with housework. This relatively stable situation changes when her mother is hospitalized with an infection, found to be contracted because her father was unable to keep the household sufficiently clean. Jackie's father is reluctant to hire outside help for housework and care for his wife, and he becomes increasingly belligerent, verbally and physically, toward his daughter, who begins to provide full time care for her parents (Brachtesende 2004; Marcell 2001). In this case, OT intervention for Jackie's parents may focus on improving physical, social, or cognitive functional performance. Additionally, OT training in proper body mechanics, energy conservation, self protection, stress reduction, adaptive self-care, and home modification techniques can assist Jackie in providing a safe and an optimal level of care for her parents, while attending to her own needs as well (Brachtesende 2004; Marcell 2001). A brief history of the development of OT will provide a context for why the profession embraces both the client and family and informal caregivers in service provision.

History and Theoretical Framework for Occupational Therapy Practice

The roots of the OT profession in the USA can be traced to the Industrial Revolution that occurred at the end of the nineteenth century and early twentieth century. The Industrial Revolution shifted the economy from a largely rural, agricultural, and crafts-based dominion to an urban, manufacturing base. The shift prompted a concurrent rise in infectious disease in more populated cities and work sites, as well as a rise in industrial injuries. The Industrial Revolution's technological, socioeconomic, and cultural shift prompted the founders of the profession, who came from a variety of professional backgrounds, to examine the role of activity or "occupation" in physical and emotional healing (Peloquin 2005). Rather than viewing healing as a passive process in which the patient played an inactive role, the founders' approach to occupational therapy provided an interactive process of purposeful activity or work effort to improve health and meaningful outcomes related to participation in daily tasks (Peloquin 2005).

World War I greatly influenced the development of the profession (Peloquin 2005). Women were encouraged to enter the fledgling profession of OT to help soldiers recover from battle wounds. Treatment emphasized the need to engage both the interest and the emotion of the patient to promote physical and emotional healing. The objective of care was to return to useful occupation after wartime injury and illness (Peloquin 2005). World War II brought technological and scientific advancements. These advancements gave the occupational therapist a more specific set of skills for practice and saw the development of specialized systems for care.

The post World War II growth of rehabilitation services increased the profession's focus on specialization or segmentation of body parts amongst various medical interventions associated with rehabilitation (Friedland 2005). For example, speech therapy increased its focus on oral structures and speech; physical therapy focused on lower extremities and walking; and OT increasingly focused on upper extremity fine motor skills and activities of daily living. The medical care model prioritized medical outcomes, such as increased strength or range of motion. Practitioners adopted a more medically oriented, paternalistic approach to treatment. The specialization reinforced the need for the therapists' expertise and the related requirement for patients to comply with prescribed therapeutic programs. This trend diminished the roles of clients, as well as informal and family caregivers, in the provision of care.

The OT profession was guided back to its holistic and inclusive roots, in part, by the World Health Organization's 1946 broad definition of health as "a state of complete physical, mental and social well-being and not merely the absence of disease or infirmity" (WHO 1946). To address this broad conceptualization of health and augment its widely used International Classification of Diseases, Injuries and Causes of Death (ICD) coding system for mortality, WHO began examining a classification system related to the consequence of diseases for coding morbidity. The WHO International Classification of Impairments, Disabilities, and Handicaps (ICIDH) was developed in the 1970s. The ICIDH linearly extended the concept of disease to address body abnormalities or impairments, and the consequences of these impairments: disability (WHO 1980).

Concerns about terminology, lack of input from persons with disabilities; and the inappropriateness of the linearity of the model, prompted WHO to revise the classification framework. In 2001, WHO approved the International Classification of Functioning, Disability and Health (ICF) after extensive worldwide testing of its cross cultural applicability. The testing enlisted input from a variety of stakeholders including persons with disabilities (Üstün et al. 2001; WHO 2001). As part of the WHO family of classifications, the ICF is designed "to provide unified and standard language and framework for the description of health and health related states" (WHO 2001, p. 3). The ICF model is depicted in Fig. 1.

The ICF classification framework complements OT practice as the ICF function codes enhance ICD codes by providing additional information about level of function within the context of the environment. ICF concepts can be captured through the collection of functional status information (FSI) that reflects an individual's ability to carry out activities of daily living and to participate in various life situations or in society (Clauser and Bierman 2003). ICD codes provide information about diagnosis. For instance, a person may be diagnosed with diabetes mellitus, with a corresponding

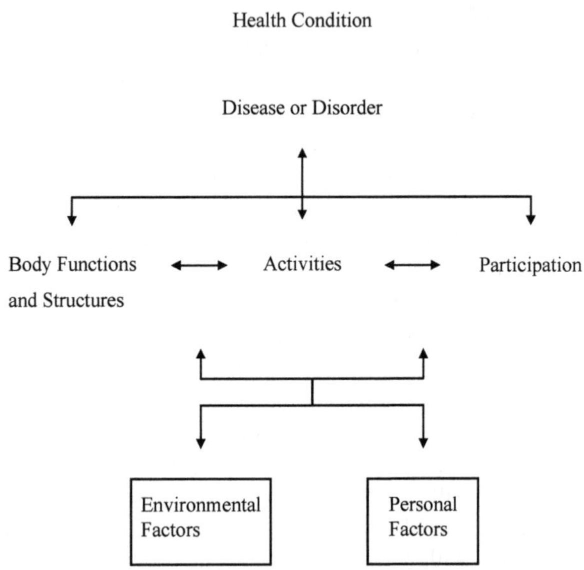

Fig. 1 World Health Organization International Classification of Functioning, Disability, and Health model (WHO 2001, p. 18)

International Classification of Diseases, 9th Revision, Clinical Modification (ICD-9-CM 1989) code of 250. However, use of ICF codes gives additional information about body function, body structure, activity level, and societal participation within the context of the environment. Continuing the example, additional insight is gained when ICF codes provide information that the person with diabetes mellitus has a change in body function; for example, blood vessel function (b415), affecting lower extremity body structure (s750). Using ICF codes, it would be possible to indicate that this limits an activity, such as walking (d450), and participation in work (d850). ICF codes also assist in identifying environmental barriers; for example, that insurance will not cover cost of a prosthesis, considered a product and technology for personal use in daily living (e115) (WHO 2001). In its 2007 report, "The Future of Disability in America," Institute of Medicine panel recommended that the ICF be adopted and refined as the conceptual framework for disability monitoring and research (Committee on Disability in America 2007).

The OT profession was an early adopter of the WHO's ICF classification framework, and has integrated the ICF into its occupational therapy practice framework: domain and process, hereafter referred to as the OT Framework (AOTA 2008). The OT Framework presents a summary of interrelated constructs that define and guide OT practice (AOTA 2008). The OT Framework focuses on: (1) the domain, or profession's purview, which is to support health and participation in life through engagement in occupation, and (2) the dynamic occupational and client-centered process used in the delivery of OT services (AOTA 2008).

As noted in the OT Framework, OT practitioners believe that occupations are multidimensional, complex, and may be shared as cooccupations (AOTA 2008). Care giving is a cooccupation that involves active participation on the part of the caregiver and the recipient of care (AOTA 2008). Consideration of cooccupation supports an integrated view of the client's engagement in relationship to significant others within context (AOTA 2008). Therefore, the OT practitioner may engage a broader view of the person who is the client and include the family and informal caregivers in intervention planning and implementation. Additionally, OT practitioners may focus primarily on the family or informal caregiver to provide the skills and knowledge, as well as environmental supports that are essential to fulfilling the caregiving role.

Findings from a qualitative research study by Franklin and Rodger (2003) illustrate this point. Franklin and Rodger explored parents' perspectives and skills related to feeding in a purposeful sample of either both parents or mothers only of eight infants and young children with chronic medical conditions who had received therapy at a tertiary children's hospital. In-depth interviews and mealtime observations indicated that parents attributed satisfaction with medical care, management of nutrition, and support from professionals, partners, and parents as contributing to their ability to cope with and adjust to provision of feeding interventions. Some feeding interventions required knowledge and skill development by these family caregiver study participants. These interventions included the physical tasks of feeding with a nasogastric (NG) or gastrostomy (G) tube, as well as managing feeding issues such as food selectivity and delayed oral motor skill development. However, study participants reported a wider range of issues affecting family life such as disruptions to family routines, concerns about the impact on parent–child relationships, and effects of feeding intervention on siblings. These concerns demonstrate the need for a client-centered focus for OT interventions that consider psychosocial aspects of caregiving for everyone involved or affected by provision of care, as well as skills and knowledge development (Franklin and Rodger 2003).

This history of client-centeredness, characterized by mutual cooperation, sets OT practice apart from other health professions that have traditionally utilized paternalistic or authoritarian approaches to care for persons with a disability (DeJong and Basnett 2001; Hubbard 2004). Client-centeredness embraces the concept of full participation or active and meaningful involvement of persons with disabilities and their families in decisions affecting them at the individual and systems level (Silverstein 2002) The concept of full participation is embraced in disability policy and may be required by law (Silverstein 2000, 2002). For example, the Older Americans Act Amendments of 2006 outline the equal opportunity of older Americans to "full participation in the planning and operation of community-based services and programs provided for their benefit." (42 U.S.C. 3001). Client-centered practice allows OT practitioners to collaboratively address informal caregiving issues from the perspective of the dyad of the care recipient and family or informal caregiver.

Status of Occupational Therapy Practice

An overview of the status of OT practice and the demographic characteristics of OT practitioners provides a basis for understanding the educational background, employment settings, regulatory environment, and continuing education requirements that equip, permit, and enhance OT practitioners' ability to provide competent care to family and informal caregivers. To implement client-centered practice, OT practitioner education includes the study of human growth and development, as supported by physiology and neuroscience, with specific emphasis on the social, cultural, emotional, and physiological effects of illness and injury. Occupational therapists enter the field with a masters or doctoral degree. Occupational therapy assistants earn an associate degree and work under the supervision of an occupational therapist. Occupational therapists and occupational therapy assistants must both complete supervised clinical internships in a variety of health-care settings, and pass a national certification examination (AOTA 2006d). The National Board for Certification in Occupational Therapy develops, administers, and continually reviews a national certification process for occupational therapy practitioners (NBCOT 2005). States regulate OT practice and licensure.

According to the U.S. Department of Labor occupational therapists held about 108,000 jobs in 2010 (DOL 2012a). Median annual earnings of occupational therapists were US$72,320 in 2010 (DOL 2012a). In 2010 occupational therapy assistants held about 36,000 jobs and had a median annual salary of US$47,490 (DOL 2012b). The AOTA has also done a series of surveys in 1990, 1997, 2000, 2006 and 2010 to monitor workforce compensation, benefits, and other workforce related issues (AOTA 2006a, 2010). These surveys supplement DOL figures and provide an overview of OT practitioners and practice settings that influence delivery of services and supports to family and informal caregivers.

In 2010, AOTA conducted its compensation and workforce study online through invitations to individuals (members, nonmembers, and former members of the AOTA) who had opted to receive AOTA related information (AOTA 2010). The online format more than tripled the responses from previous mailed versions of the survey. Results show that the ratio of women to men in occupational therapist positions has remained relatively stable. As with previous survey findings, the 2010 survey estimated that about 91.9 % of occupational therapists were women and about 8.1 % were men (AOTA 2010). However, the 2010 survey found that 8.1 % of occupational therapy assistants were men (AOTA 2010) This reflects a growth from the 2.9 % of men as occupational therapy assistants in the 2006 survey (AOTA 2006a, 2010). The high representation of females in the profession represents its historical roots, and mirrors the historically high prevalence of women in family and informal caregiver roles.

The broad range of occupational therapy practice settings permit professional focus on family and informal caregiver issues for all age groups. According to the 2010 survey, the employment settings where the largest percentage of OT practitioners (about 26.2 %) worked were categorized as nonmental health hospital settings. This category consisted of general hospitals (acute inpatients), hospice (general hospital), hospital-based outpatient services, neonatal intensive care units, pediatric units of general hospitals, freestanding rehabilitation hospitals, and rehabilitation units of general hospitals (AOTA 2010).

In the 2010 survey, approximately 21.6 % of OT practitioners work in school settings. Students with activities of daily living needs may be identified by Section 504 of the Rehabilitation Act of 1973 and its amendments. Occupational therapy practitioners in the schools may also work with students with special education needs and their families, as identified by the Individuals with Disabilities Education Improvement (IDEA) Act of 2004. The IDEA describes the processes for evaluation and receipt of special education and related services in the school settings (U.S. Dept of ED Undated). The high level of involvement of OT practitioners in school and transitional settings for high school students enhances the profession's ability to address family and informal caregiver roles for parents or adult guardians for students with disabilities. It also facilitates the profession's ability to address the needs of siblings who provide care for a person with a disability or special health care need. Involvement of the OT profession in the school setting may also assist with provision of support for students who provide care for other members of their family unit, such as an elderly grandparent or a parent with a disability.

The third largest category of identified employment settings for OT practitioners is long-term care skilled nursing and subacute services. This category represents long term care facilities, skilled nursing facilities, and subacute care units of general hospitals (AOTA 2010). About 19 % of OT practitioners were employed in facilities classified as skilled nursing or subacute care facilities in 2010. This was a slight increase from the 17 % of OT practitioners employed in freestanding skilled nursing and subacute facilities in 2006 (AOTA 2006a, 2010). This increase in employment in long term care and skilled nursing facilities contrasts with the Olmstead v. L.C. (1999) Supreme Court decision that promotes community-based care for persons with disabilities.

With respect to community-based care, OT practitioners are employed in a variety of community-based, freestanding outpatient, and hospital-based home health settings (AOTA 2010). Community based settings, employing about 2.0 % of occupational therapy practitioners, include adult day care programs, area agencies on aging, community residential care facilities, environmental modification programs, group homes, independent living centers, low vision program, prevention and wellness programs, retirement assisted living, senior centers, and supervised housing (AOTA 2010). In 2010, about 9.3 % of occupational therapy practitioner survey respondents reported practicing freestanding outpatient settings such as comprehensive outpatient rehabilitation facilities (CORFs); physician or optometrists offices; private practice, rehabilitation agencies or clinics, or nonprofit agencies (AOTA 2010). About 5.8 % of occupational therapy practitioner survey respondents reported working in home health or mobile therapy settings. As the summary of practice information demonstrates, the profession will need to continue to adjust to shifts in practice settings to provide optimal care for families and informal caregivers in the future.

OT practitioners typically demonstrate continuing competence and professional development through adherence to state licensing requirements for continuing education and through national board certification, board certification in advanced practice, and specialty certification. Board certification is an advanced practice designation for occupational therapists in a major domain of OT: pediatrics, gerontology, physical rehabilitation, or mental health (AOTA Undatedb; Glantz 2003). Specialty certification for occupational therapists and occupational therapy assistants recognizes specific specialties relevant to OT practice that possess a defined set of skills, techniques and interventions (Glantz 2003). Specialty certification includes driving and community mobility; feeding, eating, and swallowing; environmental modification; and low vision practice (AOTA 2006b). Continuing practice competence is not currently recognized for either family-centered care or caregiver practice areas. However, the 2005 Ad Hoc Workgroup on Families and Caregivers across the Lifespan report recommended that families and caregivers across the life span be recognized as an essential, and increasingly significant, domain of OT practice (Behr et al. 2005). This would be a vital and important first step in a process for certification of continuing practice competence in family and informal caregiving.

The AOTA has also organized crosscutting special interest sections (SIS) to promote continuing competence and develop professional communities with mutual areas of interest. These SIS are categorized by the type of disability, age of clients, program areas, location of practice, and roles assumed by practitioners (such as educators and administrators). The SIS focus organized efforts, such as newsletters, response to legislative concerns, or provision of technical assistance to members of the profession (AOTA 2006e). While family and informal caregiving across the life span is not currently one of the recognized special interest sections for the profession, the 2005 Ad Hoc Workgroup on Families and Caregivers across the Lifespan has recommended consideration of continuing education opportunities that incorporate evidence about the role of OT with families and caregivers (Behr et al. 2005, p. 3). A current example of this recommendation is a continuing education course entitled "Occupational Therapy for Family, Professional, and Paraprofessional Caregivers of Individuals with Dementia" that is available online for OT practitioners (Corocan 2004). This course represents an attempt to use telecommunications and distance learning methods to provide continuing education. The availability of additional continuing education offerings for family and informal caregivers is strengthening the profession's family and informal caregiving research efforts to date, as summarized in the following review of the OT literature.

Family Caregivers in Occupational Therapy Literature

OT Search is a is a bibliographic database jointly managed by the AOTA and its research foundation, the American Occupational Therapy Foundation, to electronically catalog the national and international literature of occupational therapy and related subject areas (AOTA Undateda). An *OT Search* inquiry of the term "caregivers" was performed in December, 2005 to focus on OT contributions to the family and informal caregiving specific to the OT literature. The search yielded 345 literature citations published from 1975 to 2005. The number of articles cited per year is sporadic through the late 1970s and mid-1980s, but escalates to a peak of 32 articles cited in 1993. The number of OT caregiver-related citations identified by *OT Search* decline thereafter, particularly after the year 2000, with only five articles cited in 2005. A follow up *OT Search* inquiry in December, 2012 identified 55 literature citations published from 2006 through 2012. The median number of articles related to caregiving that were cited was eight per year during the 2006–2012 timeframe.

The relatively stable level of publications is occurring as societal focus on family and informal caregiving is on the upswing. The decline in publications noted in *OT Search* on the topic of family and informal caregiving over time may reflect the profession's growing emphasis on other topics, such as evidence-based practice. Also, *OT Search* may not reflect the OT publications in journals for other disciplines that address an interdisciplinary context on family and informal caregiver-related topics. The identified *OT Search* citations are briefly summarized in the following paragraphs with respect to representation of the topics of family and informal caregivers across the life span, diagnostic conditions, diversity, OT family and informal caregiving assessment, and quality of research. This summary helps identify areas of expertise and provides direction for future study.

Much of the identified *OT Search* earlier literature focuses on specific age ranges of the care recipient, particularly the pediatric and elderly population. This trend also holds true for literature citations from 2006 to 2012. This parallels the age ranges most often represented in a U.S. Department of Health and Human Services (HHS) review of its caregiver related training, program evaluation, research, and advocacy efforts (HHS 2005). Although children and the elderly represent critical age groups, a life span approach would more broadly cover the entire age spectrum.

About one third of the articles published through 2005 identified using *OT Search* discuss caregiving related to a specific condition. Care recipient conditions cited most frequently, listed in decreasing order, are Alzheimer disease/dementia, traumatic brain injury, cerebral vascular disease, and human immunodeficiency virus (HIV)/acquired immunodeficiency syndrome (AIDS). Less than 5 % of the articles related to caregiving identified by *OT Search* during the early timeframe examined care recipients from an occupational performance perspective.

This changed during the 2006–2012 *OT Search* timeframe as the literature was more likely to examine skills and roles related to caregiving with respect to broader groups of care recipeints. For example, Colyvas et al. (2010) studied whether occupational therapists who used a participation-based approach differed in their teaching interactions with caregivers when compared with occupational therapists who used a traditional approach to provision of early intervention services. They described a participation-based approach as one in which the occupational therapist teaches the caregivers or caregiver, competence in implementing strategies with their children (Colyvas et al. 2010). Conversely, a traditional approach was described as working directly with a child rather than educating and training the caregiver (Colyvas et al. 2010). Their review of forty videotaped occupational therapy early intervention service sessions examined services provided to children with a variety of diagnoses. While 50 % of the children in the study had been diagnosed with developmental delay; other diagnoses included cerebral palsy, Down syndrome, and Prader–Willi syndrome (Colyvas et al. 2010). Their study found that occupational therapists practicing using a participation-based approach were significantly more likely to engage in joint interaction with the caregiver and child. Occupational therapists using a traditional approach were significantly more likely to model interventions for observing caregivers. The researchers concluded that neither joint interaction nor modeling were explicit teaching styles. They recommended that the profession could benefit from further research to examine caregiver learning and empowerment when explicit teaching was being performed to facilitate caregiver involvement in their child's intervention (Colyvas et al. 2010).

The literature, identified using *OT Search*, reflects several publications that address diversity issues associated with family and informal caregiving. The definition of and need for cultural competence and challenges of service provision to diverse populations is addressed in articles by Karner and Hall (2002); Kosloski et al. (2002); and Lyons (2000). A limited number of articles also address specific racial/ethnic groups or special populations, including Hispanics or Latinos (Talamantes et al. 1995; Taugher 1996), African-Americans (Malone-Beach et al. 2004), lesbians (Shelton 2001), and families with low incomes (Baum 1991). Cultural perspectives are also being expanded through international cooperation in research. For example, Caron et al. (2012) looked at the role of culture in crosscultural parental reports of sensory processing in children with autism spectrum disorders in Israel and the USA.

Because of its emphasis on client-centered care and occupation, the OT profession is uniquely positioned to conduct research to assess the role of family and informal caregivers and the impact of that role on their lives. A variety of assessment tools have been utilized to assess the family and informal caregiver role and its impact on caregiver health, well-being, and participation. For example, OT research studies for adult care utilize the role change assessment for older adults (Hogan et al. 2004; Rogers and Holm 1999), the general health questionnaire (Semlyen et al. 1998), and the functional behavior profile (Baum and Edwards 2000).

Occupational therapy's client-centered care approach also embraces assessment tools that may provide insight into the caregiving dyad of care recipient and family care provider. Potential tools for assessing the caregiving dyad in the elderly are included in a review article by Corradetti and Hills (1998) and by Carlson et al. (in press). Assessment tools that are reviewed include the Screen for the Caregiver Burden (Vitaliano et al. 1991), Zarit Burden Interview (Zarit et al. 1980); Caregiver Burden Inventory (Novak and Guest 1989); and the Patient Caregiver Functional Unit Scale (Fredman and Daly 1997). There is a need to develop standardized OT assessment tools that address family and informal caregiving issues. Ideally these would incorporate assessment of positive aspects of caregiving, such as personal or spiritual growth realized during end-of-life care or attainment of new insights into community resources and support systems and not just assessment of the *burden* of care.

The emerging discipline of occupational science, the study of human occupations, examines time spent in caregiving activities and the impact of caregiving responsibilities on daily lives (Ujimoto 1998; Zuzanek 1998). Information from time-use studies is important to inform methodologies of national surveys, such as the Bureau of Labor Statistics American Time Use Survey, which measures the amount of time people spend doing various activities such as paid work, childcare, volunteering, commuting, and socializing (DOL 2006). Measurement of time spent in family and informal caregiving is vital to economic assessments of societal benefits contributed by family and informal caregivers, as well as opportunity costs experienced by family and informal caregivers.

In general, much of the OT family and informal caregiving literature describes personal experiences, programs, training materials, or small-scale research efforts as both qualitative and quantitative in nature. However, findings from these smaller, pilot studies can be applied to larger populations to establish efficacy of educational materials, interventions, or assessment tools that can be used across settings. This brief review of the literature highlights the need for additional insight into family and informal caregiving performance and role across the life span. The review of the OT literature also calls attention to the importance of considering the diversity of racial, ethnic, and cultural backgrounds as well as lifestyle choices of family and informal caregivers in OT education, practice, research, and policy development. The need for developing and standardizing caregiver and caregiver/care recipient dyad assessment tools that incorporate an OT perspective is also highlighted through the examination of the literature. Finally, the analysis of the literature demonstrates the profession's potential contributions to scientific development of temporal concepts, measurement, and economic consequences of family and informal caregiving. An overview of current OT education provides insight into how the educational setting may prepare tomorrow's practitioners to address these topics in the future.

Occupational Therapy Education

The philosophy of OT education is "grounded in the belief that humans are complex beings engaged in a dynamic process of interaction with the physical, social, temporal, cultural, psychological, and spiritual environment" (Dickerson and Royeen 2003, p. 1). Through a collaborative and active learning process, OT educators promote competencies for practice to improve human participation and quality of life for those individuals with and without impairments or limitations (Dickerson and Royeen 2003). Education regarding individuals or populations with or without impairments or limitations is crucial as it expands the scope of preparation for OT practice to include prevention efforts that limit risk for impairment. It also expands the educational preparation to include family and informal caregivers, who may not have an impairment or limitation, within the scope of practice. The role of OT education regarding family and informal caregiver issues can be clarified in the context of developing educational standards.

In December 2012 there were 151 active accredited occupational therapy programs and 183 active accredited occupational therapy assistant programs in the USA (AOTA 2012a, b). The accreditation standards establish the critical requirements necessary to prepare individuals to become entry-level occupational therapists or occupational therapy assistants. Both the occupational therapy and occupational therapy assistant accreditation standards undergo revision through a process designed to "ensure participation by the broadest possible constituency" (ACOTE® 2005).

The ACOTE® has sought feedback on draft standards from constituency groups, including educational program representatives, fieldwork educators and coordinators, consumers, regulators, students, and the public-at-large (ACOTE® 2005).

The standards for accreditation present a curriculum framework for practice preparation in a variety of settings (i.e., schools, hospitals, community, and long-term care settings) across the life span (i.e., pediatrics, adolescents, adults, and geriatrics) (ACOTE® 2005). The August, 2006 final standards for accreditation call for foundational education content requirements that encompass the demonstration of knowledge and understanding of structure and function of the human body, such as biological and physical sciences, human development, and human behavior, including behavioral and social sciences (ACOTE® 2007). This knowledge would be supplemented by educational coursework and experiences designed to provide understanding and appreciation of the role of sociocultural, socioeconomic, diversity factors, and lifestyle choices in contemporary society (ACOTE® 2007). Skills in statistics and an understanding of the development of assessment tools and research methodology to support evidence-based practice are also required in educational curricula for occupational therapists, and an understanding of the importance of these skills is required for occupational therapy assistants (ACOTE® 2007). While the curriculum standards currently express the need for a client-centered and family-centered approach to practice, how many of the current educational programs have specific coursework associated with family caregiving supports that are consistent with the standards is unknown (S. Behr, personal communication, December 8, 2005).

The terminal degree for occupational therapists in an academic setting is a doctorate. Some faculty may have a doctorate in occupational therapy or occupational science. However, it is usual and customary to have faculty members with a doctorate in related areas of health science or social science including, but not limited to, education, neuroscience, public health, psychology, policy, or sociology. A terminal degree in any of these areas would be considered a terminal degree for occupational therapists in academia. However, the growth in doctoral programs in occupational therapy and occupational science acknowledges the profession's realization that a doctorate in the field enhances capability for research to further develop the evidence base specifically for occupational therapy practice.

Policy and Advocacy Efforts

Raising the entry requirements for the profession to a postbaccalaureate level and increasing the emphasis on doctoral-level training comes at a critical juncture for the OT profession. These standards are particularly important in light of a current policy environment that is characterized by a rising emphasis on individual and population level functional status information, legal requirements for community-based care, changing demographics of the aging population, continued need for cost containment, as well as demands for evidence to substantiate reimbursement and practice. Each of these trends heightens the need to address family caregiver issues on an individual and population level. Critical reviews of the profession are facilitating its adaptation to these and other trends in order to strengthen its ability to influence associated policy issues. A brief overview of recent steps the profession has taken to equip itself better to address policy issues assists in understanding how the profession is preparing itself and its practitioners to address family and informal caregiving at a policy level.

A key element of the profession's self-review process was an institutional ethnographic examination of issues related to power and justice development of the OT profession (Townsend 2003). In an institutional ethnographic approach, the collection, management, and analysis of data are organized to find out how conceptual practices of power (e.g., guidelines, standards, practices, policies, laws, media images, brochures, and budgets) organize the processes of ruling and subordination invisibly and unconsciously in the everyday world without the use of direct force (Townsend 2003). When viewed through this lens, the OT profession has historically held a subordinate position to what had been a traditionally male-dominated medical profession, with its emphasis on diagnosis and acute care intervention to prevent mortality. This parallels the history of family and informal caregivers, who have traditionally been predominantly female, and the traditional emphasis on the care-recipient diagnosis in family and informal caregiving training and advocacy efforts (Mintz 2002).

The OT profession in the USA is responding to the institutional ethnographic findings, as well as trends and challenges in the policy and political landscape by realigning its professional organization's strategic plan to commemorate its 100th anniversary in 2017 (AOTA 2006c). Through a multiyear process initiated in 2003, leaders in the field elicited stakeholders from around the world to assist in planning for potential changes and conditions that will create both challenges and opportunities for the profession in the years ahead. During the strategic planning process, relevant drivers of change were identified as follows: aging and longevity, health-care costs and reimbursement, prospective and preventive medicine, assistive technologies, lifestyle values and choices, stress and depression, information access/learning, universal design for active living, increasing diversity of the population, and the changing world of work (AOTA 2006c).

Each of these change drivers can be related to OT service provision to family and informal caregivers. As the population ages and lives longer, the need for family and informal caregivers is expected to increase. Efforts to limit health-care costs and constrain reimbursement can be anticipated to raise the dependence on family and informal caregivers. The emphasis on preventive health care can include the need to prevent injuries to family and informal caregivers that may be sustained when providing care (Vitaliano et al. 2003). Healthy lifestyle choices may assist in maintaining family's and informal caregivers' physical and mental health. Assistive technology or universal design may lessen the need for family or informal care. Increased competition in a global economy may hinder an employer's ability to provide employment benefits, such as telecommuting or flexible work hours, that may assist family and informal caregivers in balancing employment responsibilities with caregiving demands. These change drivers present both challenges and opportunities for the OT profession with regard to family and informal caregiver service provision and associated policy issues.

The American Occupational Therapy Association, through its strategic planning process, envisions a powerful, widely recognized, science-driven, evidence-based, globally connected, and diverse professional workforce. In this vision, the profession will enable people to improve their physical and mental health, secure well-being, and enjoy higher quality of life through preventing and overcoming obstacles to participation in the activities they value (AOTA 2006c).

Major policy trends support this vision of full participation in society for care recipients as well as family and informal caregivers. For example, the Government Accountability Office, in its review of reimbursement for inpatient rehabilitation facilities (IRF), included the recommendation that the Centers for Medicare and Medicaid Services (CMS) more thoroughly describe subgroups of patients that require IRF services, possibly using FSI or other factors, in addition to diagnosis, to assist with reimbursement processes (GAO 2005). Additionally, CMS is implementing claims-based data collection of FSI for outpatient therapy as of January, 2013 (CMS 2012). The New Freedom Initiative responds to the historic Olmstead v. L.C. Supreme Court decision by promoting community living for people with disabilities (National Council on Disability 2003).

The OT profession has progressively increased its acknowledgment of the importance of social policy in achieving its professional vision and goals. Policy changes are currently viewed as critical to enabling occupation and full societal participation, or occupational justice, for occupational therapy clients. To work toward this goal, the profession has a political action committee in the USA. The political action committee monitors federal- and state-level legislation affecting the profession and provides regular legislative, policy, and reimbursement information to members. For instance, OT professionals have provided statements to the House Committee on Ways and Means regarding Medicare services and universal assessment in postacute care settings, sponsored a web conference call to address reimbursement caps on outpatient rehabilitation services, and provided training regarding provisions in reauthorization of the IDEA. As a member of the Independence through Enhancement of Medicare and Medicaid Coalition, the AOTA provided comments to CMS regarding the Medicare national coverage determination for power mobility devices (ITEM 2005). Another example of a collaborative partnership was the involvement of AOTA staff members and OT practitioners with a Mental Health Liaison Group to support legislation regarding parity for mental health treatment (Metzler et al. 2006). These examples of policy involvement impact family and informal caregivers because they address the identification of appropriate postacute care settings for Medicare beneficiaries with disabilities and facilitate service provision to students with disabilities and their families. The profession's policy efforts have also worked toward improving access to care and reducing burden of payment for persons with disabilities and their caregivers for outpatient services and mental health services.

The OT profession's strategic planning process and policy efforts have set the stage for the profession's continued growth. The profession's vision is to empower practitioners to facilitate full participation of persons with disabilities in society to promote occupational justice. This vision provides numerous opportunities to support family and informal caregivers through future OT practice, research, education, and policy.

Future Directions

What should the future hold for OT practice with respect to family and other informal caregivers? OT practice that has traditionally been individualized to specific clients in a controlled medical setting is increasingly challenged to expand its role to a community-based, population level of assessment, prevention, intervention, and outcomes measurement. Population-based approaches to OT service provision open new avenues for intervention, including social marketing, health screening, advocacy, consumer-directed care, and environmental modification to enhance outcomes. Family and informal caregiving research, as well as practice trends, point out gaps in care for OT practitioners to address in future population and community-based practice.

Generally, early caregiving research focused on topics such as the economic impact of caregiving, the growth of family and informal caregiving in relationship with the evolution of the health-care system, demographic characteristics of caregivers and recipients, and use of services (Kinney Hoffman 2002). Later, research focused on physical, psychological, social, and financial sequelae of family and informal caregiving. Findings indicated that family and informal caregivers have been predominantly women, are unpaid for their caregiving work, and sustain negative consequences of caregiving such as depression, poor perceived health, and increased risk of mortality (Christakis and Allison 2006; Cohen et al. 2002; Kinney Hoffman 2002; Pinquart and Sorenson 2003). These findings strongly suggest the need for OT to include a population-based approach to address issues related to maintaining caregiver health, preventing caregiver injury, and developing public policy that supports informal caregivers in community-based settings.

The OT profession has demonstrated its ability to address population-based approaches to services through its cosponsorship of an annual "National School Backpack Awareness Day" that contributes to student public health by promoting backpack safety (AOTA 2005). As recommended by the profession's *Families and Caregivers across the Lifespan* report (Behr et al. 2005), lessons learned through the backpack safety social marketing and screening campaign can be translated to OT involvement in family and informal caregiving. Increased prominence of the OT profession in rehabilitation related to automobile driving also illustrates the ability of the profession to address issues on a population level. Fact sheets with information about transportation alternatives for older adults and web-based information about identification or risk factors for automobile driving developed in collaboration with the National High Traffic Safety Administration are examples of existing population-based approaches to service provision that may assist family and informal caregivers (AOTA 2004).

The need for population-based social marketing approaches that address family and informal caregivers is highlighted by a recent review of family and informal caregiving literature, public education materials, and news coverage (Eisai Inc. 2004; Kinney Hoffman 2002). It concluded that "the findings of this review of the literature, communications materials and news coverage overwhelmingly indicate that the issue of self-awareness, self-acknowledgement and their relationship to empowerment of the family caregiver has not been explored" (Kinney Hoffman 2002, p. 6). Occupational therapy practitioners can promote social marketing messages that affirm family and informal caregivers' efforts to seek balance in life roles by emphasizing the time, medication, case management, communication, injury prevention, and advocacy skills acquired by family and informal caregivers as they gain expertise in their roles (Berg 1997; Crowe et al. 2000; Ergas and Fischer 1998; Nicholson 1999; Orange and Colton-Hudson 1998). Empowering messages may also credit the values and spirituality of family caregivers in their decision to provide care; and emphasize the positive economic contribution to society that is contributed collectively by family and informal caregivers.

Current intervention and reimbursement mechanisms are beginning to recognize the need to include the perspective of the consumer in managing chronic care on a population level. "Consumer-directed health care" is intended to reduce the influence of insurance by expecting people to spend their own money through high deductibles and coinsurance at the point of service (Berenson 2005). Consumer satisfaction ratings of services, tiered reimbursement mechanisms, and "boutique medicine" emphasize consumer preference and participation in services. Occupational therapy's historical emphasis on individual level client-centered care and consumer involvement in OT assessment and care plan development provide a wealth of background for the profession to lead other disciplines in similar approaches to practice. OT's emphasis on client-centered care should enhance consideration of the family and informal caregiver role in the client/caregiver dyad in this process.

Disease management programs, a set of interventions designed to improve health by working with clients and their providers on a treatment plan that emphasizes self-management techniques, are increasingly being emphasized in diabetes mellitus (DM) care, asthma, congestive heart failure, hypertension, multiple sclerosis, HIV-AIDS, and other chronic diseases (HHS 2004b). OT practitioners have assisted clients with self-care skills that have traditionally been classified in terms of activities of daily living (ADLs) and instrumental activities of daily living (IADLs). Customarily, basic self-care ADLs have included "personal activities such as eating, grooming, hygiene, and mobility that are necessary for maintenance of one's self in the environment" (Christiansen et al. 2005, p. 543). Instrumental activities of daily living are activities related to independent living and include preparing meals, managing money, shopping for groceries or personal items, performing light or heavy housework, and using a telephone (HHS 2004d).

Technological advances may be facilitating substitution of health information technology, assistive technology, or other technological alternatives for traditional activities of daily living or instrumental activities of daily living (Agree et al. 2005).

For example, online grocery shopping services may be utilized by a family or informal caregiver who is unable to leave a care recipient unattended while going to the grocery store. OT practice is responding to these technological advances by assessing technological impact on the basic definitions of ADLs and IADLs to assist in identifying ways of assisting clients as well as family and informal caregivers in these areas of occupational performance.

The growing emphasis on consumer-directed care and disease management efforts, combined with technological advances, heightens the need for the profession to view health self-management as a self-care skill. University of Connecticut Health Center's five-week course in "health care survival skills" is an example of efforts to teach consumers about the complexity of the of the US health-care system and addresses topics such as understanding information about insurers and drug companies, how to be an advocate for a family member who is receiving health services, and how to ensure that best practices for care are being provided (AHL 2006a). In addition to leading the development of health self-care management skills for the general population, OT practitioners should provide leadership in provision of reasonable accommodations for care recipients and family or informal caregivers who may benefit from alternative formats or instructional approaches to address cognitive or intellectual disabilities, or physical or sensory impairments. Occupational therapy's high esteem for full participation emphasizes the need to practice in the context of the family and informal care provider environment—whether it be the home setting, workplace, site of spiritual support, business, or leisure pursuits.

A concern about the adoption of consumer-directed health services has been the reluctance of consumers to actively participate in their care (Berenson 2005). The participatory nature of OT intervention may assist in identifying alternative strategies for clients and their families or informal care providers to assume responsibility for their health. This will help ensure that family and informal caregiver preferences and needs at both the individual and population level are addressed and expressed in various arenas: assessment, interventions, satisfaction and quality measures; reimbursement mechanisms; and other outcomes of care at both the individual and population level.

The National Committee for Quality Assurance (NCQA) has embraced the concept of patient-centered medical homes (PCMH) as a promising model of adult- and pediatric-coordinated primary care (NCQA 2011). One objective of PCMHs is to help develop relationships between primary care providers, their patients, and patients' families, when appropriate to provide safer, higher quality of care (NCQA 2011). Metzler, Hartmann, and Lowenthal envision a future role for OT practitioners in primary care settings to provide coordinated and integrated case management services; practice in the context of family and community to conduct activity analyses within the client's home, social, and work settings; and to provide the whole-person orientation that is embedded in the OT scope of practice and skill set (Metzler et al. 2012).

Future Occupational Therapy Family Caregiver Research

As noted earlier in the review of the *OT Search* literature citations on family and informal caregivers, there has been more focus on children and the elderly in the OT caregiving literature. Emphasis on the family and informal caregiver perspective in practice settings should be facilitated by a research agenda that examines the universality of the family and informal caregiver occupational role across the life span. In this approach, commonalities and differences with respect to the caregiver role would be identified from the perspective of the family or informal caregiver, rather than by care recipient characteristics of age, diagnosis, or place of care. For example, a role or functional approach to research might look at family or informal caregiver advocacy skill development. There may be similar barriers to care recipients that require family or informal caregiver advocacy skills regardless of whether these skills are needed to address a school administration's reluctance to provide services identified in an individualized education plan to a student with a learning disability, negotiate with a physician to change the prescription of a middle-aged family member with depression, or navigate an aging parent's enrollment in Medicare's prescription medication program.

Assuring adequate sample size is often a struggle for studies of disability groups with low prevalence in the population. Utilization of a cross sectional study design that examines the role or performance of family or informal caregivers across the life span, rather than by care recipient diagnosis or age, would potentially increase sample sizes for family and informal caregiving studies. Stratification of the analysis by the gender of caregiver, the length of time involved in the family, or informal caregiver role may assist in addressing analytical issues. For example, it may help identify differences across family or informal caregivers by their own characteristics, such as communication skill level or level of assertiveness and not the care recipients' diagnosis or age. This approach may help target effective family and informal caregiver interventions and outcomes.

Conversely, there may be differences in level and type of supports that are desired by a family or informal caregiver depending on the length of time an individual has been in a family or informal caregiving role. Just as we have begun to differentiate between preventive, acute, and long-term care for care recipients, supports may vary for informal caregivers who are providing intense assistance to someone newly diagnosed or injured versus the constant nature of long-term care across a long period of the family or informal caregiver's life span. For example, a 2012 study conducted by the National Alliance for Caregiving, the National Multiple Sclerosis Society and the Southeastern Institute of Research found that the long life cycle of multiple sclerosis, a chronic and potentially disabling disease, suggests that the total number of years an individual may serve as a caregiver for an individual with multiple sclerosis will be "much, much longer than caregivers in general: 9 years for these caregivers compared to less than 5 years for all caregivers" (NAC et al. 2012, p. 61). Longitudinal research may assist with identifying caregiver supports over longer periods of time. The aging of the population, the shift to community-based care, increased cancer and HIV/AIDS survival rates, as well as the longer life expectancies of persons with developmental disabilities and complex health-care needs provide fertile ground for large scale, longitudinal, population-based research efforts, such as the Framingham Study of Cardiovascular Disease (Oppenheimer 2005) or the Women's Health Initiative (Langer et al. 2003).

A longitudinal study of caregivers could follow family and informal caregiving cohorts over an extended period of time to examine health, well-being, roles, performance, and participation in the home, the workplace, and other settings. The OT profession has a historical emphasis on involving women in the field and the foresight to develop a strategic vision to empower the profession. Given the historical predominance of women caregivers and the high proportion of females in the OT profession, the OT profession embodies the skills necessary for conceptualization, design, and development of private and public sector partnerships for longitudinal study of family and informal caregivers.

The Future of Occupational Therapy Education

Raising the entry level of the profession to the postbaccalaureate level is an important step in elevating the competence and science of practice and research. The mounting call for research competence is exemplified by the 2005 "Rehabilitation Medicine Summit: Building Research Capacity," which included representatives from professional organizations, consumer groups, academic departments, researchers, governmental funding agencies, and the private sector. Participants discussed five elements of research capacity for rehabilitation medicine: (1) researchers, (2) research culture, (3) funding, (4) partnerships, and (5) metrics. An insufficient number of quality rehabilitation researchers was identified as one of the key problem areas in rehabilitation research. Action plans for appropriate mentoring of researchers, development of rehabilitation research training curricula, and the need to fund and enhance a research environment, infrastructure, and culture were identified (Frontera et al. 2006). Collaborative efforts such as this provide the opportunity for the OT profession to enhance research capacity with other disciplines. The 2011 Occupational Therapy Research Agenda identifies major research goals for OT research. These include a basic research goal priority focusing on the "experience of disability and/or chronic health problems for individuals and their families across the lifespan" (AJOT 2011).

Multiple national efforts are calling for and supporting an interdisciplinary approach to training of future researchers to facilitate interdisciplinary research. For example, the National Institutes of Health (NIH) has been engaged in activities known as the "NIH Roadmap" with the goal of accelerating the pace of discovery of new knowledge about the prevention, detection, diagnosis, and treatment of disease and disability. Recognizing that scientific advances are increasingly being made at the interfaces of traditional disciplines and that scientific approaches are becoming more integrative, the NIH has become particularly interested in developing a new interdisciplinary research workforce (HHS 2004c). Also, the

National Research Council's Committee on National Needs for Biomedical and Behavioral Scientists notes that "enhanced oversight of research training will lead to the preparation of a workforce that better reflects the nation's needs and more scientists who are prepared for the increasingly interdisciplinary nature of research" (National Research Council 2000, p. 2).

Embracing a broader scope of educational opportunities and partnerships should be a natural extension of the historical roots and holistic approach embedded in the OT profession. What may be new and challenging is finding pathways of partnering with disciplines that, traditionally, have been less associated with the profession, including public health, statistics, economics, policy, and mass media marketing. These disciplines offer an array of opportunities to enrich and empower OT perspective of the family and informal caregiver role. New avenues for funding research, such as the NIH "Pathways to Independence Program" that supports the role of an experienced senior mentor in promoting the development of new investigators to independently perform their own research, could be used to enhance interdisciplinary research efforts (HHS 2006).

Models of interdisciplinary education from other health-related professions may serve as a template for the establishment of new partnerships with less traditional disciplines and interdisciplinary education. The population-based emphasis in public health could be critical to the OT profession's contribution to large scale clinical and survey research, as well as population-based intervention efforts. Knowledge of statistical theory and application will be vital to the enhancement and growth of OT scientific analyses for the development of assessment tools, research study design to establish efficacy, and effectiveness of care. Partnerships with economists will be critical to evaluate time spent in informal caregiving tasks and calculate economic benefits and opportunity costs for family and informal caregivers. Understanding of health and social service policy would enhance the ability to translate research into policy change and positively influence practice. The popularity of the television show "Extreme Makeover: Home Edition" demonstrated the value of the media in enhancing public knowledge of home modification and universal design for persons with disabilities and their family and informal caregivers. Increased knowledge of the use of mass media would enhance the profession's reach to the public and provide messages that empower family and informal caregivers.

Recruitment to interdisciplinary programs may be patterned on other fields' efforts. For example, the field of education has paved the way for established mathematics and science professionals who are retiring or seeking career enrichment to gain competence and credentials for teaching these subjects to elementary, middle, or high school students. The rapid growth of undergraduate health science programs that provide a fundamental education in science and health can also be used to recruit students with an interdisciplinary perspective (AHL 2006b). The OT profession may lend its professional expertise regarding topics, such as interprofessional training, task analysis, and time management, to other disciplines and employers who are seeking to add interprofessional-trained personnel into the work setting. Academic, research, and clinical settings that are accustomed to "stove-piping" employees by traditional discipline roles and duties may require assistance in adjusting personnel policies and practices, work assignments, and remuneration to accommodate individuals trained in more than one discipline.

Recognition of interprofessional learning may also apply to family and informal caregivers, who have traditionally been penalized with respect to salary and other benefits for taking time off from employment to assume higher level informal caregiving responsibilities. However, a multitude of new skills may be learned during this timeframe that benefit an employer. For example, increased awareness of time management skills required to juggle a variety of caregiving tasks may positively impact a returning employee's productivity. Learned skills in negotiating relationships with health providers and insurers may positively influence client or office relationships. Enhancing the value of interdisciplinary skills gained through family and informal caregiving could enrich the employment role of the family and informal caregiver. Assessing the workplace environment and advocating for support of family and informal caregivers would potentially decrease business costs associated with potential absenteeism, turnover, or decreased productivity of family or informal caregivers. It would also reflect the growing necessity of OT involvement in nontraditional practice settings and advance the profession's maturity and influence in policy analysis.

Occupational Therapy Growth in Policy Analysis and Influence

Much of the profession's policy-related efforts to date have been focused on care recipient needs, as well as professional practice areas. The predominance of women in the OT profession, historically higher prevalence of females in caregiver roles, and longer life expectancy will likely personalize informal caregiving policy issues to many members of the profession. Informal caregivers are more likely to not work or work part-time, resulting in lower income, loss of benefits, and lower retirement benefits. The combined personal and professional interest vested in the informal caregiver role should make family and informal caregiver policy issues a powerful practice arena for the OT profession. It provides a wealth of opportunities to advance the profession's leadership position, centennial strategic plan, and vision of occupational justice and full participation in society for persons with disabilities and their caregivers.

In his classic study of the phenomenon of stigma, Goffman noted that when an individual who is related through the social structure to a stigmatized individual, the wider society may then "treat both individuals in the same respects as one" (Goffman 1963, p. 30). Thus, many of the structural, service, attitudinal, and policy barriers that face persons with disabilities concurrently impact their caregivers as well. The National Alliance on Mental Illness recently completed its first comprehensive state-by-state analysis of mental health-care systems in 15 years. This investigation and grading of adult public mental health-care systems examined infrastructure, information access, services, and recovery and found that the national average grade for these services rated a "D" on a scale where "A" was the highest rating and an "F," failing (NAMI 2006). Issues faced by persons with disabilities, such as lack of accessible or supportive housing and access to transportation, discrimination in employment, and social isolation can markedly impact their caregivers' lives as well. Lack of accessible or supportive housing and access to transportation may require persons with disabilities and their family or informal caregivers to live in less optimal locations, hamper geographic relocation for job promotions, or create barriers to meeting basic needs such as food, clothing, or health care. Thus, evaluating the appropriateness and accessibility of resource information may be vital to enhancing access to these resources for enhanced client care and outcomes as well as increasing the level of respect for those performing the occupation of family and informal caregiving.

Environmental barriers may also impact family or informal caregivers with respect to their ability to perform their employment duties in the workplace. Caregiver bias consists of "stereotyping and bias that may be experienced by employees, men, as well as women, when the fact that they have family caregiving responsibilities becomes known at work" (Williams 2005, p. 1). In October 2005, the federal Equal Employment Opportunity Commission (EEOC) provided guidance regarding the concept of "disability by association" that may protect informal caregivers from discrimination in the workplace based on their relationship or association with an individual with a disability (EEOC 2005).

In 2007, the EEOC provided enforcement guidance for unlawful disparate treatment of workers with caregiving responsibilities (EEOC 2007). A 2012 AARP Policy Institute report found that workplace discrimination against family caregivers is becoming more commonplace and more problematic as baby boomers age and combine their work in the paid labor force and unpaid work with respect to eldercare responsibilities (Williams et al. 2012). As noted in the OT Framework, the term "occupational justice" captures the professions' concern with ethical, moral, and civic factors that can support or hinder health-promoting engagement in occupations and participation in home and community life (AOTA 2008).

OTs that practice in employment settings may potentially provide skills training to employees who are caregivers to afford the opportunity for full participation in all occupations, paid or unpaid, in which caregivers choose to engage. OT practice in the workplace may also assist employers in assessment of the workplace environment to identify policies, attitudes, or structural issues that may provide barriers to productive employment of family and informal caregivers. For example, inflexible leave policies may prohibit family or informal caregiver employees from attending to their own or care recipient needs; supervisor expressions of indifference regarding homelessness due to inaccessible housing may negatively impact employee productivity; or lack of privacy afforded to family or informal caregiver employees seated in cubicles may impede ability to communicate privately with health providers about their family members' health status. These examples provide a glimpse of prospective roles for OT practitioners to address family and informal caregiving in less traditional settings and practice arenas in order to affect future policy toward achieving the profession's vision of occupational justice for the occupation of family and informal caregivers.

Summary

This is an exciting and challenging time for the OT profession to focus on the role of family and informal caregivers. The historical roots of the profession, combined with its vision of the future, provide a sound basis for an interdisciplinary approach to practice, education, research, and policy on both the individual and population levels. The profession's leadership in the adoption of the ICF classification framework and client-centered care will enhance its ability to assess and document family and informal caregiver performance across the life span and involve persons with disabilities and their caregivers in promoting caregiver health and well-being. Avenues such as raising the entry level of the profession, implementation of educational program standards, creation of professional special interest groups, provision of continuing education opportunities, and recruitment from a variety of fields will enhance the profession's scope and development of evidence for family and informal caregiving practice. Research that focuses on the family and informal caregivers provides fresh prospects for exploration of alternative study designs, metrics, and partners. The profession's burgeoning collaborations with respect to policy and advocacy should provide stimulating opportunities to positively influence the lives and participation of persons with disabilities and their family and informal caregivers in many environments: the workplace, business, school, recreation, spiritual, and social settings.

References

Accreditation Council for Occupational Therapy Education (ACOTE®). (2005). *Draft ACOTE standards for an accredited educational program for the occupational therapist or occupational therapy assistant*. http://www.aota.org/nonmembers/area13/docs/standgd.pdf.

Accreditation Council for Occupational Therapy Education (ACOTE®). (2007). *Accreditation council for occupational therapy education standards and interpretative guidelines*. http://www.aota.org/nonmembers/area13/docs/acotestandards107.pdf.

Agree, E., Freedman, V. A., Cornman, J. C., Wolf, D. A., & Marcotte, J. E. (2005). Reconsidering substitution in long-term care: When does assistive technology take the place of personal care? *Journals of Gerontology, Series B: Psychological Sciences & Social Sciences*, *60*(5), S272–S280.

American Journal of Occupational Therapy (AJOT). (2011). *Occupational therapy research agenda, 65*, S4–S7.

American Health Line (AHL). (2006a). *Trends & timelines—Health care education: U. Conn. to offer 'patient school'*. http://elib2.cdc.gov:4671/article.aspx?s=34600.

American Health Line (AHL). (2006b). *Universities: Undergraduate health degrees gaining popularity*. http://elib2.cdc.gov:4671/article.aspx?s=34633.

American Occupational Therapy Association (AOTA). (Undateda). *About OT search*. http://www1.aota.org/otsearch/links/about.asp.

American Occupational Therapy Association (AOTA). (Undatedb). *AOTA certification. Board and specialty certification*. http://www.aota.org/Practitioners/ProfDev/Certification.aspx.

American Occupational Therapy Association (AOTA). (2004). *Occupational therapists and driving*. http://www.aota.org/olderdriver/.

American Occupational Therapy Association (AOTA). (2005). *National school backpack awareness day was a huge success!* http://www.promoteot.org/AI_BackpackAwareness.html.
American Occupational Therapy Association (AOTA). (2006a). *2006 Occupational therapy workforce and compensation report*. Bethesda: AOTA Press.
American Occupational Therapy Association (AOTA). (2006b). *Board certification, specialty certification*. (Brochure). Bethesda: Author.
American Occupational Therapy Association (AOTA). (2006c). *Centennial vision*. http://www.aota.org/nonmembers/area16/docs/vision.pdf. Accessed 20 Jan 2006.
American Occupational Therapy Association (AOTA). (2006d). *Consumer information*. http://www.aota.org/featured/area6/index.asp.
American Occupational Therapy Association (AOTA). (2006e). *AOTA's professional communities*. http://www.aota.org/nonmembers/area5/links/link05.asp#1.
American Occupational Therapy Association (AOTA). (2007a). *OT programs—accredited*. http://www.aota.org/nonmembers/area13/links/LINK28.asp.
American Occupational Therapy Association (AOTA). (2007b). *OTA programs—accredited*. http://www.aota.org/nonmembers/area13/links/link29.asp.
American Occupational Therapy Association (AOTA). (2008). *Occupational therapy practice framework: Domain and process* (2nd ed.). Bethesda: AOTA Press.
American Occupational Therapy Association (AOTA). (2010). *Occupational therapy compensation and workforce study*. Bethesda: AOTA Press.
American Occupational Therapy Association (AOTA). (2012a). *OT Master's-Level Programs—accredited*. http://www.aota.org/Educate/Schools/EntryLevelOT/38119.aspx.
American Occupational Therapy Association (AOTA). (2012b). *OTA programs—accredited*. http://www.aota.org/Educate/Schools/EntryLevelOT/38117.aspx.
Baum, C. M. (1991). Addressing the needs of the cognitively impaired elderly from a family policy perspective. *American Journal of Occupational Therapy, 45*(7), 594–606.
Baum, C. M., & Edwards, D. F. (2000). Documenting productive behaviors: Using the functional behavior profile to plan discharge following stroke. *Journal of Gerontological Nursing, 26,* 34–43.
Behr, S. K., Gray, K., Horowitz, B. P., O'Sullivan, A., Abreu, B. C., & Scott, J. B. (2005). *The American Occupational Therapy Association (AOTA) report to the executive board: Families and caregivers across the lifespan*. Bethesda: AOTA. http://www.aota.org/members/area6/links/link39.asp?PLACE=/members/area6/links/link39.asp. The American occupational therapy association. 4720 Montgomery Lane, Bethesda, MD 20824–1220.
Berenson, R. A. (2005). Which way for competition? None of the above. *Health Affairs, 24*(6), 1536–1542.
Berg, J. (1997). Strategies: Working with family members. *OT Week, 11*(1), 14–15.
Brachtesende, A. (2004). Helping caregivers cope. *OT Practice, 9,* 13–17.
Carlson, C. I., DeHay, T., & Reeves, S. (in press). Assessing 2 care needs. In R. C. Talley (Series Ed.) and R. C., N. Z. Henkin, & D. Butts (Eds.), *Intergenerational caregiving*. New York: Oxford University Press.
Caron, K. G., Schaaf, R. C., Benevides, T. W., & Gal, E. (2012). Cross-cultural comparison of sensory behaviors in children with autism. *The American Journal of Occupational Therapy, 66*(5), e77–e80.
Christakis, N. A., & Allison, P. D. (2006). Mortality after the hospitalization of a spouse. *New England Journal of Medicine, 354*(7), 719–730.
Christiansen, C. H., Baum, C. M., & Bass-Haugen, J. (2005). *Occupational therapy performance, participation, and well-being*. Thorofare: Slack, Inc.
Clauser, S. B., & Bierman, A. S. (2003). Significance of functional status data for payment and quality. *Health Care Financing Review, 24*(3), 1–12.
Cohen, C. A., Colantonio, A., & Vernich, L. (2002). Positive aspects of caregiving: Rounding out the caregiver experience. *International Journal of Geriatric Psychiatry, 17,* 184–188.
Colyvas, J. L., Sawyer, L. B., & Campbell, P. H. (2010). Identifying strategies early intervention occupational therapists use to teach caregivers. *The American Journal of Occupational Therapy, 64*(5), 776–785.

Committee on Disability in America. (2007). In M. J. Field & A. Jette (Eds.), *The future of disability in America*. Washington, DC: The National Academies Press. http://www.nap.edu/catalog/11898html

Corocan, M. A. (2004). *Occupational therapy for family, professional, and paraprofessional caregivers of individuals with disabilities*. American Occupational Therapy Association Continuing Education. http://www.aota.org/nonmembers/area3/links/link08m3.asp.

Corradetti, E. V., & Hills, G. A. (1998). Assessing and supporting caregivers of the elderly. *Topics in Geriatric Rehabilitation, 14*(1), 12–35.

Crowe, T. K., VanLeit, B., & Berghmans, K. K. (2000). Mothers' perceptions of child care assistance: The impact of a child's disability. *American Journal of Occupational Therapy, 54*(1), 52–58.

DeJong, G., & Basnett, I. (2001). Disability and health policy. In G. L. Albrecht, K. D. Seelman, & M. Bury (Eds.), *Handbook of disability studies* (pp. 610–632). Thousand Oaks: Sage.

Dickerson, A. E., & Royeen, C. B. (2003). *Philosophy of professional education*. http://www.aota.org/members/area9/docs/philoed.pdf?PLACE=/members/area9/docs/philoed.pdf.

Eisai, Inc. (25 May 2004). *Eisai, Inc. assists National Family Caregivers Association and the National Alliance for Caregiving with public education program*. http://www.eisai.com/view_press_release.asp?ID=129 & press=93.

Ergas, B. L., & Fischer, B. L. (1998). *The effects of asthma on occupational in pediatric patients with asthma and their caregivers*. New York: Touro College.

Equal Employment Opportunity Commission (EEOC). (2005). Questions and answers about the association provision of the Americans with Disabilities Act. http://www.eeoc.gov/facts/association_ada.html.

Equal Employment Opportunity Commission (EEOC). (2007). Enforcement guidance: Unlawful disparate treatment of workers with caregiving responsibilities. http://www.eeoc.gov/policy/docs/caregiving.html.

Fleming-Cottrell R. P. (Ed). (2005). *Perspectives for occupation-based practice*. Bethesda: AOTA.

Franklin, L., & Rodger, S. (2003). Parent's perspectives on feeding medically compromised children: Implications for occupational therapy. *Australian Occupational Therapy Journal, 50*(3), 137–147.

Fredman, L., & Daly, M. P. (1997). Patient-caregiver functional unit scale: A new scale to assess the patient-caregiver dyad. *Family Medicine, 29*(9), 658–665.

Friedland, J. (2005). Occupational therapy and rehabilitation: An awkward alliance. In R. P. Fleming-Cottrell (Ed.), *Perspectives for occupation-based practice*. Bethesda: American Occupational Therapy Association.

Frontera, W. R., Fuhrer, M. J., Jette, A. M., Chan, L., Cooper, R. A., Duncan, P. W., et al. (2006). Rehabilitation medicine summit: Building research capacity (executive summary). *American Journal of Occupational Therapy, 60*(2), 165–176.

Glantz, C. H. (2003). Update on AOTA certification initiatives. *OT Practice, 8*(22), 11.

Goffman, E. (1963). *Stigma: Notes on the management of spoiled identity*. Englewood Cliffs: Prentice-Hall, Inc.

Hogan, V. M., Lisy, E. D., Savannah, R. L., Kuo, F., & Fisher, G. S. (2004). Role change experienced by family caregivers of adults with Alzheimer's Disease: Implications for occupational therapy. *Physical and Occupational Therapy in Geriatrics, 22*(1), 21–43.

Hubbard, S. (2004). Disability studies and health care curriculum: The great divide. *Journal of Allied Health, 33*(3), 184–188.

Independence through Enhancement of Medicare and Medicaid Coalition (ITEM). (2005). *Comments to DMERCs regarding draft local coverage determinations for power mobility devices*. http://www.itemcoalition.org/press/comments_lcds_power_devices_(10-31-05).htm.

Individuals with Disabilities Education Improvement Act (IDEA). (2004). 20 U.S.C. 1400.

Karner, T. X., & Hall, L. C. (2002). Successful strategies for serving diverse populations. *Home Health Care Services Quarterly, 21*(3–4), 133–139.

Kinney Hoffman, M. (2002). *Self awareness in family caregiving: A report on the communication environment*. https://www.thefamilycaregiver.org/pdfs/CommEnvironmentFINAL.pdf.

Kosloski, K., Schaefer, J. P., Allwardt, D., Montgomery, R. J. V., & Karner, T. X. (2002). The role of cultural factors on clients' attitudes toward caregiving, perceptions of service delivery, and service utilization. *Home Health Care Services Quarterly, 21*(3–4), 65–88.

Langer, R. D., White, E., Lewis, C. E., Kotchen, J. M., Hendrix, S. L., & Trevisan, M. (2003). The women's health initiative observational study: Baseline characteristics of participants and reliability of baseline measures. *Annals of Epidemiology, 13*(9), S107–S121.

Law, M., Baum, C. M., & Dunn, W. (2001). *Measuring occupational performance: Supporting best practice in occupational therapy*. Thorofare: Slack.

Lyons, A. (2000). Cultural competence in occupational therapy practice. American Occupational Therapy Association (AOTA). *Home and Community Health Special Interest Section Quarterly, 7*(3), 1–2.

Malone-Beach, E. E., Skeel, R. L., & Inungu, J. N. (2004). African American women: A life course of care? *Home Health Care Services Quarterly, 23*(2), 1–18.

Marcell, J. (2001). *Elder rage, or take my father. . . please! How to survive caring for aging parents*. Irvine: Impressive Press.

Metzler, C., Jones, D., Nanof, T., & Jackson, L. (2006). Ethics and agenda (Electronic Version). *OT Practice, 11*(3), 6. http://www.aota.org/featured/area3/links/cb-022006.asp.

Metzler, C. A., Hartmann, K. D., & Lowenthal, L. A. (2012). Defining primary care: Envisioning the roles of occupational therapy. *American Journal of Occupational Therapy, 66*(3), 266–270.

Mintz, S. (2002). *Love, honor and value: A family caregiver speaks out about the choices and challenges of caregiving*. Herndon: Capital Books, Inc.

National Alliance for Caregiving and AARP. (2004) Caregiving in the U.S. Washington, D.C. http://www.caregiving.org/data/04finalreport.pdf.

National Alliance for Caregiving, National Multiple Sclerosis Society, & Southeastern Institute of Research, Inc. (2012). Multiple sclerosis caregivers. http://www.caregiving.org/pdf/research/MSCaregivers2012_FINAL.pdf.

National Alliance on Mental Illness (NAMI). (2006). *Grading the states*. http://www.nami.org/Content/NavigationMenu/Grading_the_States/Full_Report/GTS06_final.pdf.

National Board for Certification in Occupational Therapy, Inc. (NBCOT). (2005). *Mission statement*. http://www.nbcot.org/.

National Committee on Quality Assurance (NCQA). (2011). NCQA patient-centered medical home: An established model of care coordination. Washington, DC: NCQA. http://www.ncqa.org/Portals/0/PCMH2011 %20withCAHPSInsert.pdf.

National Council on Disability (NCD). (2003). *Olmstead: Reclaiming institutionalized lives. (Abr. ver.)*. Washington, DC: NCD.

National Research Council. Office of Scientific and Engineering Personnel, Committee on National Needs for Biomedical and Behavioral Scientists Education and Career Studies Unit. (2000). *Addressing the nation's changing needs for biomedical and behavioral scientists*. Washington, DC: National Academy Press. http://www.nap.edu/books/0309069815/html/

Nicholson, J. (1999). Management strategies for musculoskeletal stress in the parents of children with restricted mobility. *British Journal of Occupational Therapy, 62*(5), 206–212.

Novak, M., & Guest, C. (1989). Application of a multidimensional caregiver burden inventory. *Gerontologist, 29*(6), 798–803.

Older Americans Act and its amendments. (2006). 42 U.S.C. 3001.

Olmstead, v. L. C. (1999). 527 U.S. 581.

Oppenheimer, G. M. (2005). Becoming the Framingham Study, 1947–1950. *American Journal of Public Health, 95*(4), 602–610.

Orange, J. B., & Colton-Hudson, A. (1998). Enhancing communication in dementia of the Alzheimer's type. *Topics in Geriatric Rehabilitation, 14*(2), 56–75.

Peloquin, S. M. (2005). Occupational therapy service: Individual and collective understandings of the founders. In R. P. Fleming-Cottrell (Ed.), *Perspectives for occupation-based practice*. Bethesda: American Occupational Therapy Association.

Pinquart, M., & Sorensen, S. (2003). Associations of stressors and uplifts of caregiving with caregiver burden and depressive mood: A meta-analysis. *Journal of Gerontology: Psychological Sciences, 588*(2), P112–P127.

Rehabilitation Act and its amendments, 29 U.S.C. 794 (1973).

Rogers, J. C., & Holm, M. B. (1999). The role change assessment: An interview tool for older adults. In B. J. Hemphill-Pearson (Ed.), *Assessments in occupational therapy mental health: An integrative approach* (pp. 73–82). Thorofare: Slack, Ink.

Semlyen, J. K., Summers, S. J., & Barnes, M. P. (1998). Aspects of caregiver distress after severe head injury. *Journal of Neurologic Rehabilitation, 12*(2), 53–59.

Shelton, M. L. (2001). *Adapting with life alteration disability: Layers of adaptation and care within a lesbian community perspective*. Denton: Texas Women's University.

Silverstein, R. (2000). *Emerging disability policy framework: A guidepost for analyzing public policy* (85 Iowa L. Rev. 1691). http://www.ncwd-youth.info/assets/framework/silverstein_framework.pdf.

Silverstein, R. (2002). *Using the emerging disability policy framework to create a fully inclusive twenty-first century investment system*. http://www.nationalserviceresources.org/links/pages/563.htm?search_term=disability&m=bool.

Talamantes, M. A., Lawler, W. R., & Espino, D. V. (1995). Hispanic American elders: Caregiving norms surrounding dying and the use of hospice services. *Hospice Journal, 10*(2), 35–49.

Taugher, M. P. (1996). *Living with schizophrenia in a Hispanic/Latino community: Implications for mental health service delivery*. Milwaukee: University of Wisconsin-Milwaukee.

The international classification of diseases: Clinical modification (ICD-9-CM). (1989). *Diseases alphabetic index* (annotated, Vol. 2, 9th rev.). Ann Arbor: Edwards Brothers, Inc.

Townsend, E. (2003). Reflections on power and justice in enabling occupation. *Canadian Journal of Occupational Therapy, 70*(2), 74–87.

Ujimoto, K. V. (1998). Frequency, duration, and social context of activities in daily living: Time-budget methodology for caregiving research. *Journal of Occupational Science, 5*(1), 6–13.

U.S. Department of Education. (Undated). Building the legacy: IDEA 2004. Major topic: Evaluation and Revaluation. http://idea.ed.gov/explore/view/p/%2Croot%2Cdynamic%2CTopicalArea%2C4%2C.

U.S. Department of Health and Human Services. (2004a). *Common caregiving terms*. Washington, DC: Administration on Aging. http://www.aoa.gov/prof/aoaprog/caregiver/careprof/progguidance/resources/caregiving_terms.asp.

U.S. Department of Health and Human Services. (2004b, February 26). *Medicaid News: CMS urges states to adopt disease management programs, agency will match state costs*. Baltimore, MD: Centers for Medicare and Medicaid Services. http://www.cms.hhs.gov/apps/media/press/release.asp?Counter=967.

U.S. Department of Health and Human Services. (2004c). *Interdisciplinary training: Behavior, environment, and biology* (RFA-RM-05-010). Bethesda: National Institutes of Health. http://grants.nih.gov/grants/guide/rfa-files/RFA-RM-05-010.html.

U.S. Department of Health and Human Services. (2004d). *NCHS definitions: Instrumental activities of daily living*. Hyattsville: Centers for disease control and prevention, National Center for Health Statistics. http://www.cdc.gov/nchs/datawh/nchsdefs/iadl.htm.

U.S. Department of Health and Human Services. (2005, June). *New freedom initiative caregiver subcommittee: A descriptive analysis: Caregiver efforts for persons with disabilities within the U.S. department of health and human services*. Presented to the HHS Office on Disability New Freedom Initiative Workgroup, Washington, DC.

U.S. Department of Health and Human Services. (2006). *NIH Pathways to Independence (PI) Award* (K99/R00; PA-06-133). Bethesda: National Institutes of Health. http://grants.nih.gov/grants/guide/pa-files/PA-06-133.html.

U.S. Department of Health and Human Services. (2012). *Implementing the claims-based data collection requirement for outpatient therapy-services—Section 3005(g) of the Middle Class Tax Relief and Jobs Creation Act (MCTRJCA) of 2012*. MLN Matters Number: MM8005. Baltimore:

Centers for Medicare and Medicaid Services. http://www.cms.gov/Outreach-and-Education/Medicare-Learning-Network-MLN/MLNMattersArticles/Downloads/MM8005.pdf.

U.S. Department of Labor. (2006). *American time use survey*. Washington, DC: Bureau of Labor Statistics. http://www.bls.gov/tus/.

U.S. Department of Labor. (2012a). *Occupational outlook handbook, occupational therapists* (2012–2013 ed.). Washington, DC: Bureau of Labor Statistics. http://www.bls.gov/ooh/Healthcare/Occupational-therapists.htm.

U.S. Department of Labor. (2012b). *Occupational outlook handbook, Occupational therapy assistants and aides* (2012–2013 ed.). Washington, DC: Bureau of Labor Statistics. http://www.bls.gov/ooh/healthcare/occupational-therapy-assistants-and-aides.htm.

U.S. Equal Employment Opportunity Commission (EEOC). (2005). *Questions and answers about the association provision of the Americans with disabilities act*. http://www.eeoc.gov/facts/association_ada.html.

U.S. Government Accountability Office. (2005). *Report to the senate committee on finance and the house committee on ways and means. Medicare: More specific criteria needed to classify inpatient rehabilitation facilities* (GAO-05-366). http://www.gao.gov/new.items/d05366.pdf.

Üstün, T. B., Chatterji, S., Bickenbach, J. E., Trotter II, R. T., Room, R., Rehm, J., et al. (Eds.). (2001). *Disability and culture: Universalism and diversity*. Kirkland: Hogrefe and Huber Publishers.

Vitaliano, P. P., Russo, J., Young, H. M., Becker, J., & Maiuro, R. D. (1991). *The screen for caregiver burden. Gerontologist, 31*(1), 77.

Vitaliano, P. P., Zhang, J., & Scanlan, J. M. (2003). Is caregiving hazardous to one's physical health? A meta-analysis. *Psychological Bulletin, 129*(6), 946–972.

Wilkens Blank, C., & Finlayson, M. (2007). Exploring the impact of multiple sclerosis on couples: A pilot study. *Canadian Journal of Occupational Therapy, 74*(2), 134–142.

Williams, J. (2005). *Conversations with the experts: Caregiver bias: Work/life issues as diversity concerns* (7(4)). Boston: Sloan Work and Family Research Network, Boston College. http://wfnetwork.bc.edu/The_Network_News/10/The_Network_News_Interview10.pdf.

Williams, J. C., Devaux, R., Petrac, P., & Feinberg, L. (2012). *Protecting family caregivers from employment discrimination*. Washington, DC: AARP Public Policy Institute. http://www.aarp.org/content/dam/aarp/research/public_policy_institute/health/protecting-caregivers-employment-discrimination-insight-AARP-ppi-ltc.pdf. Accessed 30 Sept 2013.

World Health Organization (WHO). (1946). *Preamble to the constitution of the world health organization as adopted by the international health conference, New York, 19–22 June, 1946; signed on 22 July 1946 by the representatives of 61 States* (official records of the World Health Organization, no. 2, p. 100, and entered into forces on 7 April 1948). http://www.who.int/about/definition/en/.

World Health Organization (WHO). (1980). *International classification of impairments, disabilities, and handicaps*. Geneva: Author.

World Health Organization (WHO). (2001). *International classification of functioning, disability, and health*. Geneva: Author.

Zarit, S. H., Reever, K., & Bach-Peterson, J. (1980). Relatives of the impaired elderly: Correlates of feelings of burden. *Gerontologist, 20*(6), 649–655.

Zuzanek, J. (1998). Time use, time pressure, personal stress, mental health, and life satisfaction from a life cycle perspective. *Journal of Occupational Science, 5*(1), 26–39.

Education: A Model of Schools as Caregiving Communities

K. Leigh Baldwin

Education: A Model of Schools as Caregiving Communities

Educators are the embodiment of caregiving, as perceived by students. Typically, recollection of one's favorite teacher produces thoughts and feelings centered in concern, attention, and caring that was provided by the teacher, as well as the curricular content that was imparted. Although instruction occurs in everyday interactions through modeling and, increasingly, via formal programmatic supports, many of the caregiving elements that educators model are learned vicariously. Educators typically teach students about ethics, relationships, communication, and respect, in addition to the educator's particular content area expertise (math, science, etc.). Educators teach students how to both *be* caring and to *provide* care (i.e., caregiving) through their own daily example in the classroom. Ultimately, educators represent the models of self-respect, integrity, and genuineness that they eventually want to be expressed in their students. This expectation is clearly delineated by the National Board for Professional Teacher Standards:

> Accomplished teachers are models of educated persons, exemplifying the virtues they seek to inspire in students—curiosity, tolerance, honesty, fairness, respect for diversity and appreciation of cultural differences—and the capacities that are prerequisites for intellectual growth: the ability to reason and take multiple perspectives to be creative and take risks, and to adopt an experimental and problem-solving orientation. (2002, p. 4)

Overall, a defining characteristic of educators as caregivers is that they conceptualize each student from the "whole child" percept. Specifically, educators see past barriers to learning and their own barriers to caregiving, regardless of magnitude, and work steadily toward a child's potential. In this process, the educator's vision incorporates social, emotional, biological, educational, familial, and cultural dimensions relevant to understanding and reaching each child.

K. L. Baldwin (✉)
Blanchfield Army Community Hospital, Department of Defense,
Building 6988, 30th Street, Ft. Campbell, KY, USA
e-mail: kathryn.l.baldwin.civ@mail.mil

R. C. Talley, S. S. Travis (eds.), *Multidisciplinary Coordinated Caregiving*,
Caregiving: Research • Practice • Policy, DOI 10.1007/978-1-4614-8973-3_7,

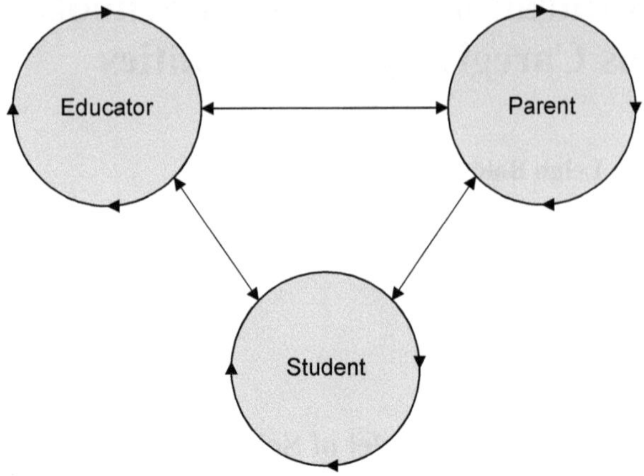

Fig. 1 Reciprocal caregiving triad in education. (Adapted from Haigler et al. 2004)

Defining Schools as Caregiving Communities

Relatedly, when defining caregiving in education, it is important to view the school community from a systems perspective. For instance, historical understanding of caregiving has focused on the informal provision of assistance from one individual to another within the context of a personal relationship. For example, common notions of the term "caregiving" involve images of family members caring for medically ill individuals. However, the act of caregiving within professional fields is becoming increasingly formalized, and efforts are being made to teach, monitor, and assess this process. Haigler et al. (2004) describe how the Rosalynn Carter Institute for Caregiving (RCI) extended the conceptualization of caregiving to incorporate *both* personal and professional dimensions. Specifically, the RCI advances the field of caregiving by promoting the family member-recipient of care dyad, and by recognizing the pivotal role of the medical and other professionals as vital sources of caregiving.

Applied to education, this model can be adapted to refer to parents and educator working collaboratively for the enhancement of student outcomes. Figure 1 illustrates the triangular nature of caregiving in educational communities, with an interdependence between parents, students, and educators. Caregiving in educational contexts often includes peer-to-peer supports (represented by the feedback loop within each circle in Fig. 1) and interdependent relationships. For example, educators often provide caregiving and support to each other via consultation. Parents support each other via formal and informal networks, and students are a valuable source of caregiving for each other. In this sense, caregiving in education is a very dynamic endeavor that extends well beyond traditional conceptualizations of a hierarchical, personal caregiving dyad.

Finally, paradigms for educational caregiving must distinguish "caregiving" from "caretaking" and "caring." Whereas "caretaking" has *social* implications, connoting a dependency in the relationship (Prillaman et al. 1994), "caring" is a more *affective* trait or characteristic that an individual possesses. This chapter is specifically oriented to the *behavior* of "caregiving," referring to the formal, conscious act of facilitating the growth and development of another individual. In this respect, traditional theories of learning and motivation offer insight into the fundamental basis of caregiving in educational institutions.

Theoretical Foundations

The "whole child" concept (DuCharme 1995) refers to the importance of accounting for a child's social, emotional, biological, spiritual, familial, cultural, and financial development in addition to their academic growth. This holistic perspective is essential to educator's caregiving efforts and is a common theme of many educational theories. For instance, Bloom's discussion of educational objectives, one of the most often cited paradigms in educational research, addresses cognitive, affective, and psychomotor domains (Bloom 1956; Krathwohl et al. 1973). Furthermore, as noted in his edited works (Vygotsky and Kozulin 1986; Vygotsky et al. 2007), Vygotsky emphasizes the role of the educator in advancing a student's understanding beyond that which he or she could achieve alone (i.e., zone of proximal development). And, John Dewey (1997a, b reprints), often cited as one of the most influential educational theorists of the twentieth century, stressed community, democracy, and experience in his theories of education. His works illustrate the fact that learning does not occur in isolation and that one's experiences have a strong impact on the ability to learn. In fact, a theme among many prominent theories of this era centers on the notion that new learning is incorporated into existing schemas, as stated by Jean Piaget (Piaget and Inhelder 2000; Singer and Revenson 1996).

Furthermore, throughout the twentieth century, there has been a progressive recognition of the broader environmental context in which children learn and develop. For example, the dynamic social context of children's lives is addressed by Bronfenbrenner's (1979) ecological model, which includes concentric circles representing various levels of influence in an individual's life. Bronfenbrenner recognized the interdependence of individuals, families, and systems (such as educational communities), as reflected in his statement, "No society can long sustain itself unless its members have learned the sensitivities, the motivations, and skills involved in assisting and caring for other human beings" (1979, p. 53, as cited in McDermott 2003).

Finally, applying the "whole child" and ecological approaches to motivating students, one begins to see the manner in which educators frequently act as caretakers. For instance, a child who arrives to school malnourished or lacking adequate shelter or care at home demonstrates the primacy of these needs when he or she is unable to focus on learning due to poverty, hunger, or stress. Self-actualization (including higher order thinking and learning) will only occur when lower order, basic physiological needs are first met, according to Maslow (1987, 1999). When educators facilitate the recognition of and appropriate responses to a child's needs, they are demonstrating the art of caregiving via a "whole child" approach to learning.

Modern Conceptualizations

While the aforementioned traditional epistemology (Vygotsky and Kozulin 1986; Dewey 1997a, b; Maslow 1987, 1999) does not explicitly refer to "caregiving," modern scholars are beginning to formalize our understanding of exactly what defines educators as caregivers. For example, a growing body of literature utilizes Gilligan and Noddings' theories on moral development and ethics, respectively, as a foundation for understanding the caregiving aspects of the education profession (Gilligan 1982; Gilligan et al. 1990, 1988; Noddings 1984, 1986, 1988, 1992, 1995). These theoretical positions, although grounded in feminist theory, are particularly suited to the present analysis given the prominent foci of caring and caregiving dominant in both. A basic illustration of this point is Noddings' differentiation of aesthetic caring (which tends to be objective and systematic) from authentic caring (addressing more of the interpersonal, subjective qualities) in educational practices (Noddings 1988, 1992). Noddings (1995) has written extensively on the necessity of care as a moral imperative for educators, stating that, "developing people with a strong capacity for care is a major objective of responsible education."

Further, Fisher and Trondo (1990) distinguish between "taking care of" (aesthetic, objective elements) and "caregiving" (i.e., the authentic caring model articulated by Noddings). These advances in our understanding of the "art" and "science" of education provide a rich context in which to further delineate the caregiving dimensions in educational practices.

Table 1 represents this dichotomy, with an extension to incorporate many of the broader concepts found in the academic leadership literature. Specifically, Table 1 illustrates the technical and relational aspects of caregiving in education. Whereas the *technical* stresses curriculum and instruction, pedagogy, and production of student outcomes, the *relational* element best represents the caregiving element in education. The relational element is much more individualized, spontaneous, and transformative. Overall, caregiving educators focus on: products *and* people; the science *and* art of teaching; subjects *and* students; systems *and* customs; evaluation *and* intuition; accountability *and* spontaneity; operationalizing *and* inspiring; absolutes *and* abstract reasoning (Table 1). It is important to stress that the two components (technical and relational) are not mutually exclusive. In order to be effective, an educator must be accountable for the technical aspects of their work (i.e., ensuring a well prepared curriculum and assessment methods) combined with a genuine caring for students that extends beyond the academic work that students produce.

Training Educators as Caregivers: Responsibility

Within teacher preparatory institutions, the college curriculum has shown an increasing focus on caregiving aspects (i.e., the relational element represented in Table 1). As such, the "caregiving" concept developed over the years from one with an internal focus (traits, characteristics) that connote "caring" to an external focus on the *act of*

Table 1 Pedagogy: The curriculum and caregiving dichotomy

Context	Curriculum: Technical	Caregiving: Relational
Traditional analogy	Science	Art
Theoretical foundations	"Taking care of"	"Caregiving"[a]
	Aesthetic	Authentic[b]
	Objective	Subjective[c]
	Subject-centered	Student-centered[d]
Performance criteria	Outputs	Inputs
	Quantitative	Qualitative
	Products	People
Areas of focus in practice	Systems	Customs
	Evaluation	Intuition[c]
	Accountability	Spontaneity
Interactions	Unilateral	Reciprocal
	Formal	Informal
	Operational	Inspirational
Type of change involved	Transactional	Transformational
	Top-down	Inside-out
	Reform	Transform
Other conceptual qualities	Rules	Circumstances[c]
	Realistic	Idealistic
	Absolute	Abstract

[a] Fisher and Trondo (1990)
[b] Noddings (1984, 1986, 1988, 1992, 1995)
[c] Prillaman et al. (1994)
[d] National Teacher Professional Standards Board (2002); Noddings (1984)

"caregiving." By focusing more on the act (caregiving) rather than the disposition (caring), the idea has evolved that caregiving behaviors can be operationalized. Educators in training, such as teachers and school administrators, are now commonly required to take courses in classroom management, behavior principles, consultation, and individual differences—all of which including caregiving components. In addition, the caregiving qualities of educators and other school personnel are being codified in professional training standards, professional codes of ethics and performance review documents. An explicit example of this is illustrated in the five core propositions outlined by the National Board for Professional Teacher Standards (NBPTS), which represent the hallmark of ethical standards for the field of education (NBPTS 2002). First, the NBPTS, in recognizing both the art and science of education, notes, "While there are principles and precepts, skills and techniques, to guide the work, teaching is also an activity with artistic aspects, a craft calling for reflection and judgment" (NBPTS 2002, p. 5). Similarly, the NBPTS (2002) advances a basic educational caregiving philosophy:

> A teacher's foremost responsibility is to the intellectual development of our youth, but they are mindful of the broad range of children's needs, including the need for guidance and the strong presence of caring and nurturing adults. This is a difficult set of obligations to fulfill. On the one hand, teachers are prepared neither by training nor by role to serve as parent surrogates or social workers. The distinctive mission of teaching is to promote learning, a complex undertaking in itself. On the other hand, education's broad and humane purposes

> do not admit any narrow specialization. Students' physical, emotional, and social well-being cannot be separated from their intellectual growth. (p. 20)

The caregiving elements contained within this phrasing is of import. Overall, the national core propositions presented by the National Board for Professional Teaching Standards hold as a central premise that education is a complex and dynamic field. Attempting to partition out various aspects of effective educational practices (including caregiving) is overly reductionistic and artificial; rather, such analysis must take a Gestalt-like perspective and consider that the "whole" of effective education is greater than each of its respective parts (technical versus relational, for instance).

Finally, it is noted that movements to recognize, monitor, and assess caregiving elements in education are present across multiple education-related disciplines. Professional training standards and ethics codes for various fields, including school social work, school psychology, and guidance counseling, contain references to "professional work characteristics." Responsibilities to students and communities are much broader than the technical application of knowledge. For example, in an attempt to operationalize the relational expectations within the school psychology profession, the National Association of School Psychologists (NASP 2000) requires that school psychology training programs assess and monitor degree candidates' ethical responsibility, interpersonal skills, communication abilities, respect for individual differences, and dependability (collectively referred to as "professional work characteristics"). In addition, school psychology, social work, and counseling professionals are evaluated in relational, caregiving domains well into their careers. By holding educators accountable for the caregiving aspects of their profession, caregiving is increasingly recognized in both research and practice as essential in helping students remove complex barriers to learning.

Overall, theories addressing the social, cognitive, and ecological influences on development and learning provide a firm foundation for our burgeoning understanding of what, exactly, constitutes caregiving in education. This has been refined in more recent discussion of the *technical* versus *relational* elements of the education profession with due recognition of both areas within professional standards for educator training and practice.

The following section expands such discussion by proposing a specific model of educational caregiving which incorporates both theoretical underpinnings and current educational practices.

A Model of Educational Caregiving in Practice

Figure 2 presents a model of education as communities of caregiving. Examples are provided of some of the primary barriers to caregiving. These are counterbalanced (by Maslow's hierarchy of needs), with supports represented on the right (Maslow 1987, 1999). Furthermore, all barriers and supports are organized according to the ecological context in which they occur (Bronfenbrenner 1979). For instance, an individual-level support is a student's resilience, while school health clinics are

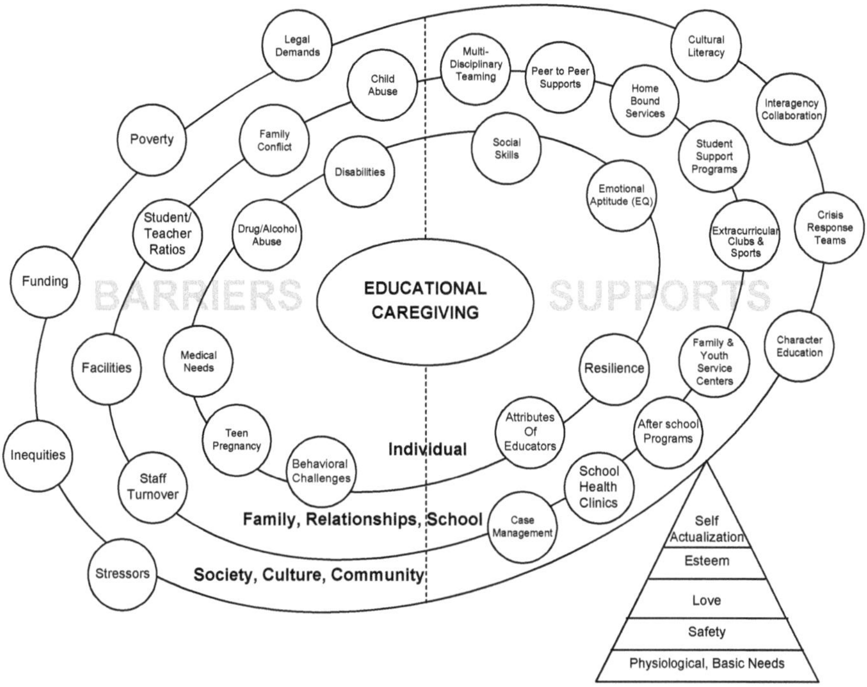

Fig. 2 Model of education as communities of caregiving

considered a school/family-level support. On the outermost circle, character education programs and crisis response teams are society/community-level support systems. Similarly, barriers to learning/teaching are listed on the left, according to whether they are individual, family/school, or society/systems-level considerations. The inclusion of Maslow's hierarchy (triangle) on the right side represents how educators facilitate each student's movement toward self-actualization by assisting the student with basic needs, and with finding safety, love and belonging in the course of the learning process. The actions in which educators engage to promote student movement toward self-actualization is what defines them as caregivers and is the foundation upon which all school-based programmatic supports are built, as represented by Fig. 2. Overall, the micro- and macro-level supports for caregiving in education collectively promote educators' and students' self-actualization, hence establishing a *community of caregiving.*

The Achievement Gap

As indicated by Fig. 2, educators provide care by both giving (e.g., an education) and by taking away (barriers to learning). Many times an educator's caregiving efforts are directed toward the latter, i.e., removing barriers to learning. For example, this might include addressing the ramifications of a student's (or their family member's) drug/alcohol use, poverty, and abuse. Therefore, it is imperative that any model of education as communities of caregiving include a thorough consideration of such barriers. In educational literature, such barriers are often referred to as contributing to an "achievement gap."

The "achievement gap," typically holds one of two connotations. First, the "gap" is used to describe the difference between the performance of students in the majority as compared to minority populations (as defined by variables such as socioeconomic status and ethnicity (Kober 2001; Morris 2002; Paige 2001). Secondly, the term "achievement gap" is also used to refer to the ipsative comparisons of a student's demonstrated academic performance, as compared to what is expected, or what is his or her potential. Interestingly, both situations are negatively effected by hardships, such as psychological, social, physical, or behavioral challenges, and are collectively referred to as barriers to learning.

Barriers to learning are often framed exclusively from the perspective of the learner. Less often cited under this theoretical model are the challenges encountered by educators (see Edelman and Taylor, this series). Educators' attempts at caregiving are sometimes hampered by considerations such as scarcity of resources, language barriers, attrition, job satisfaction, and stressors. In order to present a holistic view of what is needed to "close the achievement gap," it is essential that a student's barriers to learning be addressed in conjunction with an educator's barriers to caregiving. Ideally, once such barriers are removed, both students and educators can progress toward self-actualization, as envisioned in Maslow's (1987, 1999) aforementioned hierarchical model of motivation.

Closing the Achievement Gap: Barriers to Learning

Caregiving is critical given the current needs of school-age children. According to the U.S. Surgeon General (U.S. Department of Health and Human Services 1999), in the course of 1 year, approximately one in five school-age children present with symptoms of a DSM IV (Diagnostic and Statistical Manual of Mental Disorders) disorder, and 21 % of all children ages 9–17 actually receive mental health services in a year (American Psychiatric Association 2000). Many students arrive at school with a diverse array of psychological difficulties, including depression, anxiety, and drug and alcohol abuse. In fact, "Indications are strong that students who are affected by family strife, crime, alcohol and drug abuse, and other problems will increasingly seek mental health services from school personnel" (NASP n.d., Job Outlook section 2).

Furthermore, in the 2001–2002 academic year, 13.4 % of all students were identified as receiving special education services due to a disability interfering with the learning processes (National Center for Education Statistics 2003). Prevalence statistics demonstrate that many psychological factors impede the learning potential of our nation's children.

In addition to psychological factors, social/familial, physical, and behavioral considerations also represent a challenge to the educational process. Social/familial barriers often include divorce, poverty, and abuse. Children from abusive homes and those whose parents are divorced are at higher risk for negative educational outcomes, such as underachievement and dropping out (Dawson 1981; Hanson 1999; Nisivoccia 1997). Also, low socioeconomic status (SES), which includes factors such as family income, parental education level, and parent occupation(s), is associated with lower academic performance when compared to the performance of students from higher SES backgrounds (Lin 2001). Furthermore, physical barriers, such as health problems affect students' concentration and stamina, are directly linked to academic performance (American Academy of Pediatrics 1992). Several health-related concerns receiving considerable attention recently are childhood obesity, sexual activity/STDs, and eating disorders. Finally, behavioral challenges presented by many students include opposition to authority figures, truancy, threats and acts of violence toward educators, and fighting with peers. Such problems detract from the learning experience and add to demands on an educator for caregiving (Reid et al. 2004).

Closing the Achievement Gap: Barriers to Caregiving

To accurately assess the current status of caregiving in education, an examination of barriers in this realm is necessary. Perhaps one of the most pressing concerns is the current rate of attrition in the field of education (included as "staff turnover" in Fig. 2). For example, "Nationally, 22 % of all new teachers leave the profession in the first 3 years because of lack of support" (U.S. Department of Education n.d., 8). This is a complex problem that appears to be based in heightened demands for educator accountability and occurs at a time of declining educational resources and supports.

One particular consideration pertains to challenging student-teacher ratios in an era of increasing inclusion and diversity in the classroom. For instance, the Individuals with Disabilities Education Improvement Act (IDEA 2004) requires that all students are educated in the least restrictive environment, which often means they are mainstreamed with same-age peers to the maximum extent possible. While this is theoretically sound, delivery on this requirement sometimes falls short in practice. For instance, teachers may report that they have little time for needed collaboration with special education specialists in order to ensure the availability of adequate classroom supports (Coleman 2001; Ferguson 1999). This places increased pressure on teachers.

Furthermore, diversity-related challenges are seen in areas beyond those of differing ability levels. For example, educators are challenged to adequately prepare for a multitude of cultures and native languages that are increasingly represented among students (Lin 2001). Class enrollment often changes throughout the year with increasing populations of migrant students (Henderson and Daft 2002). Also, educators frequently express a need for classroom behavior management supports and strategies to reach culturally and racially diverse learners who present with varying motivation levels.

Overall, these caregiving challenges are compounded by current legislation, which establishes rather uniform standards for student performance (No Child Left Behind Act (NCLB) 2001). Many argue that such reform initiatives undermine progress that has been made to date in terms of understanding individual differences in human expression and learning. While it is true that "all children can learn at high levels" (NCLB 2001), a crucial distinction is that what is defined as "high" varies from student to student. Many educators argue that such "forced fit" and "teaching to the masses" compromises their ability to individualize instruction and set custom benchmarks for performance based on student ability. In this respect, some components of modern educational reform are counter to what has long been identified as best practices in education. Such a climate, which combines micro-level expectations of a relational nature with macro-level technical and outcomes-based education, heightens a dichotomy (see Table 1) that results in considerable tension for many educators (Noddings 1995).

In addition to limitations in their abilities to address diverse needs, educators often express frustration at their perceived lack of control over many of the outcomes that their students are expected to demonstrate. As represented in Bronfenbrenner's (1979) ecological model (Fig. 2), there are many dimensions of influence in a child's life, including social, familial, and cultural spheres. Current educational reform mandates require that a primary indicator of educator effectiveness consist of student outcomes. Educators are held directly accountable (including public rewards and sanctions) for student performance. This approach does not take into account the myriad of influences in a child's life external to the educational system. Similarly, as cited in Prillaman et al. (1994, p. 5), "Many educators express dissatisfaction at having their work viewed and evaluated only in terms of technical effectiveness . . .[yet] recently, the language of the technical continues to be reinforced by the notions inherent in much of the present school reform movement." Current educational reform initiatives stress the science of education to the exclusion of the more relational, caregiving elements and hold educators directly responsible for the entirety of academic outcomes. In this respect, modern reform movements ignore the Gestaltist principles that enhance development of the whole child as well as the social and ecological contexts in which learning occurs.

Closing the Achievement Gap: Supports for Caregiving

Throughout their training, educators are taught didactics as well as caregiving (technical and relational). While caregiving is most often manifested in daily classroom interactions with individual students, occasionally teachers have reason to harness resources and elevate caregiving in a manner to effect more dynamic change for students and their families. Large scale, deliberate attempts to intervene for positive change in the educational system on behalf of students and/or families are what constitutes educational advocacy. Specific examples include programs oriented toward cultural literacy, use of interagency collaboration, participation on school crisis response teams, and development of family resource/advocacy centers (Fig. 2). Many times, resources for such programs are derived through educator-initiated grant-writing or parent-driven fundraising. In this manner, educators become involved in systems-level initiatives that extend their caregiving beyond the classroom level. Thus, educational activity can encompass pedagogy, caregiving in daily interactions (the classroom), and larger-scale advocacy. This form of collective caregiving can initiate with the student, the educators, or the parents (keeping in mind a tri-part relational view of caregiving) and typically involve all three parties (Haigler et al. 2004). In this sense, *educational advocacy* is a dynamic form of caregiving involving multiple stakeholders.

In addition, research has demonstrated the efficacy of social skills training (Vaughn et al. 2003), promotion of cultural literacy (Dilworth 1998), and character education in shaping students to become caregivers. Although "character education" is somewhat controversial in contemporary educational systems (Boyd 1996), related notions of "emotional IQ," "resilience," and "social competence" are universally promoted as ideals to instill in students (Brooks and Goldstein 2001; Goleman 2005). Likewise, formal study has begun to target specific methods that educators can employ to facilitate students' development of non-academic skills that are essential for success in life. As stated eloquently by Martin Luther King, Jr., "The function of education is to teach one to think intensively and to think critically. Intelligence plus character—that is the goal of true education" (as cited in Carson et al. 1992). This sentiment is echoed by Noddings (1995), who stated that "developing people with a strong capacity for care is a major objective of responsible education." Advocating for others and respecting their diverse needs is the hallmark of effective caregiving. As applied to education, this leads to empowerment and self-sufficiency, which is the ultimate goal in the educational process.

Additional Supports for Caregiving: Schools as Full Service Sites

Given the increasing recognition of multidimensional student needs, combined with the practicality of serving students at school, full service schools exemplify educational advocacy (collective caregiving) in action. Students are required to attend school, thus are a "captive audience." These considerations make the school setting a very practical site for the delivery of services such as medical office visits, psychological services, and case management. Accordingly, there has been a growing movement toward schools as full service sites (Dryfoos 2002). The exact nature and extent of services vary by factors such as location, community need, and available resources. However, there are some commonalities across programs. For example, many school sites utilize a core cadre of education professionals involved in multidisciplinary teaming, interagency collaboration, parent participation, and case management. Additional components associated with full service schools include school clinics, support groups, therapy services (mental health, speech/language, occupational and/or physical therapy), tutoring, afterschool programs, crisis response teams, health services or clinics, and home-based services.

Additional Supports for Caregiving: Peer-to-Peer Supports

An area that has been neglected in the education-related literature is the caregiving that occurs on a peer-to-peer basis (student to student; educator to educator; parent to parent). As interactions within a school setting are reciprocal and not exclusive to the teacher-student dyad (Fig. 1), we must also address the immense support and caring that peers often receive from one another in school settings. Peer-to-peer supports take many forms. Of course, caregiving occurs within the informal nature of spontaneous interaction. However, just as there are formal programs in place for educator-to-student and/or family advocacy, most school systems now have very progressive formalized programs of caregiving that occur across all grades.

Pertaining to student-to-student caregiving, academic tutoring from peers is very common, and such a program will often pair a younger student with an older one for tutoring and mentoring, with the intention of strengthening the younger child's abilities within specific areas. Peer tutoring also occurs on a less structured (or more unplanned basis) in the classroom when informal help is offered. Another manner in which student-to-student caregiving occurs is through peer mediation programs. These programs utilize trained student mediators to arbitrate disputes and make recommendations for resolution of a contentious issue. The efficacy of peer mediation as a problem solving model in school systems has been consistently demonstrated (Mather and Rutherford 1991). Finally, extracurricular sports and clubs provide a wealth of opportunities for student-to-student caregiving. For instance, in learning to work collaboratively as a team, students are encouraged to set aside individual ambition in favor of team goals, and to demonstrate patience and reliance upon each other—all of which necessitates caregiving. Overall, considering the modeling effects, communication patterns, and nonverbal behaviors inherent in each of the student-to-student examples cited, caregiving influences can be just as prominent among peers as between students and educators.

Peer-to-peer caregiving occurs between educators, as well. Some of the related research can be found in the area of consultation (Dougherty 2005). For instance, many theories of consultation refer to the means by which an educator solicits caregiving assistance from a colleague in order to address a professional need. Additionally, there are some programs instituted in school districts that attempt to formalize a caregiving relationship (such as peer mentoring programs designed for new educators). But perhaps one of the primary forms of caregiving that occurs at this level (between colleagues), is the informal demonstration of support or encouragement, such as seen during times of stress.

Finally, relationships between parents are also a strong source of caretaking occurring in educational contexts. Consider the depth of communication that sometimes occurs as parents rely upon one another for information and encouragement when their child is struggling in school. Parents often create vast informal networks and build relationships with fellow parents that continue as their children progress through the grades. Such caregiving relationships are further solidified through parent involvement in school-based extracurricular programs, parent volunteers in the classroom, and formal organizations such as the PTA (Parent Teacher Association). Parent-to-parent caregiving significantly influences many students' school performance, since such supports can often help remove barriers to learning. Overall, peer supports (among students, teachers, and parents) have received little formal attention in models of educational caregiving that have been proposed to date.

Future Directions

Research

Several barriers to learning and to effective caregiving in education have been identified. While there is a growing body of research aimed at understanding how to most effectively reduce these barriers, particular studies aimed at "caregiving" in education remain sparse. In practice, educators are very adept at moving from advocacy (i.e., acting on behalf of another) toward empowerment (i.e., student self-sufficiency & actualization) through their example and daily interactions. Additional research is needed in order to better articulate this elusive process. The field of nursing may be considered as a point of reference, given that this specialty has amassed a considerable amount of research explicitly on the caregiving elements of the profession (Cook 2003; Sitzman 2002; Smith 2004; Watson 1985, 1994, 2002). Similarly, there is a body of literature on caregiving qualities of preschool teachers, but this needs to be expanded to a much broader understanding across the developmental spectrum (Caulfield 1997; Lee 1988; VanderVen 1989).

Furthermore, it is noted that investigation into the nature and extent of caregiving among educators in university settings is warranted. A comprehensive review of the literature reveals that there is practically no information that conceptualizes postsecondary educators as caregivers (Thayer-Bacon and Bacon 1996). Given what is known about the roles and functions of postsecondary educators, it can be inferred that there is a strong caregiving component at this educational level. Accordingly, comparable study to that which has been conducted in the general field of elementary and secondary education to date would be insightful.

Relatedly, with the increasing development of distributed learning (e.g., internet-based courses, teleconferencing) as an alternative method for delivering instruction, it is important to investigate the extent to which the caregiving aspect of educators' practices are maintained in electronic mediums (Goldstein 2003). Increasingly, both college degrees and high school-level academic instruction are being delivered through distance learning. With both relational and technical aspects essential to education (Table 1), methods for retaining caregiving in online instruction need to be identified and related investigations pursued.

Finally, as relates to student-to-student caregiving, research supports particular programmatic aspects, such as peer tutoring and mediation (Mather and Rutherford 1991). However, very little study to date exists on the manner in which caregiving facilitates programs or the effects of varying types and levels of peer caregiving on student outcomes. This is comparable to the lack of research on parent to parent supports, as well. For instance, there is very little information on the efficacy of parent-initiated education programs (such as parent advocacy centers/services).

Training

Training continues to be a need in order to enhance educational caregiving practices. First, continuing with our adaptation of the triad model of caregiving, parents are a key element in the caregiving process (Haigler et al. 2004). Yet, there are very few programs in the school system that actually teach caregiving skills to parents. Educators encourage parents to be involved in their child's school, but provide little to no instruction in how to comprehend the system, what is expected of them, and how to respond to disagreement, for example. Additionally, R. Weaver (personal communication, March 16, 2007) emphasizes the need to train parents in advocacy, especially in areas involving education-related legislation and communication with policy makers. Parent education programs would enhance the efforts of full service schools and increase compliance with educational and clinical treatment plans. Similarly, additional study is warranted in effective ways to instruct parents as caregivers in the educational process.

Additional awareness of caregiving issues is needed in teacher preparatory programs, as well. While university training programs are expected to monitor and assess a trainee's "professional work characteristics," there is wide variability in how institutions define and measure these traits. Similarly, while professional training standards stress the relational aspects of an educator's work, there is evidence to suggest that, in practice, "competence" and "commitment" elements of an educator's professional activities continue to overshadow "caregiving" aspects (Morris 2002). Furthermore, there are few opportunities for formal peer mentoring as an educator-in-training begins to transition into practice. R. Weaver (personal communication, March 16, 2007) cites this as essential to facilitate the relational, caregiving qualities that may not be directly taught in training programs. Overall, professional discourse on this matter, similar to what has occurred in the nursing profession, would greatly advance our methods for promoting relational elements (Table 1) in education. Additional research, in terms of how to empirically define and measure caregiving qualities is warranted. The definition and measurement of caregiving qualities in education are clearly delineated areas for future research.

Furthermore, outreach and training in relational components of education (caregiving) for educators practicing in rural areas is suggested (Dorrell 1992). Smaller, rural districts typically do not have access to the variety and quantity of continuing professional development opportunities as do their peers in more urban areas. In order to facilitate collegial support and enhance peer-to-peer caregiving, and to support educator-to-student caregiving (especially when rural educators are faced with burnout), updated trainings and/or peer support meetings are needed.

Policy and Practice Implications: Caring for the Caregivers

Given the rate of attrition of new educators and the shortage of qualified personnel in some teaching areas, it is critical that issues such as job satisfaction, pay, stress, and burnout are further examined in order to elucidate the reasons for turn-over (U.S. Department of Education n.d., 8). Refinement in the area of peer-to-peer (i.e., collegial) caregiving might prove a viable avenue for addressing some of these challenges. The expectations on educators as caregivers are, obviously, quite immense. As cited in the literature and reported anecdotally by educators, there is increasing pressure to produce in the technical elements of their work. As a result, many feel as though they have to sacrifice other important qualitative aspects of their teaching due to time constraints. Tension is also created by legislative demands, which tend to overemphasize universal standards and underemphasize the ecological context in which students learn. Increasing accountability combined with declining resources creates a tense work environment for many educators (Wolfgramm 1995).

Clearly, there are many demands on educators and a need for enhanced recognition of their work and contributions. Statements originally voiced by philosopher Jacques Barzun (1944), "teaching is not a lost art, but the regard for it a lost tradition," are echoed by current educational leaders. Reg Weaver, past president of the National Education Association (NEA), includes "respect for teaching" as one of the modern "3 Rs" as essential for effective schools in the twenty-first century (NEA n.d.; R. Weaver, personal communication, March 16, 2007). Additional study, legislation and school policy focusing on methods for supporting the relational, caregiving (Table 1) element of educators' work (the "art") while simultaneously upholding the technical, curricular aspects (the "science") is critically needed.

Conclusion

While society generally recognizes the caregiving qualities of educators and other school personnel, there has been considerably more empirical study on the technical elements of their work than on their relational, caregiving responsibilities. However, there is increasing recognition, both in the research literature and in practice, of the relational, care elements that are essential to successful academic outcomes. By valuing educators, parents, and students as caregivers, we are optimally positioned to address the "whole child" within an ecological context, remove barriers to learning, and promote each child's self-actualization.

References

American Academy of Pediatrics. (1992). *Health care and a child's ability to learn: A survey of elementary school teachers*. (ERIC Document Reproduction Service No. 358958).
American Psychiatric Association. (2000). *Diagnostic and statistical manual of mental disorders (text rev.)*. Washington, DC: Author.
Barzun, J. (1944). *Teacher in America*. New York: Atlantic Monthly Press.
Bloom, B. S. (1956). *Taxomony of educational objectives, handbook I: The cognitive domain*. New York: David McKay Co., Inc.
Boyd, S. M. (1996). Character education, the U.S. constitution and the U.S. supreme court. *Update on Law-Related Education, 20*(1), 23–25.
Bronfenbrenner, U. (1979). *The ecology of human development: Experiments by nature and design*. Cambridge: Harvard University Press.
Brooks, R., & Goldstein, S. (2001). *Raising resilient children: Fostering strength, hope and optimism in your child*. New York: McGraw-Hill.
Carson C., Luker, R., & Russell P. (Eds.). (1992). *The papers of Martin Luther King, Jr., Volume I: Called to serve, January 1929-June 1951*. Berkeley: University of California Press.
Caulfield, R. (1997). Professionalism in early care and education. *Early Childhood Education Journal, 24*(4), 261–263.
Coleman, M. R. (2001). *Conditions of teaching children with exceptional learning needs: The bright futures report*. Arlington: Council for Exceptional Children. (ERIC Document Reproduction Service No. 455660).
Cook, P. R. (2003). Caring as an imperative for nursing education. *Nursing Education Perspectives, 24*(4), 192–198.
Dawson, P. (1981). *The effect of the single-parent family on academic achievement: A review of related literature*. (ERIC Document Reproduction Service No. 241604).
Dewey, J. (1997a). *Experience and education (Reprint ed.)*. New York: Free Press.
Dewey, J. (1997b). *Democracy and education (Reprint ed.)*. New York: Free Press.
Dilworth M. S. (Ed.). (1998). *Being responsive to cultural differences: How teachers learn*. Thousand Oaks: Corwin Press. (ERIC Document Reproduction Service No. 415196).
Dorrell, L. D. (1992). *Just take your time and keep it between the lines: Rural education and the at-risk student*. Paper presented at the annual convention of the National Rural Education Association, Washington, DC. (ERIC Document Reproduction Service No. 355073).
Dougherty, A. M. (2005). *Psychological consultation and collaboration in school and community settings*. Belmont: Thomson Brooks/Cole.
Dryfoos, J. (2002). Full-service community schools: Creating new institutions. *Phi Delta Kappan, 83*(5), 393–399.
DuCharme, C. C. (1995). *The concept of the child: 1890–1940*. (ERIC Document Reproduction Service No. 391595).
Ferguson, D. L. (1999). *On working together: Groupwork, teamworks, and collaborative work among educators. On point ... brief discussions of critical issues in urban education*. Newton: Education Development Center, Inc., National Institute for Urban School Improvement. (ERIC Document Reproduction Service No. 437473).
Fisher, B., & Trondo, J. (1990). Toward a feminist theory of caring. In E. Abel, & M. Nelson (Eds.), *Circles of care*. Albany: SUNY Press.
Gilligan, C. (1982). *In a different voice*. Cambridge: Harvard University Press.
Gilligan, C., Ward, J. V., & Taylor, J. M. (1988). *Mapping the moral domain*. Cambridge: Harvard University Press.
Gilligan, C., Lyons, N. P., & Hanmer, T. J. (1990). *Making connections*. Cambridge: Harvard University Press.
Goldstein, L. S. (2003). Challenges enacting caring teacher education. *Journal of Teacher Education, 54*(5), 441–455.

Goleman, D. (2005). *Emotional intelligence: Why it can matter more than IQ* (10th anniversary ed.). New York: Bantam.

Haigler, D. H., Bauer, L. J., & Travis, S. S. (2004). Finding the common ground of family and professional caregiving: The education agenda at the Rosalynn Carter Institute. *Educational Gerontology, 30,* 95–105.

Hanson, T. L. (1999). Does parental conflict explain why divorce is negatively associated with child welfare? *Social Forces, 77*(4), 1283–1316.

Henderson, A., & Daft, J. (2002). *State Title I migrant participation information, 1998–1999.* Washington, DC: Department of Education. (ERIC Document Reproduction Service No. 468509).

Individuals with Disabilities Education Improvement Act. (2004).

Kober, N. (2001). *It takes more than testing: Closing the achievement gap. A report of the center on education policy.* Washington, DC: Center on Education Policy. (ERIC Document Reproduction Service No. 454358).

Krathwohl, D. R., Bloom, B. S., & Bertram, B. M. (1973). *Taxonomy of educational objectives, the classification of educational goals. Handbook II: Affective domain.* New York: David McKay Co., Inc.

Lee, M. W. (1988). *What you give is what you get.* Washington, DC: Howard University. ERIC Document Reproduction Service No. 304208).

Lin, Q. (2001). Toward a caring-centered multicultural education within the social justice context. *Education, 122*(1), 107–115.

Maslow, A. H. (1987). *Motivation and personality (3rd ed.).* New York: HarperCollins Publishers.

Maslow, A. H. (1999). *Toward a psychology of being.* New York: John Wiley & Sons.

Mather, S. R., & Rutherford, R. B. (1991). Peer-mediated interventions promoting social skills of children and youth with behavioral disorders. *Education and Treatment of Children, 14*(3), 227–242.

McDermott, D. R. (2003). Building better human connections: Parenting/caring education for children and teens in school. *Childhood Education, 80*(2), 71–76.

Morris, V. G. (2002). Caring—The missing C in teacher education: Lessons learned from a segregated African American school. *Journal of Teacher Education, 53*(2), 120–124.

National Association of School Psychologists. (2000). *NASP standards for training and field placement programs in school psychology.* Bethesda: NASP Publications.

National Association of School Psychologists. (n.d.). *FAQs—The profession of school psychology.* http://www.nasponline.org/about_nasp/sp_faq.html.

National Board for Professional Teaching Standards. (2002). *What teachers should know and be able to do: The five core propositions of the national board.* http://www.nbpts.org/about/coreprops.cfm.

National Center for Educational Statistics. (2003). *Digest of education statistics tables and Figures: United States department of education.* http://nces.ed.gov/programs/digest/d03/tables/dt052.asp.

National Education Association. (n.d.). *The three R's: NEA advertising radio commentary.* http://www.nea.org/columns/index.html.

Nisivoccia, J. D. (1997). *The influence of parental separation and divorce on adolescent academic achievement: Developmental issues.* (ERIC Document Reproduction Service No. 420819).

No Child Left Behind Act, PL 107–110. (2001).

Noddings, N. (1984). *Caring: A feminine approach to ethics and moral education.* Berkeley: University of California Press.

Noddings, N. (1986). Fidelity in teaching, teacher education, and research for teaching. *Harvard Educational Review, 56*(4), 496–510.

Noddings, N. (1988). An ethic of caring and its implications for instructional arrangements. *American Journal of Education, 96*(2), 215–230.

Noddings, N. (1992). *The challenge to care in schools.* New York: Teachers College Press.

Noddings, N. (1995). Teaching themes of care (caring and education). *Phi Delta Kappan, 76*(9), 675–670.

Paige, R. (2001). *"No child left behind": A blueprint for education reform.* Testimony before the budget committee, house of representatives. (ERIC Document Reproduction Service No. 452569).
Piaget, J., & Inhelder, B. (2000). *The psychology of the child.* New York: Basic Books.
Prillaman, A. R., Eaker, D. J., & Kendrick, D. M. (Eds.). (1994). *The tapestry of caring: Education as nurturance.* Norwood: Ablex Publishing Company.
Reid, R., Gonzalez, J. E., Nordness, P. D., Trout, A., & Epstein, M. H. (2004). A meta-analysis of the academic status of students with emotional/behavioral disturbance. *Journal of Special Education, 38*(3), 130–143.
Singer, D. G., & Revenson, T. A. (1996). *A Piaget primer: How a child thinks* (Rev. ed.). New York: Plume (Penguin Books).
Sitzman, K. L. (2002). Interbeing and mindfulness: A bridge to understanding Jean Watson's theory of human caring. *Nursing Education Perspectives, 23*(3), 118–124.
Smith, M. (2004). Review of research related to Watson's theory of caring. *Nursing Science Quarterly, 17*(1), 13–25.
Thayer-Bacon, B. J., & Bacon, C. S. (1996). Caring professors: A model. *Journal of General Education, 45*(4), 255–269.
U.S. Department of Education. (n.d.). *Survival guide for new teachers.* http://www.ed.gov/teachers/become/about/survivalguide/message.html.
U.S. Department of Health and Human Services. (1999). *Mental health: A report of the surgeon general—Executive summary.* Rockville: U.S. Department of Health and Human Services, Substance Abuse and Mental Health Services Administration, Center for Mental Health Services, National Institutes of Health, National Institute of Mental Health.
VanderVen, K. (1989). *The relationship between notions of caregiving held by early childhood practitioners and stages of career development.* (ERIC Document Reproduction Service No. ED 309860).
Vaughn, S., Kim, A., Sloan, C. V., Hughes, M. T., Elbaum, B., & Sridhar, D. (2003). Social skills interventions for young children with disabilities: A synthesis of group design studies. *Remedial and Special Education, 24*(1), 2–15.
Vygotsky, L. S., & Kozulin, A. (Ed.). (1986). *Thought and language (Rev. ed.).* Cambridge: MIT Press.
Vygotsky, L. S., Cole, M., John-Steiner, V., Scribner, S., & Souberman, E. (Eds.). (2007). *Mind in society: Development of higher psychological processes.* Cambridge: Harvard University Press.
Watson, J. (1985). *Nursing: The philosophy and science of caring.* Boulder: University Press of Colorado.
Watson J. (Ed.). (1994). *Applying the art and science of human caring.* New York: NLN.
Watson, J. (2002). *Instruments for assessing and measuring caring in nursing and health sciences.* New York: Springer.
Wolfgramm, H. F. (1995). Needed: An ethic of caring in our schools. *Education, 115*(4), 516–522.

Part III
Disciplinary Contributions to Caregiving

Health Communication and Caregiving Research, Policy, and Practice

Lisa Sparks

In the inaugural issue of *Health Communication*, Jon Nussbaum (1989) commented that evidence strongly suggests, "health communication as a legitimate field of inquiry has finally arrived." In the same issue, Gary Kreps (1989) asked, "What difference can the field of health communication make to the public?" (p. 35). Since then, health communication scholars have been contributing to the answer from a variety of perspectives. Leading health communication scholar and editor of *Health Communication,* Teri Thompson states that health communication deals with health care related environments that give meaning to health status by assuming and defining its cause (Thompson 2000). The U.S. Department of Health and Human Services (2000), in achieving the Healthy People 2010/2020 initiatives to educate the public on the nation's major health priorities, put forth this definition of health communication:

> The art and technique of informing, influencing, and motivating the individual, institutional, and public audiences about important health issues. The scope of health communication includes disease prevention, health promotion, health care policy, and the business of health care as well as enhancement of the quality of life and health of individuals within the community.

Put simply, health communication *involves creating shared meaning about health care and conditions*. Health communication covers a wide-ranging array of topics, including disease control and prevention, emergency preparedness and response, injury and violence prevention, environmental health, workplace safety, and general communication behavior as it relates to well-being and leading healthy lives. Health promotion efforts at the national level often take a developmental life-span perspective with a focus on adolescent health, aging, women's health issues, men's health issues, school health, and minority health (Parrott 2004; Sparks and Villagran 2010).

L. Sparks (✉)
M.S. Health and Strategic Communication, Chapman University,
Orange, CA 92866, USA
e-mail: sparks@chapman.edu

Chao Family Comprehensive Cancer Center, NCI Designated,
University of California, Irvine, CA 92697, USA
e-mail: lsparks1@UCI.edu

R. C. Talley, S. S. Travis (eds.), *Multidisciplinary Coordinated Caregiving,*
Caregiving: Research • Practice • Policy, DOI 10.1007/978-1-4614-8973-3_8,

Health communication as a field has certainly arrived and is thriving with applications to many important health contexts, especially caregiving research, policy, and practice.

Objectives and Organization

The purpose of this chapter is to provide an evidence-based approach to health communication and caregiving research, policy, and practice. By conveying a sense of the broadened scope of recent communication theory and research, the purpose of this chapter is to propose an evidence-based framework through which health communication as applied to caregiving research, policy, and practice might occur. To achieve this goal, I begin with a brief introduction to health literacy followed by the state of the science of health communication and caregiving research, policy, and practice including health communication in the health information age and health messaging. This section includes an overview of the major variables in health communication research, including the significant body of literature on message framing. To exemplify the issue of health message framing, I offer a case study to explore the impact that message frames can have on receivers' perceptions of health-related information. The third section is devoted to a discussion of the major theoretical and conceptual frameworks utilized in health communication, health education, and health behavior fields, which can be utilized as effective teaching tools and provide an important introduction to the major theoretical frameworks guiding health communication interventions that are crucial to health behavior change in caregiving and related contexts. Exposure to such health theories in one comprehensive chapter provides a logical transition to how evidence-based health messages translate into health policy and practice. The final section of the chapter outlines the proposed SMILE-HCCM model of health care interventions. The SMILE-HCCM is an evidence-based model that draws from recent theory and research in the field of communication to create a flexible framework for health communication and caregiving research, policy, and practice and implications. The goal is to further translate existing research into practice by providing a model that can be tested and applied in health care settings with target populations to achieve more effective and appropriate decision-making and better health outcomes (Sparks and Nussbaum 2008; Sparks and Villagran 2010).

Health Literacy and Caregiving Research, Policy, and Practice

Effective health communication is a central component in the provision of health care and the promotion of public health information. Health literacy refers to an individual's competence or knowledge in the field of public health and their ability to read, understand and use provided information in order to make intelligent health-related decisions. A 2006 American Medical Association Foundation and American

Medical Association report on health literacy identified these obstacles to efficient communication: "(1) difficulty obtaining, processing, and understanding health information, (2) health care system complexity, (3) practice pressures, (4) cultural and language issues, and (5) lack of clinician training on effective communication strategies." It also stated that, "at least 50 % of adults in the USA are at increased risk for serious consequences due to low health literacy." (p. 1) An individual's health literacy is dependent upon and determined by a number of factors; including literacy level, the sentence structure and complexity of the material given, linguistic barriers, differing cultural contexts, and the efficacy of the method in which health messages are communicated (Kreps and Sparks 2008). In order to address this issue and make health care more "patient centered," the health care reform law has designated funds for the creation and dissemination of "patient decision aids" in the form of handouts, videos, and computer programs that will help patients understand their treatment options (Sparks and Villagran 2010).

Presently, large disparities exist between individuals and basic health care knowledge, resulting in generally low health literacy levels. Yet, while this general lack of health literacy is prominent in many sectors of the population, it is particularly disproportionate among certain demographic groups, showing that certain populations are marginalized under current health education techniques (Sparks and Nussbaum 2008). Those who are more vulnerable to health risks, due to lower levels of health literacy, include ethnic minorities, recent immigrants, the elderly, those who suffer from a limited formal education, are socio-economically deprived and have poor access to relevant health care information (Kreps and Sparks 2008; Sparks and Nussbaum 2008). This also gives evidence that opportunities to increase health literacy may provide a way to lessen inequities in health concerns. Considering health care is a public and personal issue, discrepancies over health literacy in terms of patient treatment may also translate into discrepancies over knowledge of the public health care system, health care reform law, and health care decision-making (Sparks 2008), all of which can greatly impact caregiving as well as caregiving research, policy, and practice.

For example, the recently passed health care legislation contains over 2,000 pages of complex, legal language. With some 25 % of the USA population being functionally illiterate, it may be assumed that those who receive a limited formal education may have increased difficulty in information acquisition, having to navigate a complex system of health care reform law. Therefore, these groups may fall into a perpetual cycle of inequity with low health literacy levels, and increased vulnerability to personal health risks and confusion in a complex health care system. Health literacy has vast implications for health communication researchers and practitioners interested in health information delivery, comprehension, and subsequent medical adherence issues that may arise.

Consider for a moment the history of healthcare and healthcare reform in the US, from placing the new healthcare reform law into context with landmark legislation in 1935 that created Social Security and the legislation in 1965 that enacted Medicare and Medicaid. The landmark Patient Protection and Affordable Care Act (PPACA) and the Health Care and Education Reconciliation Act of 2010, which comprised the healthcare reform legislation in 2010 are real and impacting our healthcare delivery systems and patient care in unique, complex, and radical ways that we have yet to fully understand.

A New York Times report on July 29, 2012 summarized that in March 2010, Congress passed the healthcare bill put forth by President Obama. The law put in motion the creation of a nationwide insurance system that would provide most Americans with basic healthcare coverage, a goal that had been on the Democratic agenda for 75 years. In 2012, the Supreme Court in a 5–4 vote largely upheld the proposed legislation after considering several challenges to much of the law's key provisions. The healthcare law seeks to extend insurance to more than 30 million people, primarily by expanding Medicaid and providing federal subsidies to help low- and middle-income Americans to purchase private coverage. It will create insurance exchanges for those buying individual policies and prohibit insurers from denying coverage on the basis of pre-existing conditions. To reduce the increasing cost of Medicare, it puts together a panel of experts to limit government reimbursement to only those treatments shown to be effective, and creates incentives for providers of package services rather than charge by individual procedure.

The Congressional Budget Office claims that the law will cost the government about $ 938 billion over 10 years, and also estimates that it will reduce the federal deficit by US$ 138 billion over a decade (see Crowley 2012). This legislation is not without controversy, as it has components involving significant disagreement among politicians, corporate stakeholders, physicians, citizens, and the insurance industry. If you have not paid much attention to healthcare in America, it is time to do so because it will very likely impact you and your loved ones in the future.

Information quality, information seeking, and uncertainty can greatly impact patients and caregivers. For instance, Bevan et al.'s (2012) exploration of healthcare reform information sources in relation to information quality, information seeking, and uncertainty found that magazines are the preferred source for such quality information and decreased uncertainty. In particular, when magazines were employed as a source of healthcare reform information, individuals employed information seeking, and revealed that this information was satisfying and easier to obtain, and were more certain about their understanding of healthcare reform (Bevan et al. 2012). Further, when newspapers were rated the most important healthcare reform information source, participants sought more information. These findings are particularly consistent with Dutta-Bergman's (2004) research, which found that those who obtained health information from newspapers or magazines were more health-oriented than individuals who did not.

Both newspapers and magazines can provide active, cognitively involved, in-depth coverage of a health issue and can also be archived for future information seeking (Bevan et al. 2012). These qualities may make magazines, and to a lesser extent, newspapers, particularly appealing as an information source to new caregivers who are learning about healthcare reform. The growth of magazines as a health information source (Gill and Babrow 2007) means that this media channel has the potential to be an invaluable resource for individuals seeking healthcare reform information (Bevan et al. 2012), particularly caregivers.

When healthcare reform information was obtained from interpersonal sources such as family or friends, participants felt that knowledge was less satisfying, more difficult to obtain, and felt more uncertain about healthcare reform than those who did not. This pattern aligns with Pecchioni and Sparks' (2007) health information sources research on family caregivers who reported more satisfaction with Internet sources of health information, but differs from their findings related to patient satisfaction and preferences for interpersonal-based health information sources (i.e., doctors and nurses). In addition, when family or friends were selected as the most important healthcare reform information source, less information seeking occurred. However, the authors suggest that the Internet is still a frequently used and important source of healthcare reform information, and should also be considered by those who have invested in the continuation and success of the healthcare reform legislation.

Health literacy, therefore, is an important construct for understanding patients' and caregivers' needs for health information, as well as their abilities to access and utilize such health information and messages for critical health decision-making. Health literacy currently is defined by the National Academy of Sciences, National Library of Medicine (NLM), Healthy People 2010/2020, and the Institute of Medicine (IOM) as "the degree to which individuals have the capacity to obtain, process, and understand basic health information and services needed to make appropriate health decisions that may affect the health of Americans and the ability of the healthcare system to provide effective, high quality care." As such, patients and their caregivers need to be able to competently evaluate and locate health information for credibility and quality, analyze relative risks and benefits, calculate dosages, interpret test results, etc. Health literacy includes the concepts of accessing and understanding information and services, with a comprehensive skill set of literacy that potentially includes visual (graphs and charts), computer (operate and search), information (obtain and apply relevant information), and numeracy (calculate and reason numerically) skills required to make appropriate health decisions (see e.g., Nielsen-Bohlman et al. 2004; Ratzan et al. 2000). Further, patients and their caregivers need strong oral communication to adequately and accurately describe their symptoms, concerns, and must be able to competently search for and understand health information for stronger decision-making skills. According to the American Medical Association, poor health literacy is "a stronger predictor of a person's health than age, income, employment status, education level, and race" (Report on the Council of Scientific Affairs, Ad Hoc Committee on Health Literacy for the Council on Scientific Affairs, American Medical Association, *JAMA*, Feb 10, 1999). In *Health Literacy: A Prescription to End Confusion*, the Institute of Medicine reports that 90 million people in the USA, nearly half the population, have difficulty understanding and using health information. As a result, patients often take medicines on erratic schedules, miss follow-up appointments, and do not understand instructions like "take on an empty stomach". It is clear that health literacy and communication have huge implications for health communication-based research, policy, and practice (Parker et al. 2003). Patients and their family members clearly need help accessing and navigating the health care maze in order to have the tools to provide the best care possible for loved ones.

An individual's health literacy is dependent upon and determined by a number of factors; including literacy level, the sentence structure and complexity of the material given, linguistic barriers, differing cultural contexts, and the efficacy of the method in which health messages are communicated (Kreps and Sparks 2008). Presently, large disparities exist between individuals and basic health care knowledge, resulting in generally low health literacy levels. Yet, while this general lack of health literacy is prominent in many sectors of the population, it is particularly disproportionate among certain demographic groups, showing that certain populations are marginalized under current health education techniques (Sparks and Nussbaum 2008). Those who are more vulnerable to health risks, due to lower levels of health literacy, include ethnic minorities, recent immigrants, the elderly, those who suffer from a limited formal education, are socio-economically deprived and have poor access to relevant health care information (Kreps and Sparks 2008; Sparks and Nussbaum 2008; Sparks and Villagran 2010).

Health literacy is an important component of health information acquisition, understanding, and processing and plays a key role in health information seeking behaviors for patients and caregivers. Becoming health literate can lead to better health outcomes through improved cultural competence, oral and written communication, and numeracy. Patients and caregivers alike must become literate consumers of health information by increasing their knowledge and ability to communicate about important health issues for more informed decision-making (e.g., Sparks et al. 2010).

The State of Health Communication Research and Caregiving Research, Policy, and Practice

The field of health communication has grown exponentially over the last 25 years or so (Beck et al. 2004; Thompson et al. 2003; Sparks and Villagran 2010; Wright et al. 2013), with research in health communication becoming one of the most highly regarded contexts of communication study among communication professionals. There are currently two journals devoted to the topic of health communication in the US, including *Health Communication,* published since 1989 by Lawrence Erlbaum Associates, and *Journal of Health Communication,* published since 1996 by Taylor and Francis, with an emerging international interest including *Journal of Communication in Healthcare*, published by Maney Publishing, UK since 2008. Scholars have also discussed the history, future trends, and specific contexts in health communication in several overview books (see e.g., Beck 2001; du Pré 2000, 2005a; Geist-Martin et al. 2003; Jackson and Duffy 1998; Kreps and Thornton 1992; O'Hair et al. 2008; Sparks et al. 2008a; Thompson et al. 2003; Sparks and Villagran 2010; Wright et al. 2013), special issues of journals (see e.g., Kreps et al. 2010a; Kreps et al. 2008a; Parrott 2004a; Ratzan 1994; Sparks 2003a) as well as hundreds of journal articles, book chapters, and invited TED talks (see Sparks 2011). All have provided important outlets for the study and dissemination of health communication research, policy, and practice. Through these works, health communication scholars are dramatically increasing attention to pertinent health communication issues and contributing in important ways by translating such research into policy and practice. Because of the inherent complexities of contemporary health communication and the potential to impact society, we must continue to clearly disseminate the most important theoretical and methodological orientations of the health communication field. There is no better way to inform the health care and research community than to engage in translating such research efforts into practice.

At its core, the health communication field focuses on two major elements: (1) message production and processing and (2) the creation of shared meaning about health issues in relationships. Communication researchers and professionals address health care issues from a variety of perspectives, including interpersonal and relational issues in provider—patient communication (Beck 2001; Beck et al. 1997; Burgers et al. in press; Donohew and Ray 1990; du Pré 2000, 2005a; Harzold and Sparks 2007; Kreps and Thornton 1992; Pomerantz et al. 1997; Ragan and Glenn 1990; Robinson 1998; Robinson and Stivers 2001; Roter and Hall 1992; Sharf and Street 1997; Smith-du Pré and Beck 1996; Sparks et al. 2012a; Sparks and Villagran 2010; Thompson et al. 2003; Vanderford et al. 1997; Whaley 2000), communication and skills training (Rowan 2000, 2003, 2004), conflict and argument issues (Bevan and Sparks, in press; Bevan et al. 2012), disclosure issues (Sparks et al. 2005), caring for special populations such as older adults (Giles et al. 1990; Hummert and Nussbaum 2001; Nussbaum et al. 2003; Sass 2000; Sparks et al. 2008b; Sparks 2003b; Sparks 2007; Sparks and Nussbaum 2008), broader social and community health issues such as promotion and prevention (Joseph 2010; Kreps and Thornton 1992; O'Hair et al. 2008; Kreps et al. 2010b), health risk communication and health PR (Kreps et al. 2005; Rowan et al. 2003; Rowan et al. 2008), cultural issues and disenfranchisement (Mokros and Deetz 1996; Nussbaum et al. 1996; Nussbaum et al. 1996; Pecchioni et al. 2008; Pecchioni et al. 2004; Sparks and Mittapalli 2004), social support (Adelman and Frey 1997; Cawyer and Smith-du Pré 1995; du Pré and Ray 2008; Jones 1997; Robinson and Turner 2003; Sarason et al. 1997), intergroup communication and social identity issues (Harwood and Sparks 2003; Sparks and Harwood 2008; Sparks et al. 2012a; Villagran and Sparks 2010), health organizations and decision making (du Pré 2005a; O'Hair and Sparks 2008; O'Hair et al. 2005; O'Hair et al. 2003), health information sources (Bevan et al. in press; Mirkiani Thompson 2011; Pecchioni and Sparks 2007; Rakovski et al. 2012; Sparks-Bethea et al. 2000), health information quality (Bevan et al. 2011a), health campaigns (Sparks and Turner 2008; Witte et al. 2001), the role of spirituality (du Pré 2002; du Pré and Lepper 2008; Egbert et al. 2008), the role of humor, narratives, interviewing and message strategies in health care (Anderson and Martin 2003; Bellet and Maloney 1991; du Pré 1998; Frankel 1990; Harzold and Sparks 2007, 2008; Marshall 1993; Sparks 2001; Sparks et al. 2005; Sparks-Bethea et al. 2000; Suchman et al. 1997; Sparks and Turner 2008; Wanzer et al. 2009), health literacy, information technologies, e-health, and telemedicine (Kreps and Sparks 2008; Kreps et al. 2008b; Query and Wright 2003; Robinson and Turner 2003; Sparks and Nussbaum 2008; Sparks and Villagran 2010; Villagran et al. 2010), social media and social aggregates/networks and health (Kee et al. in press), as well as broader health policy issues (Bevan et al. in press; Gordon et al. in press; Mirkiani Thompson et al. 2011; Thompson et al. 2003; Thompson 1984). (For detailed account of the history of health communication, see Thompson et al. 2003). Relatively recent research has investigated a variety of health communication variables as applied to the unique distance caregiving context (Bevan et al. 2011a; Bevan et al. 2011; Bevan and Sparks 2011; Bevan et al. 2012; Sparks et al. 2012b).

Health Communication in the Health Information Era

The advent of the Internet has provided health information seeking opportunities that were previously unimaginable. Just doing a simple Google search for the term "Health Information" produces nearly a billion hits and with the pervasiveness of Internet access anyone within arms distance of a web browser can access more health information than they could consume in a lifetime.

One major reason researchers have become interested in health communication messaging and health information seeking behavior is due to the recent explosions of technology and easy access to health messages and information. Fox (2006) suggests 80 % of adults surveyed have searched for health information online and 53 % of them indicated they used the information found in health decisions. Similarly, Madden and Fox (2006) found that 58 % of the caretakers surveyed reported that the Internet was an important tool for making health decisions. Research supports the notion that patient satisfaction information is connected to service quality and serves as a predictor of health-related behavior (Pascoe 1983), which may indicate that certain patient characteristics are predictors of health efficacy. Further, research has indicated that patients who perceive their physicians as caring and competent were more likely to be satisfied with the medical treatment and the health information (Guldvog 1999). Prior research from the NCI 2005 Health Information National Trends Survey indicates that when participants were asked "Where would you go for cancer information" 50 % stated they would go to their provider followed by Internet (34 %), library (5 %), family (4 %), and print media (4 %). Research has revealed that family members of patients reported being significantly more satisfied with the Internet in terms of health information sources, whereas patients themselves reported more satisfaction with doctors and nurses as health information sources (Pecchioni and Sparks 2007). Time constraints, competing demands for attention, and a lack of training in effective communication impair physician's communication with patients (Sparks et al. 2007), which most certainly influences patient health information seeking behaviors (Sparks and Villagran 2010), and can greatly impact medical adherence and decision-making for patients (Tinley et al. 2004). Health care providers are accustomed to processing highly complex medical information while their patients and family members are typically not as familiar with such highly technical medical information.

In an era in which access to health information has a profound effect on longevity (see e.g., Sparks 2007; Sparks 2003b; Sparks and Nussbaum 2008), one important health communication research goal, especially of the National Network of Libraries of Medicine, has centered on improving health care provider access to health information, especially in rural, underserved, and minority communities (see Kreps and Sparks 2008; Witte 1998). Access to health information should, arguably, be broadened to include access for both formal and informal health care providers. For example, the conundrum in community-based long-term care is that formal and informal caregivers have what some theorists have come to acknowledge as contradictory structures (Litwak 1985); the potential for conflict always exists. At the same time, they have complementary roles in that the two networks must be able to coordinate their efforts on a regular basis (see e.g., Travis and Sparks-Bethea 2001). For contemporary long-term shared health care to be successful for all involved, there must be a comfortable distance between formal and informal providers that is still close enough to coordinate the caregiving goals, while not leading to destructive conflict (Litwak 1985). Litwak and Meyer (1966) refer to successful negotiation of this experience as "balanced coordination" and note its apparent essential role in successful health care communication efforts. As Thompson (1984) acknowledged, it is important to investigate variables that moderate processes discovered in prior research and then build upon those studies in new investigations rather than starting from scratch. In addition to foci on messages and relationships, health communication scholars focus on evaluating the effectiveness of patient–provider interaction, health information, and health campaigns. Research has generated increasing understanding of how to stimulate desired health behaviors via communication (see Sparks and Villagran 2010; Witte 1998). Evidence-based approaches involving evaluation efforts best assess health communication interventions, particularly when it comes to our most vulnerable at-risk populations. If such evaluations reveal that certain variables are not receiving the consideration needed, then new and better evidence-based outreach interventions can be developed in order to achieve better health outcomes for patients and those caring for them.

Designing Effective Theory-Based Health Messages

Health behavior, health communication, and public health communication scholars study messages and interventions that encourage patients to be active participants in health communication contexts. In addition to designing mediated health messages, we need to focus on effective evidence-based message strategies that will prove effective for the unique complexities and barriers that the patients and their family members often face (see e.g., Sparks 2007; Sparks 2011; Sparks and Nussbaum 2008; Sparks and Turner 2008); that said, such a goal must be pursued by paying attention to the unique cognitive and emotional processes that different populations often deal with, followed by particular interpersonal message framing that will more likely reach such specific populations—one patient and one family at a time and paying close attention to the linguistic and communicative cues enacted (Burgers et al. in press; Sparks et al. 2005).

In recent years, health communication scholars and health practitioners have utilized prospect theory by using message framing to understand the communication involved in risky decisions (see e.g., Kahneman and Tversky 1979; Kahneman and Tversky 2000; Tversky and Kahneman 1981; Sparks 2007, 2011; Sparks and Villagran 2010). The landmark essays of Amos Tversky and Daniel Kahneman describe prospect theory, which suggests that individuals will react differentially to information presented as gains or losses. People encode information relevant to choice options in terms of potential gains or potential losses. Thus, factually equivalent information can be presented to people differently so they encode it as either a gain or a loss (framing). A framing effect is demonstrated by constructing two transparently equivalent versions of a given problem, which nevertheless yield predictably different choices. The standard example of a framing problem is the "lives saved, lives lost" question, which offers a choice between two public health programs proposed to deal with an epidemic that is threatening 600 lives. One program will save 200 lives; the other has a 1/3 chance of saving all 600 lives and a 2/3 chance of saving none. In this version, people prefer the program that will save 200 lives. In the second version, one program will result in 400 deaths; the other has a 2/3 chance of 600 deaths and a 1/3 chance of no deaths. In this formulation, most people prefer the gamble. Of course, these formulations present identical situations. The only difference is that in the first formulation, the problem is framed in terms of lives saved and in the second, the situation is framed as a matter of lives lost. Thus, the message frame that a decision-maker adopts is controlled partly by *the formulation of the problem* and partly by the norms, habits, and personal characteristics of the decision-maker (Tversky and Kahneman 1981, p. 453). In essence, individuals tend to select some aspects of a perceived reality and make them more salient during interaction.

In an effort to empirically test message framing in the provider and patient interaction, Burgers et al. (in press) recently investigated the role of specific linguistic and communication formulations in a doctor's bad news delivery. The author's focused on the effects of negations and message framing on patients' immediate responses to the message and the doctor, and long-term consequences including quality of life and medical adherence intentions. Specifically, two lab experiments were set up with 2 (language use: negations (e.g., not good, not bad) vs. affirmations (e.g., good, bad)) × 2 (framing: positive vs. negative) between subject designs. After reading a transcription (experiment 1) or seeing a film clip (experiment 2), participants rated their evaluation of the message and the doctor, expected quality of life, and medical adherence intentions. Results indicated that positively framed bad news with negations scored more negative on these dependent variables than positively framed affirmations for both experiments. However, for negatively framed negations, these results are reversed (experiment 2). Furthermore, the evaluations of the message (experiment 1) and the doctor (both experiments) mediate the interaction of framing and language use on medical adherence intentions. As such, small linguistic variations (i.e., negations vs. affirmations) in breaking bad news can have a significant impact on the health message, doctor evaluation, and medical adherence intentions. Providers, at least in the bad news context, should refrain from using negations to break positively framed news, and employ negation language when breaking negatively framed news.

Nearly all health-related information can be construed in terms of either gains (benefits) or losses (costs) (Sparks 2011). But which frame works better? The answer typically depends on whether the target health behavior is an illness detection behavior or an illness protection behavior (Rothman et al. 1993). Detection behaviors (e.g., prostate exam) involve uncertainty (i.e., You may have a health problem). Prevention or protection behaviors (e.g., using sunscreen) typically lead to relatively certain outcomes (i.e., You keep your healthy status).

Prospect Theory predicts that loss-framed information leads to preference for uncertainty, whereas gain-framed information leads to preference for certainty. Research findings indicate that loss-framed messages were effective in promoting mammography, BSE, and HIV testing. Gain-framed messages were effective in promoting infant car restraints, physical exercise, smoking cessation, and sunscreen. The message-framing component of prospect theory has been utilized in health risk studies dealing with the uncertainty and risks involved in disease detection (see e.g., Banks et al. 1995a; Meyerowitz and Chaiken 1987; Rothman et al. 1993). Meyerowitz and Chaiken's (1987) research suggests that female participants were more convinced to conduct breast self-examinations after being exposed to negatively framed messages than positively framed messages. Negatively framed messages have also been found to be more effective in persuading persons to engage in detection behaviors, such as seeking health information or discovering a lump or mole (see Rothman et al. 1993). Another recent empirical study examined the joint effect of message framing and time perspective in adherence promoting communication targeting patients with chronic diseases (Zhao et al. 2011). Results indicated that among high consideration of future consideration (high-CFC) patients, gain-framed adherence messages generated stronger intentions and more favorable attitudes toward future adherence than loss-framed messages. High CFC participants also rated gain-framed messages as stronger, more likable, and less irritating than loss-framed messages. Among patients of low or medium levels of CFC, there was no clear advantage for either frame across the outcome variables (Zhao et al. 2011).

Health messages differ in whether they recommend preventing a health risk or hazard (e.g., wearing seatbelts) or recommend detecting a health risk or hazard (e.g., breast self examinations) (see Sparks 2011). Seeking out health information can be a frightening and even risky endeavor. Knowledge gained from information seeking strategies will not cure disease, but it can help in finding out if one is at risk for cancer; thus, such strategies are considered detection behaviors (see e.g., Mitchell 2000; Mitchell et al. 2001; Sparks and Turner 2008; Sparks and Villagran 2010). Detecting a health problem is viewed as more risky, though, because in the process of gathering health information about particular symptoms, individuals may find out they have a serious health problem. Not knowing allows for a state of blissful ignorance. Prevention is less risky because you are taking measures to ensure not becoming sick or hurt. That said, negatively framed messages are more likely to smooth the progress of detection behaviors, largely because risky options are preferred when individuals are considering losses (Rothman et al. 1993; Sparks 2011). Let's explore this idea via the following case study:

Case Study: Message Framing Gone Bad

Carlo is a 50-year-old Hispanic male who is an active professional in his field, a loving father and husband, an avid mountain climber, and marathon runner. He works for 50–60 h in a week, but regularly exercises most of the time (i.e., running and weights). His diet is normal and typically healthy, consisting of fish, pasta, some meat, vegetables, grains, some fruit, wine or beer, coffee, and as often as possible, chocolate. Carlo says he did not fully understand the importance of message framing until he had a personal encounter with its subtleties during a health care encounter. He relates his experience in his own words:

> A couple of months ago I developed some unusual symptoms, and a quick web check indicated that a possible explanation for the symptoms could be ALS (amytrophic lateral sclerosis aka: Lou Gehrig's disease). The websites I visited did indicate that other causes were possible, but there was little clarity as to how to distinguish ALS from more benign syndromes. Additionally, there was no indication of how likely one diagnosis was versus another. What I quickly learned was that if I was going to see a doctor, (s)he would probably look for signs of hyper reflexivity (reflexes abnormally brisk) and for a particular reaction of my toes when stimulating the nerves on the bottom of my foot.
>
> Through a neurologist friend, I was given the name of a doctor who is supposedly one of the best clinicians in the field. I then visited the doctor and he did, in fact, test my reflexes and my toes. At the end of the visit, despite my obvious anxiety (which he had acknowledged), he delayed his conversation with me for several minutes. First he scribbled in his folder for a long time, then he went to his office for 5 min (was he reading up about my symptoms and proper tests to be performed), then he came back and kept scribbling, though occasionally glanced at me.
>
> Finally, after about 10–15 excruciatingly long minutes, he was able to render his opinion. He started with an unpleasant comment: "there are a few question marks in your neurological examination." This was taken by me as a negative sign, that something was wrong. He then continued by saying that in fact I was hyper reflexive in four limbs! This really set me thinking that maybe I needed to get my affairs in order as soon as possible (i.e., create a will and prepare myself for death). What is amazing, however, is what he said right after that. He told me that, in fact, my reflexes were 'within the norm', though 'on the brisk side'.

This brings us to the first comment on message framing. Here are two ways one could frame the information (or messages).

1. There are a few question marks in your neurological examination. You have hyper reflexivity in four limbs, though one could say that your reflexes are within the norm, though on the brisk side. [What happened at the doctor's office.]
2. Your reflexes are within the norm, somewhat on the brisk side, though this could easily be a result of your state of stress. [What should have happened.]

The outcome of #1 is that the patient immediately senses that something is wrong (the 'question marks' comment), and this sensation is then followed by the clarification that there is hyper reflexivity (one of the KEY symptoms for a clinical diagnosis of ALS). The state of mind of the patient is now a highly stressed and emotional one, making it quite difficult to consider the subsequent qualification ('the reflexes are within the norm') with the extreme importance it has. Arguably, this is a scenario where one's emotional state is likely impacting the ability to cognitively process the important components of the message(s) being delivered by the physician.

Had the patient been exposed to message #2, it is much more likely that he would have had a lower emotional response and thus, would have been more capable of cognitively processing the message by hearing "your reflexes are within the norm." In essence, this likely would have translated into something entirely different and positive such as "you do not exhibit hyper reflexivity," which was a much more accurate description of the actual diagnosis.

The second issue concerning message framing has to do with the fact that the doctor never explained what the 'couple question marks' were. The patient and his wife inferred that the hyper reflexivity was one of them (but, there was NO hyper reflexivity, and so they were worrying for no good reason), and since he mentioned 'couple' (which typically means 'two' and most certainly more than one), they assumed that the toes test gave bad results as well. The patient (and primary caregiver aka: 'wife')should have asked for further clarification, but likely did not because of the severe levels of stress and worry at that time (i.e., high emotion levels likely impacting ability to think clearly).

Now, let us go to the final moments of the visit.

1. Well, there is a 10–15 % chance you have ALS [He did not explain where or how he got that number and what it meant.], and the only way to find out is to do an electromyography (EMG). If I were to bet, I would bet you don't have ALS, but I certainly would not bet the farm on it! [What happened at the doctor's office.]
2. I am 90 % sure you only have a benign syndrome. I'd be willing to bet on it. To make completely sure, we should probably run an EMG. [What should have happened.]

Though the 'content' of #1 and #2 is the same, the way the patient is able to cognitively process it (or hear it and then process it) is totally different. In the first case, the patient is faced with a substantial chance of ALS. Further, 10–15 % is actually pretty high, especially if one considers that ALS is an extremely rare disease. Thus, for the doctor to think that the likelihood is so high, it leaves the patient thinking that he must have seen something to lead him to say that percentage. His apparently reassuring comment on the 'bet', however, is quickly tempered and turned ominous, by the qualification about the 'farm.'

In case #2, the patient hears that he is most likely fine, and the only reason for the test is because there is no absolute way to rule out ALS otherwise. In this case study, the patient does an excellent job of explaining how message framing affected his perception of his condition. I am sure we all either have experienced some healthcare communication frustrations either ourselves or through family or friends. Effective evidence-based health communication interventions can help. Future research should give practitioners feedback on their messages to patients and caregivers so that the insights gained from prospect theory and message framing of vital health information can help providers, patients, and caregivers understand medical conditions and avoid unnecessary anxiety.

Theories Used in Creating Messages to Stimulate Health-Related Behavior Change

Prospect theory has shown that message features affect the ways health and illnesses are perceived. Another focus of health communication research has been on exploring the ways in which communication affects peoples' attitudes. Can a change in attitude move people from *thinking* about a prevention or detection behavior to *acting on their beliefs*? What causes individuals to change their health-related behavior? How do the accounts patients and informal caregivers present about a health condition, impact their management of that condition? Such questions are at the heart of a significant amount of health communication research. Prospect theory, message framing, health communication, and the research it has spawned have been particularly fruitful. More research needs to be done in terms of the impact of health message framing in particular and unique health contexts such as caregiving as well as targeted messaging for at-risk populations with lower health literacy levels and varied cultural backgrounds, so we can truly make a difference in decision-making and related health outcomes. Now, let's turn to some of the most widely utilized theoretical frameworks to guide health interventions for behavior change.

The Health Belief Model

The health belief model (HBM) (Janz and Becker 1984; Rosenstock 1974) is one of the most commonly used models of health behavior change and is probably the most frequently taught model in outreach intervention courses. Many have used it to guide the development of intervention and evaluation efforts, and its influence on health communication research is enormous. It was developed as an overarching framework on how to promote preventive behaviors (such as immunizations) by a group of social psychologists in the early 1950's (Janz and Becker 1984). The HBM suggests that preventive health behavior is influenced by five factors: (a) perceived barriers to performing the recommended response, (b) perceived benefits of performing the recommended response, (c) perceived susceptibility to a health threat, (d) perceived severity of a health threat, and (e) cues to action.

HBM suggests that individuals weigh the potential benefits of the recommended response against the psychological, physical, and financial costs of the action (the barriers) when deciding to act. For example, a patient may realize the benefit of having up-to-date information but may lack access, the skills, or even the transportation needed to get to a library. In this case, the barriers would outweigh any benefits and the patient probably would not seek out up-to-date information. Similarly, the HBM suggests that individuals evaluate whether or not they are really susceptible to a threat and whether or not the threat is truly severe. Rosenstock (1974) has noted that the combination of perceived susceptibility and severity provide the motivation for action, and the comparison of perceived benefits to perceived barriers provides the means or pathway to action. Thus, the stronger the perceptions of severity, susceptibility, and benefits, and the weaker the perception of barriers, the greater the likelihood that health-protective actions will be taken.

Demographics and prior experiences are said to affect the four variables just described (i.e., perceived susceptibility, severity, benefits, and barriers), as are "cues to action." There can be external cues (such as television shows or mass mailings) and internal cues (such as symptoms), which are suspected to increase perceptions of susceptibility and severity. This in turn triggers the decision-making process, whereby perceived barriers and benefits are weighed against each other.

The HBM has been empirically tested as the basis for educational campaigns on a number of health behaviors, including bicycle helmet use (Witte et al. 1993), vaccination for infectious diseases, adolescent fertility control (Eisen et al. 1985), and risky sexual practices (Vanlandingham et al. 1995). Overall, perceived barriers have been the strongest predictor of whether or not individuals engage in health-protective behaviors, followed by perceived susceptibility (Janz and Becker 1984). Janz and Becker (1984) found that the perceived severity was the weakest predictor across studies employing the HBM. The HBM may be viewed as the grandmother of most modern health education theories. As such, its variables and principles can be seen in many of the other models.

The Theory of Reasoned Action

Messages created for outreach efforts are very often based on intuitive appeal, rather than sound methodology (Fishbein and Ajzen 1981). Even if a theory is used to develop messages, campaigners tend to use the variables in the theory as guidelines without carefully considering the concrete content or words in a message. For instance, campaign designers might address theoretical variables in a message by looking at the severity of a threat and the audience's susceptibility to that threat, but the verbal and nonverbal cues used to address these variables are not systematically chosen. Fishbein and Ajzen (1981) go so far as to conclude that "the general neglect of the information contained in a message and its relation to the dependent variable is probably the most serious problem in communication and persuasion research" (p. 359).

Fishbein and Ajzen (1975, 1981) suggest specific message construction and evaluation techniques based on their theory of reasoned action (TRA). In TRA, Fishbein and Ajzen (1975) propose that a person's behavior is predicted by intentions, which in turn are predicted by attitudes toward the behavior and subjective norm. These attitudes are predicted by behavioral beliefs and evaluations of those beliefs. Subjective norms are predicted by normative beliefs and the motivation to comply with those normative beliefs. Fishbein and Ajzen (1975) state that two sets of beliefs must be altered prior to behavior change: (1) beliefs about the consequences of performing a certain behavior and the evaluation of those consequences (attitude), and (2) beliefs about what other people or referents think about the behavior to be performed and the motivation to comply with those referents (subjective norm). Only when a message targets the salient beliefs of these variables do attitudes and subjective norms, and subsequently, behavioral intentions and behavior, change.

Overall, TRA is one of the few theories to offer a systematic approach to the construction of the content of a health education message. It has been applied to a number of health-related behaviors, including the impact of health risk messages about tap water (Griffin et al. 1995), sexual practices and AIDS related-behaviors (Fishbein and Middlestadt 1989; Fishbein et al. 1991; Vanlandingham et al. 1995), childbearing intentions (Crawford and Boyer 1985), testicular cancer prevention (Brubaker and Wickersham 1990), exercise in schoolchildren (Ferguson et al. 1989), alcoholism (Fishbein et al. 1980), cigarette smoking (Norman and Tedeschi 1989), and many others.

Social Cognitive Theory

Bandura's social cognitive theory or social learning theory has been used extensively for interventions and evaluation efforts. The Stanford 5-Cities project used social cognitive theory to prevent heart disease. Social cognitive theory has also been used in a number of AIDS prevention projects. The thrust of the theory focuses on perceived self-efficacy. Bandura (1989) defines self-efficacy as "people's beliefs that they can exert control over their motivation and behavior and over their social environment" (p. 128). Bandura (1977) views self-efficacy as the driving force of human behavior. "Efficacy expectations are a major determinant of people's choice of activities, how much effort they will expend, and of how long they will sustain effort in dealing with stressful situations" (Bandura 1977, p. 194). In other words, perceived self-efficacy is your perceived self-effectiveness or what you believe about your capability to perform a certain action.

Another important construct in Bandura's theory centers on outcome expectations. Outcome expectations refer to an individual's belief that a certain behavior will lead to a certain outcome. For example, "I believe that if I search the Internet for credible and current health information I will get the information needed to effectively treat a patient" is an outcome expectation. Outcome expectations are different from efficacy expectations in that the latter is an individual's belief on whether he or she is able to "successfully execute the behavior required to produce the outcomes" (Bandura 1977, p. 193). For example, even if outcome expectations are high, efficacy expectations may be low (e.g., "I don't know how to search for credible sites on the Internet."). In short, according to social cognitive theory, a person can believe that certain actions lead to a particular outcome, but this individual may doubt his or her ability to perform the action. According to Bandura (1977), only when efficacy expectations are high will people perform certain behaviors. Efficacy expectations can vary on dimensions of magnitude (level of difficulty of task; people may have different efficacy expectations for simple tasks than for difficult tasks), generality (specific to general), and strength (weak to strong; Bandura 1977).

Stages of Change Model

One of a number of stage models of behavior change, the transtheoretical model allows educators to determine which stage the majority of their target audience members are in, along a continuum of no action to consistent action (DiClemente and Prochaska 1985). The model, also referred to as the stages of change model (SOC), suggests there are five stages to the performance of a behavior : *Precontemplation, Contemplation, Preparation, Action, and Maintenance*. In the *Precontemplative* stage, individuals do not intend to change their behavior because they are completely unaware of the behavioral options available to them. They may not realize they are engaging in a risky behavior or they may deny that their behavior puts them at risk for harm. In the second stage, however, this risk becomes apparent to the individual. *Contemplation* is the stage in which individuals begin to think about the behavior that is putting them at risk and contemplate the need for change. In this stage, for example, an individual recognizes the need for more information. In the third stage, *Preparation*, individuals make a commitment to change and take some action to prepare for the behavioral change, such as taking a class on how to speak a foreign language or making an appointment to secure a medication. It is in the *Action* stage that individuals perform the new behavior. In this stage, for example, a person might continue to improve his or her foreign language skills or sign up for additional informational resources on keeping up with various medicines. Of course, it is in the *Maintenance* stage that individuals consistently continue to carry out the learned behavior over time.

The SOC model is useful to campaign designers for several reasons. First, individuals in different stages exhibit distinct behavioral characteristics (Weinstein 1988). Thus, researchers can effectively analyze and segment a target audience according to their different stages of change. Then, practitioners can strategically design messages to move individuals through the stages (Maibach and Cotton 1995). For example, if campaigners wish to design a campaign to promote a new service, and they determine that the majority of the members of the target population are in the contemplation stage, they can design messages to systematically move audience members through the preparation, action, and maintenance stages. Similarly, if the majority of the target audience is in the maintenance stage, educators can provide messages which reinforce and support the desired behavior. This model has been empirically tested with numerous health topics, including cancer prevention behaviors, smoking cessation, sunscreen use, addictive behaviors, pregnancy prevention, and risky sexual behaviors (e.g., Grimley et al. 1993; Prochaska et al. 1992).

Integrative Model of Health Information Seeking

Dutta-Bergman (2006) proposed the Integrative Model of Health Information Seeking (IMHIS) in an effort to explain the conditions under which people employ the mass media to seek out health information. In the model he suggests that health orientation or the motivation to seek out health information and efficacy or the individual's perceptions of their ability to find and understand health information they find are the primary predictors of health information seeking. Bodie and Dutta (2008) state "a health motivated consumer actively participates in health-related issues, actively searches out relevant health information, and is better able to recall this information when appropriate (Celsi and Olson 1988; Dutta-Bergman 2004a; Maclnnis et al. 1991; Moorman and Matulich 1993; Park and Mittal 1985)" (p. 190).

The concept health orientation is used to refer to those factors influencing the motivation of the individual to seek health information. Within the concept health orientation, variables such as the individual's general interest in health issues, their specific interest in gaining health information on a particular topic that is often born out of a need for that information, and the individual's willingness to process health information were identified by Dutta-Bergman as being important. Research generally supports this component of the model. Patients who are highly health motivated are more likely to seek out health information on their own, more likely to be involved in health decisions, and are more successful at recalling health information when tested (Celsi and Olson 1988; Dutta-Bergman 2004a; Maclnnis et al. 1991; Moorman and Matulich 1993; Park and Mittal 1985). They are also more likely to search for health information from sources other than their primary care physician (Dutta-Bergman 2004a) and more likely to actively seek out such information from the Internet than their less highly health oriented counterparts (Dutta-Bergman 2004a, 2004b). Bodie and Dutta (2008) state that people who have a reason for acquiring health information (e.g., having been diagnosed with an illness, severity of the illness symptomology, or caretaking someone with an illness) are more likely to be motivated to seek out health information. In an effort to explain health information seeking behavior, Bodie and Dutta (2008) propose the Integrated Model of eHealth Use. The term health orientation is within the IMeHU to describe the factors related to and predictive of the motivation to seek out health information. Based on the extant literature, Dutta-Bergman suggests health orientation includes factors such as a general interest in health information, a particular interest or need for specific health information, and willingness to process health information.

The Extended Parallel Process Model

Fear appeals are defined as persuasive messages that attempt to frighten an audience into implementing a recommended response and are used frequently by politicians, advertisers, parents, and even professors. Fear appeal research is used in studying effective risk messages often focusing on health, physical, or social risks.

The extended parallel process model (EPPM) (Witte 1992a, 1992b, 1994, 1998; Witte et al. 1993) is based on Leventhal's danger control/fear control framework and builds on previous fear appeal approaches (Janis 1967; Leventhal 1970; Rogers 1975, 1983). According to the EPPM, the evaluation of a threat brings about either danger control or fear control processes (Witte 1998). First, individuals determine whether they believe the threat is serious and whether they think they are susceptible to the threat. The higher the perception of the threat, the more motivated individuals are to then evaluate the efficacy of the recommended response. When people think about the recommended response, they evaluate its level of response efficacy in terms of getting appropriate and useful information about the threat. They also evaluate their level of self-efficacy in terms of perceived ability to, for example, ask a knowledgeable health care provider the "right" questions to get the needed information to solve the problem. When the threat is perceived as low, trivial, or simply is not perceived as important to consider, the efficacy of the recommended response is typically not evaluated, often resulting in no response to the risk message. In other words, if people do not feel at-risk for a threat in some way, they tend to ignore information about the threat.

When both perceived threat and perceived efficacy are high, then individuals will be motivated to control the danger and adopt the recommended response (Witte 1998). Danger control processes are generally cognitive processes in which individuals perceive a high threat and believe they are at risk for experiencing negative consequences from the threat. Individuals who also perceive high efficacy tend to be scared of the severe threat, and because of their fear, they become motivated to protect themselves. This combination results in individuals effectively deterring the threat and facing the danger. The cognitions or thoughts that arise in the danger control processes bring about increased protection motivation, which stimulates adaptive actions such as attitude, intention, or behavior changes that control the danger (e.g., cancer prevention, reducing risky sexual encounters, or another relevant health, risk, or crisis condition).

Studies have shown that fear appeals with high levels of threat and low levels of efficacy result in message rejection, and often result in boomerang effects because people do the opposite of what is advocated (Witte 1998). Thus, when people believe they are vulnerable to a significant threat but believe that there is nothing that can be done to deal with the threat then they deny they are at risk, defensively avoid the issue, or react in unpredictable ways. In such cases, fears about a threat get in the way of taking appropriate action, and risk messages may not work (Witte 1998).

Not surprisingly, as Witte (1998) points out, for campaigns to successfully implement EPPM, high threat messages should be accompanied by high efficacy messages. If it is difficult to promote high efficacy, then one should use fear-arousing messages with extreme caution, if at all, because they may not work. Fear appeals messages are only potent persuasive devices in certain conditions.

Social Marketing

One approach to campaigns that has been widely used by health educators in both the public and private sector is that of social marketing. Social marketing involves the design, implementation, and control of campaigns aimed at altering the acceptability of the social ideas or behaviors of a specific target group or groups (Kotler 1984; Kotler and Roberto 1989). It is the application of for-profit management and marketing technologies to pro-social, non-profit programs (Meyer and Dearing 1996).

Wallack (1989) suggests that one of the keys to this approach is the reduction of psychological, social, economic, and practical distance between the target of the campaign and the behavior.

Kotler and Roberto (1989) outline five basic steps in the social marketing management process. The first step is an analysis of the social marketing environment immediately surrounding the particular campaign. Next, the social marketer must research the target-adopter population and segment the audience into groups with common characteristics. The third step involves the careful design of the campaigns objectives and strategies. It is in this step that the social marketer must consider four concerns basic to every campaign—the four 'P's.

The four "P's" are *product, price, promotion,* and *place,* also known as the marketing mix. The *product* is the behavior or the product that the target audience must change or adopt. Campaigns have targeted a number of health behavior products including condom use, contraception, and alcohol and drug use. For instance, in the Stanford Heart Disease Prevention Program (SHDPP), the products that were promoted included regular exercise, smoking cessation, dietary changes, and stress reduction. *Price* includes any physical, social, or psychological cost related to campaign compliance. In the case of the SHDPP's Smokers' Challenge, the costs of joining the challenge included the money, time, and energy spent in accepting the challenge, as well as any additional psychological costs of giving up smoking. *Promotion* deals with how the product is packaged or presented to compensate for the costs of adopting it. The Smokers' Challenge promoted the contest by removing or reducing the financial cost of the program to make it more appealing to target audiences (Lefebvre and Flora 1988). *Place* involves the availability, or often at times the accessibility, of the recommended response. The designers of Smokers' Challenge attempted to make information about the program easily accessible. They also mailed information on smoking cessation to households participating in the study. Social marketing is a well-known campaign approach with widespread adoption and allows campaigns to target their persuasive materials carefully.

PRECEDE-PROCEED Planning Model

The PRECEDE theoretical framework was developed in the 1970's by Green and colleagues (Green et al. 1980; www.lgreen.net/precede/preapps.htm). PRECEDE-PROCEED stands for the acronym Predisposing, Reinforcing, Enabling Constructs in Educational/Environmental Diagnosis, and Evaluation and is based on the premise that in the same way that a medical diagnosis precedes a treatment plan, the educational diagnosis should precede an intervention plan. In 1991, PROCEED, which is the acronym for Policy, Regulatory, and Organizational Constructs in Educational and Environmental Development, was also added to recognize the importance of environmental influences on health and health behaviors. The PRECEDE-PROCEED planning model takes the following steps: (1) social assessment (quality of life); (2) epidemiological assessment (overall health); (3) behavioral and environmental assessment (behavior, lifestyle, environment); (4) educational and ecological assessment (predisposing, reinforcing, and enabling factors); (5) administrative and policy assessment (health promotion, health education, policy, regulation, organization); (6) implementation (health promotion, health education, policy, regulation, organization); (7) process evaluation (predisposing, reinforcing, and enabling factors); (8) impact evaluation (behavior, lifestyle, environment); and (9) outcome evaluation (health and quality of life; see Gielen and McDonald 2002; Green and Kreuter 1999, p. 34).

Precaution Adoption Process Model

The Precaution Adoption Process Model (PAPM) is a stage theory similar to other stage theories (stages of change model) that question whether changes in health-relevant behaviors are describable via a single prediction equation. According to Weinstein et al. (1998), stage theories comprise four major elements: a category system to define the stages, an ordering of the stages, common barriers to change that people face in the same stage, and different barriers to change that people face in different stages. Weinstein and Sandman (2002) state that adopting a new precaution or ceasing a risky health behavior requires purposeful action. Thus, PAPM explains the psychological processes involved in how an individual decides to take action and how that decision is then translated into action through the following stages: (1) unaware of health issue; (2) learn about the health issue but unengaged in health issue; (3) decision-making process; (4) decide not to act (PAPM ends here for the time being if this step is taken); (5) deciding to act in terms of adopting the precaution or cessation; (6) acting or initiating the health behavior; and (7) maintenance of the health behavior over time. The PAPM suggests that individuals typically go through the stages in sequence, without skipping any steps.

Diffusion of Innovations

Diffusion of innovations theory spans more than five thousand publications utilizing the approach in a variety of fields, from agricultural research and rural sociology to health communication campaigns, education, and promotion, to name a few (Oldenburg and Parcel 2002; Rogers 2003). "Diffusion is the process through which an innovation, defined as an idea perceived as new, spreads via certain communication channels over time among the members of a social system" (Rogers 2004, p. 13). Rogers (1995) defines an innovation as an idea perceived as new by the adopter. Such information is most often disseminated from opinion leaders to the public in order to bring about social change surrounding a particular adoptive issue (e.g., health behavior). Social change, including decisions affecting health care communication, can happen due to certain consequences via the invention, diffusion, and adoption or rejection of new ideas (i.e., innovations). Thus, diffusion of innovations involves an innovation, communication channels, social systems, and time with the actual innovation process. It involves the five main steps of knowledge, persuasion, decision, implementation, and confirmation, which can be used in any health care communication campaign. According to DOI, the knowledge phase (phase 1) introduces an innovation by capitalizing on the spread of information by appropriate channels (e.g., mediated channels). The persuasion phase (phase 2) focuses on the diffusion of the innovation via interpersonal channels in order to potentially convince late adopters and laggards to adopt. The *decision* phase (phase 3) involves a change agent or opinion leader who influences decisions in a direction desired by a change agency. The change agent can either secure the adoption or slow the diffusion process to prevent adoption of certain innovations that have undesirable effects. Change agents typically play out several roles in the process of introducing the innovation, including: developing a need for change, establishing an information-exchange relationship, diagnosing problems, creating an intent in the client to change, translating an intent to action, stabilizing the adoption and preventing discontinuance, and achieving a terminal relationship (Haider and Kreps 2004). The implementation phase (phase 4) occurs when a person utilizes an innovation and engages in health behavior change as the new idea is put into practice. The *confirmation* phase (phase 5) occurs when a person looks for reinforcement of the already implemented innovation-decision. The adoption here is often modified or even reversed if the person is exposed to conflicting messages about the innovation. The DOI model explains that individuals typically fall into one of the following five categories reflecting a normal distribution: innovators (2.5 %), early adopters (13.5 %), early majority (34 %), late majority (34 %), and laggards (16 %; Rogers 2003).

In a recent article published in a special issue of *Journal of Health Communication,* Rogers (2004) concludes: "the diffusion process displays consistent patterns and regularities, across a range of conditions, innovations, and cultures" (p. 19). For example, adopters take on different characteristics depending upon when they choose to adopt a new way of doing something (e.g., sunscreen protection, seatbelt safety, diet, exercise, smoking cessation, new technology). Certainly, the generalizability of the diffusion model suggests that the theoretical framework can indeed be applied to a variety of real world problems and useful results, particularly in applied health care settings, health policy, and practice. By 2003, since the diffusion of innovations model was initially developed 40 years ago, the public health and health communication fields represented nearly 10 % of all diffusion publications (Rogers 2004). After Rogers' first diffusion book was published in 1962, several important additions have been made to the original model, including: the critical mass of an adoption to the point where it becomes self-sustaining; a focus on the social networks, particularly in terms of understanding how a new idea spreads via interpersonal channels; and re-invention, or how adopters change the innovation during the diffusion process.

Information-Motivation-Behavioral Skills Model

The Information-Motivation-Behavioral Skills Model (IMB) was initially used to understand human immunodeficiency virus (HIV) risk and prevention behaviors across a variety of populations, but it has broad applications in a number of health promotion contexts (Fisher and Fisher 2002). In the context of HIV, the IMB model specifies that prevention information and motivation work influence prevention behavioral skills to bring about preventative behavior. According to Fisher and Fisher (2002), the IMB model approach to health behavior promotion has the following three major components: *elicitation* of existing levels of health promotion information, motivation, behavioral skills, and health promotion behavior; *intervention* in the design and implementation of an empirically targeted intervention addressing the same components; and *evaluation* of intervention impact. In addition to HIV health promotion campaigns, the IMB has also been implemented for breast self-examinations and motorcycle safety.

Elaboration Likelihood Model of Persuasion

The Elaboration Likelihood Model of Persuasion was initially developed to explain how persuasion processes move through two major routes (central and peripheral) to change attitudes (Petty et al. 2002). The central route refers to thinking about the desirability of the communication's consequences and the likelihood that they will occur. The central route is a thoughtful and cognitively effortful route that occurs when the person is motivated and has the ability to think about the merits of the health issue being considered. Alternately, thinking under the peripheral route includes reliance on simple communication cues, such as the likeability of the message source (see e.g., Azjen and Fishbein 2000). The peripheral route is a less thoughtful route that occurs when motivation or ability is low (Petty et al. 2002). When people lack expertise about a topic, they are more likely to employ the peripheral route as they consider a health message, which helps to explain why health claims unsupported by research are often appealing. ELM has been used in many studies to understand health communication efficacy and message tailoring in health behavior change efforts.

Each of the theories outlined has guided numerous health communication interventions and campaigns over the last several decades. However, there is an important aspect of health communication that seems to be under-addressed by these theories. Specifically, current health communication theories frequently do not adequately address the interpersonal nature of health care encounters (see Becker et al. 1992; Rogers 2003, 2004), which is an essential component of caregiving for formal and informal caregivers. Further, interaction with family and friends is known to have an important impact, both for good and for ill, on health behavior (Nussbaum et al. 2000; Sparks 2007; Sparks-Bethea 2002; Sparks and Villagran 2008; Sparks and Villagran 2010). For example, we know that the health of married people is generally better than the health of single individuals. Additionally, we know that African American males who are active in the social activities of their churches are generally healthier than those not involved in church social activities (Ferraro 2004). To address the lack of a theoretical framework for effective and appropriate health care communication contexts, the SMILE health care communication (SMILE-HCCM) is put forth.

The SMILE Health Care Communication Model (SMILE-HCCM)

As political psychologist Harold D. Lasswell (1948) stated, in studying communication processes one must ask, "Who says what in which channel to whom with what effect?" Lasswell identified the central components of communication including the sender (who encodes and transmits), the content or message (communication substance), the channel (the medium through which information is transmitted), the receiver or audience (who decodes the communication to derive meaning), and the effect (a measurable outcome of the communicative process). In 1960, Berlo put forth the S-M-C-R model (sender, message, channel, receiver), which can be adapted and extended to modern day health care communication contexts. Berlo's approach places great emphasis on dyadic communication, hence emphasizing the role of the *relationship* between the source and the receiver as an important variable in the communication process (see also Sparks 2011).

Berlo's emphasis on the relationship between the communicative source and receiver is a key component of the SMILE Health Care Communication Model. The central features of the SMILE (Satisfaction, Modification-Mirroring, Identification, Listen, and Enact-Evaluate) Health Care Communication Model depict the communication challenges surrounding interpersonal and small group communication in health care settings. *Satisfaction* centers on the extent to which the health care communication encounter leaves patients feeling they have the cognitive and behavioral tools to deal with potential health issues. *Modification* suggests that health care communicators stay on message while making *modifications* to the way messages are delivered, while *mirroring* the communicative style that emerges during the health care interaction. *Identity* deals with the importance people ascribe to their *identities*, the ways in which they protect them, and the ways in which they respond when their identities are threatened. *Listening* refers to paying close attention to communicative cues that arise during each health care interaction. *Enacting* patient action and *evaluating* the current health care communication encounter occur while remembering that each interaction is based on a history of prior interaction with the patient.

The HCCM extends prior theoretical research by focusing on two distinctive features: (1) interpersonal-based message framing; and (2) reframing of message based on feedback cues during the health care communication encounter. Such subtle and natural approaches to health campaigns are very important to consider in health care interactions and can be found within the SMILE Health Care Communication Model theoretical framework. The SMILE-HCCM model says that communicators who anticipate and address the issues identified by SMILE are more apt to improve the health care communication encounter than those who are unaware of and unresponsive to these issues. The SMILE-HCCM is meant to provide a theoretical guideline for health care professionals and their interactions in health care settings.

S: Satisfaction in SMILE

Satisfaction with the health care communication encounter indicates that patients feel they have the cognitive and behavioral tools to deal with potential health issues. Research in the medical setting reveals that when patients feel empowered satisfaction ratings soar (see e.g. du Pré 2005b). In the cancer health context, Facione (2002) found that perception of risk is believed to be a significant predictor of cancer treatment and prevention measures; thus, it is important to examine how patient decision-making is affected by risk messages. For cancer survivors, risk perception is defined as a belief that the cancer will return (Mullens et al. 2004). Such beliefs are often provoked by satisfaction with claims or evidence presented by health care providers about the likelihood that the particular health issue (e.g., cancer) will remain a persistent problem or go away with proper treatment.

As explained earlier in the discussion on message framing, theoretical models that attempt to explain how and why individuals adopt a health-protective behavior are based on evidence that stresses the importance of perceived susceptibility and health risk (Witte et al. 2001). These approaches examine how patient attitudes affect decisions based on *satisfaction* with evidence about the potential risk of cancer based on demographic, socio-economic, and behavioral factors. Perceived susceptibility is combined with factors including outcome estimates, difficulty of potential action, and potential cost of noncompliance (Katapodi et al. 2004).

Based on these ideas, there is often an inverse relationship between level of perceived health risk and cognitive *satisfaction* with options to reduce risk factors. Although patient attitudes are a primary factor in health risk decision-making, particularly when it comes to cancer, the dyadic interaction between patient and provider also plays a significant role in risk assessments (Whelan et al. 2004).

Satisfaction increases when patients seek more information about their cancer through a relationship with their health care provider, although they still make risky personal decisions to reject risk information based on lifestyle, behavioral choices, or other preferences (Brashers et al. 1999). *Satisfaction* with risk claims also includes a sense of satisfaction with treatment options presented by providers based on perceived risk (Whelan et al. 2004). For instance, women whose providers used decision aids to help them make choices about treatment options were more satisfied with their decisions. Prior research also encourages physicians to develop mutual decision-making processes with patients that reflect goal-oriented rather than problem-oriented approaches (Mold 1995; Sparks et al. 2007; Sparks and Villagran 2010). However, this could pose a number of challenges as well.

Even patients who understand cancer risk statistics may still have optimistic or pessimistic biases when interpreting this information for their own lives (Facione

2002). People suffer from optimistic bias when they view themselves as less susceptible to diseases than research data reveals them to be (Thompson et al. 1998); these individuals are the "worry free" (Kreuter and Strecher 1995). Low estimations of risk are often driven by a need for control over uncontrollable health concerns. (Facione 2002; Thompson et al. 1998). For example, even heavy smokers with other personal risk factors did not perceive themselves at an elevated risk for cancer (Ayanian and Cleary 1999). In this case, dissatisfaction with evidence of elevated cancer risk for smokers was driven by their need for control over their addiction to cigarettes.

People underestimate risk factors that seem familiar and voluntary, such as smoking and diet (Fischhoff 1999; Sandman 1993; Weinstein 1999), and underestimation lessens the desire to take action (Sandman 1993; Weinstein 1999). To encourage reconsideration, physicians should present information to patients highlighting the relationship between personal choice and risk. Risk is controllable when the risk agent is a personal choice of the patient.

Conversely, some individuals suffer from pessimistic biases, or overestimation of risk. In this scenario, persons with the abilities to reduce their risk wrongly believe that cancer prevention is beyond their control. Further, a significant amount of research reports people with higher levels of worry or anxiety are more likely to overestimate their risk of cancer (e.g., Katapodi et al. 2004), and therefore choose inaction.

Research indicates that people are more apt to take action to improve their health when they view themselves as both vulnerable to a health threat and powerful enough to take action against such threats (Witte 1998). Health care communicators, therefore, need communication options for both helping patients to understand their vulnerability to health risks and their capacity for its prevention. Several tools are available to help patients correctly estimate their health risks. Risk communication strategies for public health preparedness often concern agriculture, food, water issues; infectious disease and vaccines; mental health, and general public health; as well as chemical, biological, nuclear, and radiological threats (see jhsph.edu/preparedness) (http://www.bt.cdc.gov/cerc/pdf/CERC-SEPT02.pdf) for detailed information). The Centers for Disease Control (see cdc.gov) have prioritized Risk Communication and Health Information Dissemination since 2004. Another web site, www.yourcancerrisk.harvard.edu, helps patients determine their vulnerability to a dozen cancers as "average, below average, or above average." In addition, when possible, it lists steps individuals can take to minimize their risk (e.g., such as taking a multivitamin tablet or increasing servings of leafy green vegetables). Kreuter and Strecher (1995) found that people who had such personalized feedback were more apt to overcome optimistic or pessimistic biases. Thus, personalized feedback about ways to reduce risk increases patient satisfaction with health care (Sparks and Villagran 2010).

The health care communication encounter is the key mechanism through which these types of messages should be exchanged. To successfully approach patients about risk and benefits of screening, physicians should consider using "loss framed messages" rather than "gain framed" messages when recommending cancer screening (Sparks and Turner 2008). Banks et al. (1995b) note that "loss framing" may be more persuasive because the perceived greater loss of not participating in the screening process may seem more important to patients than the smaller losses associated with taking these tests (e.g., discomfort and fear).

Testable Propositions

1. Patients who perceive more health risks will be more likely to overestimate the number and severity of their personal risk factors and be less satisfied with contradictory risk information.
2. Health care communicators who use decision tools will be associated with higher levels of communication satisfaction among patients after a health care interaction.
3. Individuals who mindfully do not engage in healthy behaviors (e.g., check-ups, preventive diet, seek treatment) are more likely to underestimate their health risk.
4. Health care communicators who can reduce patient anxiety in health care interactions will have more satisfaction among patients who comply with their specific health behavior requests (e.g., cancer screening tests, dietary changes).

M: Modification-Mirroring in SMILE

Health care professionals often fail to communicate effectively due to a lack of clear communication goals. Key messages are often framed in ways to support the goals and then *modified* according to the feedback received during interaction. Due to the continuous changes that occur during patient care, setting goals and identifying support messages are decisions that should be made prior to the interaction with the patient and the family and then *modified* with each subsequent interaction.

Modification and *mirroring* of verbal and nonverbal messages is a very important yet often overlooked communication component during the health care interaction. Health care communicators must stay on message while making *modifications* to the way messages are delivered. The key is to communicatively mirror the emotional state of the patient while staying on message and modifying the key messages to match the mood of the patient and his or her family members. The goals and messages should still be simple, straightforward, and realistic, but should be articulated on a similar emotional level as the diagnosis or health problem is being understood and digested by the patient and family. If information is not available or known, then the health care provider must be honest with the patient (Pecchioni and Sparks 2007; Sparks 2007; Sparks et al. 2007; Sparks and Villagran 2010).

Tetradic Model of Relational Adjustment. The *modification* element of health care communicative processes may also be understood through the lens of a tetradic model (O'Hair and Sparks 2008; Sparks and Hill 2005). A tetrad could characterize a diagnosed individual as being in a varying state of intensification, obsolescence, retrieval, and *modification* depending upon each relationship within the individual's network. For example, as a diagnosed individual progresses and adjusts to living with cancer, the patient *modifies* his or her relational interactions to account for the impact of the disease on each relationship in the patient's life (e.g., spouse, children, friends, health care workers, colleagues, etc.). As patients' provide information about their relational networks, health care providers can learn about how health care will likely be handled and managed. Such valuable information potentially gives the health care team a bigger picture of the health care efforts that will be needed for the patient and his or her family and can adjust treatment options accordingly. Health care communicators can also build credibility by *modifying* their communication according to the needs of the patient. Caregivers should build a relationship with their patients and get to know them as individuals by learning more about their occupations, skills, families, and support networks. The more attention health care communicators pay toward getting to know the interests of patients, the easier it will be to *modify* the key messages that are important to get across to them.

Another way to modify one's messages based on patient cues is to ask questions or make statements that elicit patients' emotions in a supportive manner. Marshall (1993) offers the "NURS" mnemonic to help physicians "get a true sense of what is going on" with patients (p. 21). "N" stands for naming the emotion, "U" for understanding/legitimating it, "R" for respecting/praising, and "S" for supporting the elicited emotion with statements such as, "I admire how you're holding up" (pp. 21–22). Use of the "NURS" formula may encourage honesty. According to the National Cancer Institute, some patients say activities they most enjoy are associated with elevated cancer risks (NCI (1998). Physicians can acknowledge the understandability of such views while encouraging patients to consider what they value most. If time is short, tell patients, but also let them know their agenda is important. *Mirroring* can be a powerful communicative tool. Learning how to *mirror* the verbal and nonverbal communicative cues of the patient can be an effective communicative strategy, particularly when the diagnosis is a difficult one. People have different communicative styles. Some individuals are highly emotional, while others show emotion less in the health care environment than they do in the comfort of their own home. Some individuals make eye contact, while others are uncomfortable making eye contact, especially with strangers. Some people generally feel uncomfortable in the health care setting, and others are not impacted by the chaos of the numerous interactions that take place when a patient enters the health care environment. In sum, health care providers should aim to match or mirror the communication style of the patient and each individual family member during each conversation. But it is important to remember that mirroring is different from imitating, and if not done naturally, a patient may suspect insincerity. *Mirroring* may help pave the way in initial interactions, but it is not meant to be a panacea for every health care interaction.

Testable Propositions

1. Health care communicators who repeat key messages (modifying each message) in health care interactions will have greater patient comprehension of available treatments for informed decision-making.

2. Health care communicators who are able to mirror nonverbal and verbal patient messages will be perceived as more credible (competent communicators) in the health care setting.

I: Identification in SMILE

Patient *identity* is important. A health care provider may gain additional insight by understanding an individual's social *identification*. Understanding where patients have come from in terms of their social *identity* and the relational networks with which they have been or currently are connected can impact health outcomes. Shifts in an individual's social *identity* occur through communication.

Social Identity Theory and Health

In recent years, Harwood and Sparks (2003), Sparks and Harwood (2008), Villagran and Sparks (2010) have argued for the general applicability of Social Identity Theory (SIT) (e.g., Tajfel and Turner 1986) to health communication literature, and most specifically to issues surrounding cancer diagnosis, treatment, and recovery. SIT is a broad socio-psychologically grounded theory of intergroup relations, which focuses particularly on the importance people ascribe to their *identities*, the ways in which they protect them, and the ways in which they respond when their identities are threatened. It deals primarily with *identification* with large social groups (age, culture, sexuality, etc.), but can also be applied to smaller and more specialized groups (an alma mater, a family, a victim of a particular disease).

Harwood and Sparks (2003) specified three levels of identity. At the primary level, individuals identify with large-scale social groups, and those identifications influence their susceptibility to and ability to cope with cancer. For instance, highly identified women might, under some circumstances, be more likely to attend to breast cancer risks and engage in appropriate prevention strategies. At the secondary level, identifications with particular behaviors will influence cancer communication processes. For example, identifying strongly as a smoker will likely make it harder to quit. At the tertiary level, identification with cancer-specific identities come into play (e.g., patient, victim, survivor, etc.). As individuals identify more strongly with being a survivor rather than a victim (and in spite of perhaps very similar prognoses), we might predict a better outcome for the survivor. In all cases, the issue here is that particular conceptualizations of self within the cancer realm have the capacity to change psychological orientation and behaviors related to cancer, and hence to influence concrete outcomes. Thus, savvy health care communicators should pay attention to changes in a patient's health status (i.e., shifts in a patient's social identity) and adjust accordingly.

Testable Propositions.

1. Health care communicators who can pay attention to changes in a patient's health status (i.e., identity shifts) during health care interactions will have increased patient communication satisfaction, thus achieving greater health outcomes.

L: Listening in SMILE

It is important to listen to patients. Using "active listening" techniques help to show interest and concern. Marshall (1993) writes that open-ended questions "show patients they will have some control over the interaction and that their concerns are important" (p. 19).

Listening for Communicative Cues During Interviews. Health care communicators who learn to identify unique and subtle communicative cues from their patients are likely to more fully understand the nature of the health care problem and related health and family issues, which contribute to information seeking, decision-making and a host of other concerns that may arise (e.g., medication administration issues, caregiving concerns, treatment options, etc.).

During interviews and conversations in healthcare environments, respondents often convey information in a humorous fashion, self-disclose something very personal, or tell detailed stories that consist of emotional content that is difficult to decipher and interpret. Words and gestures are composed of ambiguous signals and require interpretation (Sillars et al. 2000). The humorous delivery of these signals often disguises their importance. Because conversations such as these tend to occur rapidly, and the interviewer may be distracted by the humor, it is easy for the uninformed interviewer to miss information cues about problems or concerns that should be followed up with additional questions or probes.

Long-term family caregivers are frequently asked to talk about topics such as bowel movements, loneliness, personal safety, and intimate care. Such socially taboo and sensitive topics can cause periods of awkwardness and embarrassment. Previous work indicates that humor and laughter functioned as "cues" that family caregivers were approaching topics that needed a type of communication safety valve to relieve the stress, tension, or embarrassment associated with discussing the topic (Sparks-Bethea et al. 2000, Sparks-Bethea 2001; Sparks et al. 2005). To appreciate the subtlety and complexity of this communication strategy in the interviewing situation, it is vital to understand that the humorous anecdote is not the end point. Humor instead is most often the cue that sensitive probing may now need to be used in order to fully comprehend what the caregiver is experiencing.

Meta-humorous Interaction Theory (MetaHIT) MetaHIT has been utilized as a guiding conceptual framework in prior research on family caregiving and communication and the use of humor in caregiving situations (see Sparks-Bethea 2000, 2001). This theoretical approach moves beyond previous stimulus-response approaches to humorous interaction and embraces a relational or process oriented approach.

This conceptualization of humor is used on the relational or meta-communicative level as a way of safely communicating difficult issues, where cues about important aspects of one's story can be conveyed in implicit, humorous ways. The MetaHIT taxonomy extends arousal-relief theory by recognizing the typical functions of humor (i.e., cognitive, affective, and behavioral) while incorporating important relational elements that exist in the interaction. In other words, humor is often used as a cue that something of "deeper meaning" is going on in the relationship(s) involved in the story. Humor in this context is not always "funny," but instead is often used in coping or relief responses cognitively, affectively, or through behavior.

Listening: Relational Agency Model O'Hair and Sparks' (2008) research on relational agency in life-threatening illnesses further emphasizes the importance of relationships in health care communication. They identify the role of the relational partner in the management of care and refer to numerous relational challenges that caregivers face in the context of LTIs. Through the empowerment of relational resources, patients and their partners elevate their prospects for exerting *agency*, or a choice created through strategic communication, in the conduct of their interactions with each other and with the healthcare system. Partners begin to feel that their perceptions and behaviors of one another are in sync and can focus on intimacy building and strategizing how they both will manage the LTI. For example, partners may insist on second-opinions when they are faced with a disappointing prognosis report, or they may appeal insurance restrictions against participating in a clinic trial. Communication efforts such as these represent the ability to expand choices. Agency also entails having the faculties and resources necessary for making competent decisions based on a wider range of choices. Health care communicators can work closely with patients by listening carefully to the patient agent.

Testable Propositions

1. Health care communicators who listen for communicative cues in health care interactions will obtain more patient information, thus achieving better decision-making (e.g., diagnoses).
2. Patients (agents) who are given multiple choices for treatment will have greater satisfaction with the health care system.

E: Enactment and Evaluation in SMILE

Building on the Rowan et al. (2003) CAUSE model, *enactment* requires action on the part of the patient. Once a health risk has been identified and made salient to the patient, in order to optimize health outcomes, the patient needs to make an informed decision based on the best medical advice. Two substantial barriers to action, however, create challenges to behavioral change: initiating changes to longstanding habits and maintaining those changes across the life span.

Motivating patients to change is often difficult, even when patients are aware that behavioral changes are not only desirable, but necessary for their health. Health-related behaviors that individuals have been *enacting* are strongly embedded in their lives (Booth-Butterfield 2003). For instance, changing one's diet or quitting smoking are not simple actions. Instead, these changes require considerable time, determination, and persistence. Patients must feel the need to make changes and, perhaps most importantly, they must see the salience of the potentially negative outcomes of not making the desired change. For example, most people are aware that smoking increases one's chances of developing mouth, throat, or lung cancer, but are unaware that smoking also increases one's likelihood of developing other cancers as well (Moyad 2003). While most people are aware that exposure to the sun can lead to skin cancer, most are not aware of the cumulative damage that can occur over time and thus minimize estimates of their own risk (Chakrabarty and Geisse 2004).

Helping patients to understand their risk factors is an important part of this process. Therefore, while taking the patient's medical history, health care providers should spend considerable time exploring lifestyle choices and family history that put the patient at risk for a wide array of health risks as well as those that might create barriers to changing behaviors. Providers can use any opportunities that arise in these interviews to discuss the individual's risk factors. Further, health care providers need to be alert to moments when patients might be highly motivated to make a behavior change (Dracup et al. 1994).

Receiving a cancer diagnosis raises the salience of these issues for patients, and they are often more highly motivated to make changes (Patterson et al. 2003). Once patients feel the need and are motivated to make changes, they may resist making desired changes because they seem too difficult (e.g., quitting smoking). As with any seemingly overwhelming project, identifying small steps helps to make the task seem more manageable. For example, start by asking the patient to read a brochure or quit smoking for an hour and then move toward longer-term goals (Dolin and Booth-Butterfield 1995). Developing a detailed written plan that sets realistic goals, provides incentives and support, as well as planning for slips or relapses into old behavior patterns, helps patients feel in greater control of their behavior and then they are more likely to maintain changes over time (Luszczynska and Schwarzer 2003).

After patients have initiated the desired changes, maintaining these changes can continue to be a challenge, especially when embedded within a social support network that may reinforce undesirable behaviors. Health care communicators can undertake a number of strategies to help patients maintain desired changes. Regular discussions with patients should occur to provide opportunities to talk about and support successes in getting rid of embedded behaviors. Health care communicators can look for communicative cues and create opportunities in which to praise patients for any successes. In addition, helping patients see they have the ability to succeed in carrying out the health behavior is very important. The physician should note the patient's successes in other contexts and assure the patient of the physician's belief in his or her ability to succeed in this domain as well (Witte 1998). Acknowledging the likelihood of failures by developing a relapse management plan helps patients to get back on track more quickly after a failure (Luszczynska and Schwarzer 2003).

Multiple messages in a variety of forms must also be considered. For instance, while face-to-face meetings are often the best approach, this is not the only strategy available for providing support to patients. A cost and time efficient method is to send "tailored" postcards, email messages, or phone calls that remind individual patients of appointments for cancer screenings (Lantz et al. 1995). These mediated means of communication can also be used to acknowledge and provide social support for successes and offer words of encouragement.

The most effective behavioral changes occur in a web of supportive relationships (Dean 1989; Jones 1997; Sarason et al. 1997), therefore, health care professionals should involve patients' families in all stages of the process and recruit them as allies in making the needed health behavior changes. Conversely, the support network can create obstacles to making changes by continuing to support poor choices (Rook 1995), and this should be taken into account.

Evaluation requires action on the part of the health care communicator or provider. Once a health risk has been identified and made salient to the patient, in order to optimize health outcomes, the health care communicator now needs to navigate and negotiate the outcome with the patient. Health care communicators must constantly reflect and *evaluate* the current health care communication encounter while remembering that each interaction is based on a history of prior interaction with the patient. A communication goal of "educating the patient and family on every aspect of the medical complexities involved" may not be realistic; *informing them of the problem and specific dangers, providing guidance on appropriate treatments, and easing concerns* are achievable communicative goals. Messages in support of these goals must also be directly and effectively translated to the audience via more than one communication channel. After goals and messages have been established, the challenge becomes one of delivery and ensuring that messages and goals are achieved.

If the goal is to ease concern and the message in support of that is, "the risk to the patient is low," that message should be clearly stated at the outset and returned to as often as naturally possible:

> "I want to begin by first saying that the risk is very low...."
> "As I said a few minutes ago, the risk is very low...."
> "That is an important question, but before answering it I want to again let you know that the risk is very low...."
> "Before we finish here I want to remind you that the risk is indeed low."

The point is that health care communicators need to bring up the main message in multiple ways so that the audience leaves with a solid understanding of the key message(s).

Testable Propositions

1. Raising the salience of negative consequences of health-related behaviors will increase compliance with medical advice.
2. Patients who are carefully guided through the change process by using small steps and developing specific written plans to change will be more likely to comply with medical advice than those not having such support.

3. Patients who receive more supportive messages from their physicians through more than one channel of communication (i.e., interpersonal-mediated) will be more likely to comply with medical advice.
4. When health care communicators actively involve patients' family members in the change process, the patients will be more likely to comply with medical advice.
5. When health care communicators use more than one communication channel to stay on message in terms of informing them of the problem and specific dangers, the patients will be more likely to comply with medical advice.
6. When health care communicators use more than one communication channel to stay on message in terms of providing guidance on appropriate treatments, the patients will be more likely to comply with medical advice.
7. When health care communicators use more than one communication channel to stay on message in terms of easing patient concerns, the patients will be more likely to comply with medical advice.

Finally, health care communicators (caregivers) must also remember to smile, when appropriate, during health care encounters. Just as not all diagnoses are alike, not all health care interactions are alike. Adjust and tailor each health care interaction accordingly.

Implications for Practice, Education, and Research

To influence entrenched caregiving situations and patient health behaviors with targeted specialized populations, messages need to be relevant and compelling considering unique experiences, background characteristics, and preferences of the vulnerable, at-risk, or underserved audience, with health information providing direction and rationale for making the best health-related decisions and adopting health-preserving behaviors (Kreps and Sparks 2008; Maibach et al. 1996; Sparks 2007; Sparks and Turner 2008). Careful consideration must be taken to coordinate content and relational aspects of communication to inform and care for loved ones and family members and their treatment regimen without confusing or upsetting them (Buckman 1996; Gillotti et al. 2002; Pecchioni and Sparks 2007; Sparks 2003a; Sparks et al. 2007; Sparks and Villagran 2010).

By understanding nuances in evidence-based message exchanges, researchers, practitioners, and family members involved in caring for patients will be able to deliver relevant and compelling messages to at-risk populations and better health outcomes will be achieved. Designing and delivering health care communication messages to match the specific communication skills, needs, and pre-dispositions of varied patient populations is a crucial component of health care delivery (Kreps and Sparks 2008; Sparks 2007; Sparks and Nussbaum 2008; Sparks and Villagran 2008, 2010). Health communication scholars must do a better job of translating communication theories and literature into the lives of patients, caregivers, and health care provider teams. Communication theories provide sound building blocks for those interested in using reliable, research-based empirical evidence to aid in explaining the critical features of various health diagnoses to patients. Understanding how varying health literacy levels and subsequent communicative interactions play out in the construction and processing of such messages across the health communication continuum (e.g., interpersonal, small group, organizational, public, mass) is an essential step for improved health outcomes for our vulnerable populations. To influence entrenched health behaviors, evidence-based health messages (from interpersonal to mediated) need to be relevant and compelling and targeted to at-risk populations, with health information that provides direction and a rationale for making the best health-related decisions and adopting health-preserving behaviors.

References

Adelman, M. B., & Frey, L. R. (1997). *The fragile community: Living together with AIDS*. Mahwah: Erlbaum.

Anderson, J. O., & Martin, P. G. (2003). Narratives and healing: Exploring one family's stories of cancer survivorship. *Health Communication, 15*(2), 133–143.

Ayanian, J. Z., & Cleary, P. D. (1999). Perceived risk of heart disease and cancer among cigarette smokers. *Journal of the American Medical Association, 281,* 1019.

Azjen, I., & Fishbein, M. (2000). Attitudes and the attitude-behavior relation: Reasoned and automatic processes. In W. Stroebe & M. Hewstone (Eds.), *European review of social psychology* (Vol. 11, pp. 1–33). New York: Wiley.

Bandura, A. (1977). *Social learning theory*. Englewood Cliffs: Prentice Hall.

Bandura, A. (1989). Perceived self-efficacy in the exercise of control over AIDS infection. In V. M. Mays, G. W. Albee, & S. S. Schneider (Eds.), *Primary prevention of AIDS: Psychological approaches* (pp. 128–141). Newbury Park: Sage.

Banks, S., Salovey, P., Greener, S., Rothman, A. J., Moyer, A., Beauvais, J., et al. (1995a). The effects of message framing on mammography utilization. *Health Psychology, 14,* 178–184.

Banks, A. T., Zimmerman, H. J., Ishak, K. G., & Harter, J. G. (1995b). Diclofenac-associated hepatotoxicity: Analysis of 180 cases reported to the Food and Drug Administration as adverse reactions. *Hepatology, 22*(3), 820–827.

Beck, C. S. (2001). *Communicating for better health: A guide through the medical mazes*. Boston: Allyn & Bacon.

Beck, C. S., Ragan, S. L., & DuPre, A. (1997). *Partnership for health: Building relationships between women and health caregivers*. Mahwah: Erlbaum.

Beck, C. S., Benitez, J. L., Edwards, A., Olson, A., Pai, A., & Torres, M. B. (2004). Enacting "health communication:" The field of health communication as constructed through publication in scholarly journals. *Health Communication, 16,* 475–492.

Becker, T., Rogers, E., & Sopory, P. (1992). *Designing health communication campaigns: What works*? Newbury Park: Sage.

Bellet, P. S., & Maloney, M. J. (1991). The importance of empathy as an interviewing skill in medicine. *Journal of the American Medical Association, 266,* 1831–1832.

Berlo, D. K. (1960). *The process of communication*. New York: Holt, Rinehart and Winston, Inc.

Bevan, J., & Sparks, L. (in press). The relationship between accurate and benevolently biased serial argument perceptions and individual negative health perceptions. *Communication Research*.

Bevan, J., & Sparks, L. (2011). Communication in the context of long-distance family caregiving. An integrated review and practical applications. *Patient Education and Counseling, 85,* 26–30.

Bevan, J., Jupin, A., & Sparks, L. (2011a). Information quality, uncertainty, and quality of care in long distance caregiving. *Communication Research Reports, 28*(2), 190–195.

Bevan, J., Rogers, K., Andrews, N., & Sparks, L. (2011b). Topic avoidance and negative health perceptions in the distant caregiving context. *Journal of Family Communication*.

Bevan, J., Vreeburg, S. K., Verdugo, S., & Sparks, L. (2012). Interpersonal conflict and health perception in long-distance caregiving relationships. *Journal of Health Communication* 1–15. DOI:10.1080/10810730.2011.650829.

Bevan, J. L., Sparks, L., Ernst, J., Francies, J., & Santora, N. (in press book chapter, anticipated 2013). Information sources in relation to information quality, information-seeking, and uncertainty in the context of healthcare reform. In R. Ahmed & B. R. Bates (Eds.), *Health communication and mass media: Applying research to public health policy and practice*. Farnham: Gower Publishers.

Bodie, G., & Dutta, M. (2008). Understanding health literacy for strategic health marketing: e-health, literacy, health disparities, and the digital divide. *Health Marketing Quarterly, 25,* 175–203.

Booth-Butterfield, M. (2003). Embedded health behaviors from adolescence to adulthood: The impact of tobacco. *Health Communication, 15,* 171–185.

Brashers, D. E., Haas, S. M., & Neidig, J. L. (1999). The patient self-advocacy scale: Measuring patient involvement in health care decision making interactions. *Health Communication, 11,* 97–121.

Buckman, R. (1996). Talking to patients about cancer. *British Medical Journal, 31,* 699–700.

Brubaker, R. G., & Wickersham, D. (1990). Encouraging the practice of testicular self-examination: A field application of the theory of reasoned action. *Health Psychology, 9,* 154–163.

Burgers, C. F., Buekeboom, C. J., & Sparks, L. (in press). How the doc should (not) talk: When breaking bad news with negations influences patients' immediate responses and medical adherence intentions. *Patient Education and Counseling*.

Cawyer, C., & Smith- duPré, A. (1995). Communicating social support: Identifying supportive episodes in an HIV/AIDS support group. *Communication Quarterly, 43,* 243–258.

Celsi, R. L., & Olson, J. C. (1988). The role of involvement in attention, and comprehension processes. *Journal of Consumer Research, 15,* 210–224.

Chakrabarty, A., & Geisse, J. K. (2004). Medical therapies for non-melanoma skin cancer. *Clinics in Dermatology, 22,* 183–188.

Collins, D., Villagran, M. M., & Sparks, L. (2008). Crossing borders, crossing cultures: Barriers to cancer prevention and treatment along the U.S./Mexico border. *Patient Education and Counseling, 71*(3), 333–339.

Crawford, T. J., & Boyer, R. (1985). Salient consequences, cultural values, and childbearing intentions. *Journal of Applied Social Psychology, 15,* 16–30.

Crowley, S. (2012). Health care reform and the Supreme Court (Affordable Care Act). *New York Times*, July 29. http://topics.nytimes.com/top/reference/timestopics/organizations/s/supreme_court/affordable_care_act/index.html. Accessed 1 Aug 2012.

Dean, K. (1989). Self-care components of lifestyles. *Social Science and Medicine, 29,* 137–152.

DiClemente, C. C., & Prochaska, J. O. (1985). Processes and stages of change: Coping and competence in smoking behavior change. In S. Shiffman & T. A. Willis (Eds.), *Coping and substance abuse* (pp. 319–334). San Diego: Academic Press.

Dolin, D. J., & Booth-Butterfield, S. (1995). Foot-in-the-door and cancer prevention. *Health Communication, 7,* 55–64.

Donohew, L., & Ray, E. B. (Eds.). (1990). *Communication and health*. Hillsdale: Erlbaum.

Dracup, K., Baker, D. W., Dunbar, S. B., Dacey, R. A., Brooks, N. H., Johnson, C. C., et al. (1994). Counseling, education, and lifestyle modifications. *Journal of the American Medical Association, 263,* 1816–1819.

du Pré, A. (1998). *Humor and the healing arts: Multimethod analysis of humor use in health care*. Mahwah: Erlbaum.

du Pré, A. (2000). *Communicating about health: Current issues and perspectives*. Mountain View: Mayfield.

du Pré, A. (2002). Accomplishing the impossible: Talking about body *and* mind *and* soul during a medical visit. *Health Communication, 14,* 1–21.

du Pré, A. (2005a). *Communicating about health: Current issues and perspectives* (2nd ed.). New York: McGraw-Hill.

du Pré, A. (2005b). Making empowerment work: Medical center soars in satisfaction ratings. In E. B. Ray (Ed.), *Case studies in health communication*. Mahwah: Erlbaum.
du Pré, A., & Ray, E. B. (2008). Comforting episodes: Transcendent experiences of cancer survivors. In L. Sparks, D. O'Hair, & G. L. Kreps (Eds.), *Cancer communication and aging* (pp. 99–114). Cresskill: Hampton.
Dutta-Bergman, M. (2004a). Developing a profile of consumer intention to seek out additional health information beyond the doctor: Demographic, communicative, and psychographic factors. *Health Communication, 17,* 1–16.
Dutta-Bergman, M. J. (2004b). Primary sources of health information: Comparisons in the domain of health attitudes, health cognitions, and health behaviors. *Health Communication, 16,* 273–288.
Dutta-Bergman, M. (2006) Media use theory and internet use for health care. In M, Murero & R, Rice (Eds.), *The internet and health care: Theory, research, and practice* (pp. 83–103). Mahwah: Erlbaum.
Egbert, N., Kreps, G. L., Sparks, L., & du Pré, A. (2008). Spirituality and the aging patient. In L. Sparks, H. D. O'Hair, & G. L. Kreps (Eds.), *Cancer communication and aging* (pp. 277–292). Cresskill: Hampton Press.
Eisen, M., Zellman, G. I., & McAllister, A. L. (1985). A health belief model approach to adolescents' fertility control: Some pilot program findings. *Health Education Quarterly, 12,* 185–210.
Facione, N. C. (2002). Perceived risk of breast cancer. *Cancer, 10,* 256–261.
Ferguson, K. J., Yesalis, C. E., Pomrehn, P. R., & Kirkpatrick, M. B. (1989). Attitudes, knowledge, and beliefs as predictors of exercise intent and behavior in schoolchildren. *Journal of School Health, 59,* 112–115.
Ferraro, K. F. (2004). Next steps in understanding the prayer/health connection. In K. W. Schaie, N. Krause, & A. Booth (Eds.), *Religious influences on health and well-being in the elderly* (pp. 96–103). New York: Springer.
Ferraro, K. F. (2005). Health and aging. In R. H. Binstock, L. K. George, S. Cutler, J. Hendricks, & J. Schulz (Eds.), *Handbook of aging and the social sciences* (6th ed.). Burlington: Elsevier.
Fishbein, M., & Ajzen, I. (1975). *Belief, attitude, intention, and behavior: An introduction to theory and research*. Reading: Addison-Wesley.
Fishbein, M., & Ajzen, I. (1981). Acceptance, yielding and impact: Cognitive processes in persuasion. In R. E. Petty, T. M. Ostrom, & T. C. Brock (Eds.), *Cognitive responses in persuasion* (pp. 339–359). Hillsdale: Erlbaum.
Fishbein, M., & Middlestadt, S. E. (1989). Using the theory of reasoned action as a framework for understanding and changing AIDS-related behaviors. In V. M. Mays, G. W. Albee, & S. S. Schneider (Eds.), *Primary prevention of AIDS: Psychological approaches* (pp. 93–110). Newbury Park: Sage.
Fishbein, M., Ajzen, I., & McArdle, J. (1980). Changing the behavior of alcoholics: Effects of persuasive communication. In I. Ajzen & M. Fishbein (Eds.), *Understanding attitudes and predicting social behavior*. Englewood Cliffs: Prentice-Hall.
Fishbein, M., Middlestadt, S. E., & Hitchcock, P. J. (1991). Using information to change sexually transmitted disease related behaviors: An analysis based on the theory of reasoned action. In J. N. Wasserheit, S. O. Aral, & K. K. Holmes (Eds.), *Research issues in human behavior change and sexually transmitted diseases in the AIDS era* (pp. 243–257). Washington, DC: American Society for Microbiology.
Fisher, J. D., & Fisher, W. A. (2002). The information-motivation-behavioral skills model. In R. J. DiClemente, R. A. Crosby, & M. C. Kegler (Eds.), *Emerging theories in health promotion practice and research: Strategies for improving public health* (pp. 40–70). San Francisco: Josey-Bass.
Fischhoff, B. (1999). Why (cancer) risk communication can be hard. *Journal of the National Cancer Institute Monographs, 25,* 7–13.
Fox, S. (2006). Online health search 2006. PEW Internet and American Life Project. http://www.pewinternet.org/pdfs/PIP_Online_Health_2006.pdf. Accessed 31 Aug 2007.

Frankel, R. (1990). Talking in interviews: A dispreference for patient initiated questions in physician- patient encounters. In G. Psathas (Ed.), *Interaction competence* (pp. 231–262). Lanham: University Press of America.
Geist-Martin, P., Ray, E. B., & Sharf, B. F. (2003). *Communicating health: Personal, cultural, and political complexities*. Belmont: Wadsworth.
Gielen, A. C., & McDonald, E. M. (2002). Using the precede-proceed planning model to apply health behavior theories. In K. Glanz, B. K. Rimer, & F. M. Lewis (Eds.), *Health behavior and health education: Theory, research, and practice* (3rd ed., pp. 409–436). San Francisco: Josey-Bass.
Giles, H., Coupland, N., & Wiemann, J. (Eds.). (1990). *Communication, health, and ageing*. Manchester: Manchester University Press.
Gill, E. A., & Babrow, A. S. (2007). To hope or to know: Coping with uncertainty and ambivalence in women's magazine breast cancer articles. *Journal of Applied Communication Research, 35,* 133–155.
Gillotti, C., Thompson, T., & McNeilis, K. (2002). Communicative competence in the delivery of bad news. *Social Science and Medicine, 54,* 1011–1023.
Gordon, A., Miller, G., Sparks, L., & Tedesco, J. (under contract). *Beyond tea parties and death panels: Understanding the rhetoric and reality of health care reform in the U.S.* Rowman & Littlefield.
Green, L. W., & Kreuter, M. W. (1999). *Health promotion planning: An educational and environmental approach* (2nd ed.). Mountain View: Mayfield.
Green, L. W., Kreuter, M. W., Deeds, S. G., & Partridge, K. B. (1980). *Health education planning: A diagnostic approach*. Mountain View: Mayfield.
Griffin, R. J., Neuwirth, K., & Dunwoody, S. (1995). Using the theory of reasoned action to examine the health impact of risk messages. *Communication Yearbook, 18,* 201–228.
Grimley, D. M., Riley, G. E., Bellis, J. M., & Prochaska, J. O. (1993). Assessing the stages of change and decision-making for contraceptive use for the prevention of pregnancy, sexually transmitted diseases, and acquired immunodeficiency syndrome. *Health Education Quarterly, 20,* 455–470.
Guldvog, B. (1999). Can patient satisfaction improve health among patients with angina pectoris? *International Journal for Quality in Health Care, 11*(3), 233–240.
Haider, M., & Kreps, G. L. (2004). Forty years of diffusion of innovations: Utility and value in public health. *Journal of Health Communication, 9,* 3–12.
Harwood, J., & Giles, H. (2005). *Intergroup communication: Multiple perspectives*. New York: Lang.
Harwood, J., & Sparks, L. (2003). Social identity and health: An intergroup communication approach to cancer. *Health Communication, 15,* 145–170.
Harzold, E., & Sparks, L. (2007). Adult child perceptions of communication and humor when the parent is diagnosed with cancer: A suggestive perspective from communication theory. *Qualitative Research Reports in Communication, 7,* 67–78.
Harzold, B., & Sparks, L. (2008). When the parent has cancer: A life span developmental approach to adult child perceptions of communication competency, humor orientation, and relational satisfaction in the older adult parent-adult child relationship. In L. Sparks, H. D. O'Hair, & G. L. Kreps (Eds.), *Cancer communication and aging* (pp. 215–235). Cresskill: Hampton Press.
Hummert, M. L., & Nussbaum, J. F. (Eds.). (2001). *Aging, communication, and health: Linking research and practice for successful aging*. Mahwah: Erlbaum.
Jackson, L., & Duffy, B. (1998). *Health communication research: A guide to developments and directions*. Westport: Greenwood Press.
Janis, I. L. (1967). Effects of fear arousal on attitude change: Recent developments in theory and experimental research. In L. Berkowitz (Ed.), *Advances in experimental social psychology* (Vol. 3, pp. 166–225). New York: Academic Press.
Janz, N. K., & Becker, M. H. (1984). The health belief model: A decade later. *Health Education Quarterly, 11,* 1–47.

Jones, C. M. (1997). "That's a good sign:" Encouraging assessments as a form of social support in medically related encounters. *Health Communication, 9,* 119–153.

Joseph, R. M., Sparks, L., & Robinson, J. D. (2010). Diabetes, foot health education and amputation prevention. *Health Communication, 25*(6), 607–608.

Kahneman, D., & Tversky, A. (1979). "Prospect theory:" An analysis of decision under risk. *Econometrica, 47,* 263–291.

Kahneman, D., & Tversky, A. (2000). *Choices, values, and frames*. Cambridge University Press.

Katapodi, M. C., Lee, K. A., Facione, N. C., & Dodd, M. J. (2004). Predictors of perceived breast cancer risk and the relation between perceived risk and breast cancer screening: A meta-analytic review. *Preventive Medicine, 38,* 388–403.

Kee, K., Mannucci, M., Sparks, L., & Struppa, D. C. (in press). Social groups, social media, and higher dimensional social structures: Towards a simplicial model of social aggregation for computational communication research. *Communication Quarterly*.

Kotler, P. (1984). Social marketing of health behavior. In L. W. Frederikson, L. J. Solomon, & K. A. Brehony (Eds.), *Marketing health behavior* (pp. 23–39). New York: Plenum Press.

Kotler, P., & Roberto, E. (1989). *Social marketing*. New York: Free Press.

Kreps, G. L. (1989). Setting the agenda for health communication research and development: Scholarship that can make a difference. *Health Communication, 1,* 11–15.

Kreps, G. L., & Sparks, L. (2008). Meeting the health literacy needs of vulnerable populations. *Patient Education and Counseling, 71*(3), 328–332.

Kreps, G. L., & Thornton, B. C. (1992). *Health communication: Theory and practice*. Prospect Heights: Waveland.

Kreps, G. L., Alibek, K., Bailey, C., Neuhauser, L., Rowan, K., & Sparks, L. (2005). Emergency/risk communication to promote public health and respond to biological threats. In M. Haider (Ed.), *Global public health communication: Challenges, perspectives, and strategies* (pp. 349–362). Sudbury: Jones and Bartlett Publishers.

Kreps, G. L., Neuhauser, L., Sparks, L., Villagran, M. (Eds.). (2008a). Translational community-based health communication interventions to promote cancer prevention and control for vulnerable audiences [Special Issue] *Patient Education and Counseling, 71*(3), 315–350.

Kreps, G. L., Neuhauser, L., Sparks, L., Villagran, M. (2008b). The power of community-based health communication interventions to promote cancer prevention and control for at-risk populations. *Patient Education and Counseling, 71*(3), 315–318.

Kreps, G. L., Sparks, L. & Villagran, M. (Eds.). (2010a). Editor's introduction: Communication education and health promotion. *Communication Education, 59*(3), 215–219.

Kreps, G. L., Sparks, L., & Villagran, M. (Eds.). (2010b). Communication education and health promotion. [Special Issue]. *Communication Education, 59*(3).

Kreuter, M. W., & Strecher, V. J. (1995). Changing inaccurate perceptions of health risk: Results from a randomized trial. *Health Psychology, 14,* 56–63.

Lantz, P. M., Stencil, D., Lippert, M. T., Beversdorf, S., & Jaros, L. (1995). Breast and cervical cancer screening in a low-income managed care sample: The efficacy of physician letters and phone calls. *American Journal of Public Health, 85,* 834–836.

Lasswell, H. D. (1948). The structure and function of communication in society. In L. Bryson (Ed.), *The communication of ideas*. New York: Institute for Religious and Social Studies.

Lefebvre, R. C., & Flora, J. A. (1988). Social marketing and public health intervention. *Health Education Quarterly, 15,* 299–315.

Leventhal, H. (1970). Findings and theory in the study of fear communications. In L. Berkowitz (Ed.), *Advances in experimental social psychology* (Vol. 5, pp. 119–186). New York: Academic Press.

Litwak, E. (1985). *Helping the elderly: The complementary rules of informal networks and formal systems*. New York: Guilford Press.

Litwak, E., & Meyer, H. (1966). A balanced theory of coordination between bureaucratic organizations and community primary groups. *Administrative Science Quarterly, 11,* 31–58.

Luszczynska, A., & Schwarzer, R. (2003). Planning and self-efficacy in the adoption and maintenance of breast self-examination: A longitudinal study on self-regulatory cognitions. *Psychology and Health, 18,* 93–108.

Madden, M., & Fox, S. (2006). Finding answers online in sickness and in health. http://pewinternet.com/~/media/Files/Reports/2006/PIP_Health_Decisions_2006.pdf.pdf. Accessed 31 Aug 2010.

Moorman, C., & Matulich, E. (1993). A model of consumers preventive health behaviors: The role of health motivation and health ability. *Journal of Consumer Research, 20,* 208–229.

Maibach, E. W., & Cotton, D. (1995). Moving people to behavior change: A staged social cognitive approach to message design. In E. W. Maibach & R. L. Parrott (Eds.), *Designing health messages: Approaches from communication theory and public health practice* (pp. 41–64). Newbury Park: Sage.

Maibach, E. W., Kreps, G. L., & Bonaguro, E. W. (1996). Developing strategic communication campaigns for HIV/AIDS prevention. In S. Ratzan (Ed.), *AIDS: Effective communication for the 90s* (pp. 15–35). Washington, DC: Taylor and Francis.

Marshall, A. A. (1993). Whose agenda is it anyway?: Training medical residents in patient-centered interviewing techniques. In E. B. Ray (Ed.), *Case studies in health communication* (pp. 15–30). Hillsdale: Erlbaum.

Meyer, G., & Dearing, J. W. (1996, Winter). Respecifying the social marketing model for unique populations. *Social Marketing Quarterly*, 44–52.

Meyerowitz, B. E., & Chaiken, S. (1987). The effect of message framing on breast self-examination attitudes, intentions, and behaviors. *Journal of Personality and Social Psychology, 52*(3), 500–511.

Mitchell, M. M. (2000). Motivated, but not able? The effects of positive and negative mood on persuasive message processing. *Communication Monographs, 67,* 215–225.

Mitchell, M. M., Brown, K. M., Morris Villagran, M., & Villagran, P. D. (2001). The effects of anger, sadness and happiness on persuasive message processing: A test of the negative state relief model. *Communication Monographs, 68,* 347–359.

Mirkiani Thompson, N., Bevan, J., & Sparks, L. (2011). Healthcare reform information-seeking: Relationships with uncertainty, undertainty discrepancy, and health self-efficacy. *Journal of Communication in Health Care, 5,* 56–66.

Mokros, H. B., & Deetz, S. (1996). What counts as real? A constitutive view of communication and the disenfranchised in the context of health. In E. B. Ray (Ed.), *Communication and the disenfranchised: Social health issues and implications* (pp. 29–44). Hillsdale: Erlbaum.

Mold, J. W. (1995). An alternative conceptualization of health and health care: Its implications for geriatrics and gerontology. *Educational Gerontology, 21,* 85–101.

Moyad, M. A. (2003). Bladder cancer prevention. Part I: What do I tell my patients about lifestyle changes and dietary supplements? *Current Opinion in Urology, 13,* 363–378.

Mullens, A. B., McCaul, K. D., Erickson, S. C., & Sandgren, A. K. (2004). Coping after cancer: Risk perceptions, worry, and health behaviors among colorectal cancer survivors. *Psycho-Oncology, 13,* 367–376.

National Cancer Institute. (1998, June). *How the public perceives, processes, and interprets risk information: Findings from focus group research* (Report No.: POS-T086). Bethesda: Office of Cancer Communications.

Nielsen-Bohlman, L. (2004). Understanding health literacy: Implications for medicine and public health. In J. G. Schwartzberg, J. B. VanGeest, & C. Wang (Eds.), (p. 253) Chicago: American Medical Association.

Norman, N. M., & Tedeschi, J. T. (1989). Self-presentation, reasoned action, and adolescents' decisions to smoke cigarettes. *Journal of Applied Social Psychology, 19,* 543–558.

Nussbaum, J. F. (1989). Directions for research within health communication. *Health Communication, 1,* 35–40.

Nussbaum, J. F., Bergstrom, M., & Sparks, L. (1996). The institutionalized elderly: Interactive implications of long-term care. In E. Ray (Ed.), *Communication and disenfranchisement: Social health issues and implications* (pp. 219–232). Mahwah: Erlbaum.

Nussbaum, J. F., Sparks, L., & Bergstrom, M. (1996). Elder care: Different paths within an extended American family. In E. Ray (Ed.), *Case studies in communication and disenfranchisement: Applications to social health issues* (pp. 99–108). Mahwah: Erlbaum.

Nussbaum, J. F., Pecchioni, L., Robinson, J. D., & Thompson, T. (2000). *Communication and aging* (2nd ed.). Mahwah: Erlbaum.

Nussbaum, J. F., Baringer, D., & Kundrat, A. (2003). Health, communication, and aging: Cancer and older adults. *Health Communication, 15,* 185–192.

O'Hair, H. D., & Sparks, L. (2008). Relational agency in life threatening illnesses. In K. Wright & S. D. Moore (Eds.), *Applied health communication* (pp. 271–289). Cresskill: Hampton Press.

O'Hair, H. D., Villagran, M. M., Wittenberg, E., Brown, K., Ferguson, M., Hall, H., et al. (2003). Cancer survivorship and agency model: Implications for patient choice, decision making, and influence. *Health Communication, 15,* 193–202.

O'Hair, H. D., Thompson, S., & Sparks, L. (2005). Negotiating cancer care through communication. In E. B. Ray (Ed.), *Health communication in practice: A case study approach* (pp. 81–94). Mahwah: Erlbaum.

O'Hair, H. D., Kreps, G. L., & Sparks, L. (2007a). Conceptualizing cancer care and communication. In H. D. O'Hair, L. Sparks, & G. L. Kreps (Eds.), *Handbook of communication and cancer care* (pp. 1–12). Cresskill: Hampton Press.

O'Hair, H. D., Sparks, L., & Kreps, G. L., (Eds.). (2007b). *Handbook of communication and cancer care*. Cresskill: Hampton Press.

Oldenburg, B., & Parcel, G. S. (2002). Diffusion of innovations. In K. Glanz, B. K. Rimer, & F. M. Lewis (Eds.), *Health behavior and health education: Theory, research, and practice* (3rd ed., pp. 312–334). San Francisco: Josey-Bass.

Pascoe, G. C. (1983). Patient satisfaction in primary health care: A literature review and analysis. *Evaluation and program planning, 6,* 185–210.

Park, C. W., & Mittal. B. (1985). A theory of involvement in consumer behavior: Problems and issues. In J. N. Seth (Ed.), *Research in consumer behavior* (Vol. 1, pp. 201–231). Greenwich: JAI Press. http://faculty.washington.edu/tlumley/survey of the R statistical software platform version 2.11.1 http://www.r-project.org.

Parker, R. M., Ratzan, S. C., & Lurie, N. (2003). Health literacy: A policy challenge for advancing high-quality health care. *Health Affairs, 22*(4), 147–153.

Parrott, R. (Ed.). (2004a). Religious faith, spirituality, and health communication [Special Issue]. *Health Communication, 16*(1), 1–130.

Parrott, R. (2004b). Emphasizing "communication" in health communication. *Journal of Communication, 54,* 751–757.

Patterson, R., Neuhouser, M., & Hedderson, M. (2003). Cancer survivor's lifestyle changes. *Nutrition Research Newsletter, 22,* 5–6.

Pecchioni, L., & Sparks, L. (2007). Health information sources of individuals with cancer and their family members. *Health Communication, 21,* 143–151.

Pecchioni, L., Ota, H., & Sparks, L. (2004). Cultural issues in communication and aging. In J. F. Nussbaum & J. Coupland (Eds.), *Handbook of communication and aging research* (pp. 167–207). Mahwah: Erlbaum.

Pecchioni, L., Krieger, J. C., Sparks, L., Pitts, M., & Ota, H. (2008). Investigating cancer and ageing from a cultural perspective. In L. Sparks, H. D. O'Hair, & G. L. Kreps (Eds.), *Cancer communication and aging* (pp. 239–257). Cresskill: Hampton Press.

Petty, R. E., Barden, J., & Wheeler, C. M. (2002). The elaboration likelihood model of persuasion: Health promotions that yield sustained behavioral change. In R. J. DiClemente, R. A. Crosby, & M. C. Kegler (Eds.), *Emerging theories in health promotion practice and research: Strategies for improving public health* (pp. 71–99). San Francisco: Josey-Bass.

Pomerantz, A. M., Fehr, B. J., & Ende, J. (1997). When supervising physicians see patients: Strategies used in difficult situations. *Human Communication Research, 23*(4), 589–615.

Prochaska, J. O., DiClemente, C. C., & Norcross, J. C. (1992). In search of how people change. *American Psychologist, 47,* 1102–1114.

Query, J. L., & Wright, K. B. (2003). Assessing communication competence in an online study: Toward informing subsequent interventions among older adults with cancer, their lay caregivers, and peers. *Health Communication, 15,* 203–218.

Ragan, S. L., & Glenn, L. D. (1990). Communication and gynecologic health care. In H. D. O'Hair & G. Kreps (eds.), *Applied communication theory and research* (pp. 313–330). Hillsdale: Erlbaum.

Rakovski, C., Sparks, L., Robinson, J. D., Kee, K., Bevan, J., & Agne, R. (2012). A regression-based study using jackknife replicates of HINTS III data: Predictors of the efficacy of health information seeking. *Journal of Communication in Healthcare*.
Ratzan, S. (Ed.). (1994). Health communication: Challenges for the 21st century. *American Behavioral Scientist, 38*(2), 197–380.
Robinson, J. D. (1998). Getting down to business: Talk, gaze, and body orientation during openings of doctor-patient consultations. *Human Communication Research, 25,* 97–123.
Robinson, J. D., & Stivers, T. (2001). Achieving activity transitions in primary-care encounters: From history taking to physical examination. *Human Communication Research, 27,* 253–298.
Robinson, J. D., & Turner, J. (2003). Impersonal, interpersonal, and hyperpersonal social support: Cancer and older adults. *Health Communication, 15,* 227–234.
Rogers, E. M. (1995). *Diffusion of innovations* (4th ed.). New York: Free Press.
Rogers, E. M. (2003). *Diffusion of innovations* (5th ed.). New York: Free Press.
Rogers, E. M. (2004). A prospective and retrospective look at the diffusion model. *Journal of Health Communication, 9,* 13–20.
Rogers, R. W. (1975). A protection motivation theory of fear appeals and attitude change. *Journal of Psychology, 91,* 93–114.
Rogers, R. W. (1983). Cognitive and physiological processes in fear appeals and attitude change: A revised theory of protection motivation. In J. Cacioppo & R. Petty (Eds.), *Social psychophysiology* (pp. 153–176). New York: Guilford.
Rook, K. (1995). Support, companionship, and control in older adults' social networks: Implications for well-being. In J. F. Nussbaum & J. Coupland (Eds.), *Handbook of communication and aging research* (pp. 437–463). Mahwah: Erlbaum.
Rosenstock, I. M. (1974). Historical origins of the health belief model. *Health Education Monographs, 2,* 328–335.
Roter, D. L., & Hall, J. A. (1992). *Doctors talking with patients/Patients talking with doctors*. Westport: Auburn House.
Rothman, A. J., Salovey, P., Antone, C., Keough, K., & Martin, C. D. (1993). The influence of message framing on intentions to perform health behaviors. *Journal of Experimental Social Psychology, 29*(5), 408.
Rowan, K. E. (2000). Mass media explanations of illness: The problem-solving perspective. In B. B. Whaley (Eds.), *Explaining illness: Theory, research, and applications* (pp. 69–100). Mahwah: Erlbaum.
Rowan, K. E. (2003). Informing and explaining skills: Theory and research on informative communication. In J. O. Greene & B. R. Burleson (Eds.), *The handbook of communication and social interaction skills* (pp. 403–438). Mahwah: Erlbaum.
Rowan, K. E. (2004). *Risk and crisis communication: Earning trust and productive partnering with media and public during emergencies*. Washington, DC: Consortium of Social Science Associations.
Rowan, K., Sparks, L., Pecchioni, L., & Villagran, M. (2003). The CAUSE model: A research supported aid for physicians communicating about cancer risk. *Health Communication, 15,* 239–252.
Rowan, K. E., Kreps, G. L., Botan, C. H., Sparks, L., Samoilenko, S., & Bailey, C. (2008). Responding to terrorism: Risk communication, crisis communication, and the CAUSE model. In H. D. O'Hair, R. L. Heath, K. J. Ayotte, & G. R. Ledlow (Eds.), *Terrorism: Communication and rhetorical perspectives*. Cresskill: Hampton Press.
Sandman, P. M. (1993). *Responding to community outrage: Strategies for effective risk communication*. Fairfax: American Industrial Hygiene Association.
Sarason, B. R., Sarason, I. G., & Garung, R. A. F. (1997). Close personal relationships and health outcomes: A key to the role of social support. In S. Duck (Ed.), *Handbook of personal relationships* (2nd ed., pp. 547–573). New York: Wiley.
Sass, J. S. (2000). Emotional labor as cultural performance: The communication of caregiving in a nonprofit nursing home. *Western Journal of Communication, 64*(3), 330–358.
Sharf, B. F., & Street, R. L. (1997). The patient as a central construct: Shifting the emphasis. *Health Communication, 9*(1), 1–11.

Sillars, A., Roberts, L. J., Leonard, K. E., & Dun, T. (2000). Cognition during marital conflict: The relationship of thought and talk. *Journal of Social and Personal Relationships, 17,* 479–502.
Smith-duPré, A., & Beck, C. S. (1996). Enabling patients and physicians to pursue multiple goals in health care encounters: A case study. *Health Communication, 8,* 73–90.
Sparks, L. (2003a). An introduction to cancer communication and aging: Theoretical and research insights. *Health Communication, 15,* 123–132.
Sparks, L. (Ed.). (2003b). Cancer communication and aging [Special Issue]. *Health Communication, 15*(2), 123–258.
Sparks, L. (2007). Cancer care and the aging patient: Complexities of age-related communication barriers. In H. D. O'Hair, L. Sparks & G. L. Kreps (Eds.), *Handbook of communication and cancer care* (pp. 233–249). Cresskill: Hampton Press.
Sparks, L. (2008). Family decision-making. In W. Donsbach (Ed.) The *International Encyclopedia of Communication, 4,* (pp. 1729–1733). Oxford: Wiley-Blackwell.
Sparks, L. (2011). Health messages and decision-making. TED talk on health message framing and decision-making at TEDx Orange Coast. http://www.youtube.com/watch?v=d4JNyyuonko. Accessed 9 July 2012.
Sparks, L., & Harwood, J. (2008). Cancer, aging, and social identity: Development of an integrated model of social identity theory and health communication. In L. Sparks, H. D. O'Hair, & G. L. Kreps (Eds.), *Cancer communication and aging* (pp. 77–95). Cresskill: Hampton Press.
Sparks, L., & Hill, L. B. (2005). Personal relationships across the lifespan: A suggestive perspective from communication theory. *Intercultural Communication Studies, XIV,* 158–171.
Sparks, L., & Mittapalli, K. (2004). To know or not to know: The case of communication by and with older adult Russians diagnosed with cancer. *Journal of Cross Cultural Gerontology, 19,* 383–403.
Sparks, L., & Nussbaum, J. F. (2008). Health literacy and cancer communication with older adults. *Patient Education and Counseling, 71*(3), 345–350.
Sparks, L., & Turner, M. M. (2008). Cognitive and emotional processing of cancer messages and information seeking with older adults. In L. Sparks, H. D. O'Hair, & G. L. Kreps (Eds.), *Cancer communication and aging* (pp. 17–45). Cresskill: Hampton Press.
Sparks, L., & Villagran, M. (2010). *Patient and provider interaction: A global health communication perspective.* Cambridge: Polity Press.
Sparks, L., Travis, S. S., & Thompson, S. (2005). Listening for the communicative signals of humor, narratives, and self-disclosure in the family caregiving interview. *Health and Social Work, 30,* 340–343.
Sparks, L., O'Hair, H. D., & Kreps, G. L. (Eds.). (2008a). *Cancer communication and aging.* Cresskill: Hampton Press.
Sparks, L., O'Hair, H. D. & Kreps, G. L. (2008b). Cancer communication and aging: An introduction. In L. Sparks, H. D. O'Hair, & G. L. Kreps (Eds.), *Cancer communication and aging* (pp. 1–14). Cresskill: Hampton Press.
Sparks, L., Hershman, D., Neugut, A., Hillyer, G. (2012a). Reducing health disparities through evidence in action from cells to society: Co-creating text health messages to improve patient adherence to adjuvant hormonal therapy. In B. Whaley (Ed.) *Health Methods.*
Sparks, L., Bevan, J. & Rogers, K. (2012b). An intergroup communication approach to understanding the function of compliance, outgroup typicality, and honest explanations in distant caregiving relationships from an intergroup approach: Validation of a health care communication scale. *Journal of Communication in Healthcare, 5,* 12–22.
Sparks-Bethea, L. (2001). The function of humor within the lives of older adults. *Qualitative Research Reports in Communication, 2,* 49–56.
Sparks-Bethea, L. (2002). The impact of an older adult parent on communicative satisfaction and dyadic adjustment in the long-term marital relationship: Adult children and spouses' retrospective accounts. *Journal of Applied Communication Research, 30,* 107–125.
Sparks-Bethea, L. S., Travis, S. S., & Pecchioni, L. (2000). Family caregivers' use of humor in conveying information about caring for dependent older adults. *Health Communication, 12,* 361–376.

Suchman, A., Markakis, K., Beckman, H. B., & Frankel, R. (1997). A model of empathic communication in the medical interview. *Journal of the American Medical Association, 277,* 678–682.
Tajfel, H., & Turner, J. C. (1986). The social identity theory of intergroup behavior. In S. Worschel & W. G. Austin (Eds.), *The social psychology of intergroup relations* (2nd ed., pp. 7–24). Chicago: Nelson-Hall.
Thompson, T. L. (1984). The invisible helping hand: The role of communication in the health and social service professions. *Communication Quarterly, 32*(2), 148–163.
Thompson, T. L. (2000). The nature and language of illness explanations. In B. B. Whaley (Ed.), *Explaining illness: Research, theory, and strategies* (pp. 3–40). Mahwah: Erlbaum.
Thompson, S. C., Armstrong, W., & Thomas, C. (1998). Illusions of control, underestimation, and accuracy: A control psychological explanation. *Psychological Bulletin, 123,* 143–161.
Thompson, T. L., Dorsey, A. M., Miller, K. I., & Parrott, R. (Eds.). (2003). *Handbook of health communication.* Mahwah: Erlbaum.
Travis, S. S., & Bethea (Sparks), L. (2001). Medication administration by family members of dependent elders in shared care arrangements. *Journal of Clinical Geropsychology*, *7*(3), 231–243. Project Supported by a Grant from the Nursing Research Program, Clinical Applications Research, Glaxo-Wellcome, Inc.
Tversky, A., & Kahneman, D. (1981). The framing of decisions and the psychology of choice. *Science, 211,* 453–458.
U.S. Department of Health & Human Services. (2000). *Healthy people 2010.* Atlanta: CDC. http://www.healthypeople.gov/. Accessed 30 Sept 2005.
Vanderford, M., Jenks, E., & Sharf, B. (1997). Exploring patients' experiences as a primary source of meaning. *Health Communication, 9*(1), 13–26.
Vanlandingham, M. J., Suprasert, S., Grandjean, N., & Sittitrai, W. (1995). Two views of risky sexual practices among northern Thai males: The health belief model and the theory of reasoned action. *Journal of Health and Social Behavior, 36,* 195–212.
Villagran, M. M., & Sparks, L. (2010). Social identity and health contexts. In H. Giles, S. Reid, & J. Harwood (Eds.), *The dynamics of intergroup communication* (pp. 235–248). New York: Lang.
Villagran, M. M., Weathers, M., Keefe, B., & Sparks, L. (2010). Medical providers as global warming and climate change health educators: A health literacy approach. *Communication Education, 59*(3), 312–327.
Wanzer, M., Sparks, L., & Frymier, A. B. (2009). Humorous communication within the lives of older adults: The relationships among humor, coping efficacy, age, and life satisfaction. *Health Communication, 24,* 1–9.
Wallack, L. (1989). Mass communication and health promotion: A critical perspective. In R. E. Rice & C. K. Atkin (Eds.), *Public communication campaigns* (2nd. ed., pp. 353–367). Newbury Park: Sage.
Weinstein, N.D. (1988). The precaution adoption process. *Health psychology, 7,* 355–386.
Weinstein, N. D. (1999). What does it mean to understand a risk? Evaluating risk comprehension. *Journal of the National Cancer Institute Monographs, 25,* 15–20.
Weinstein, N. D., & Sandman, P. M. (2002). The precaution adoption process model. In K. Glanz, B. K. Rimer, & F. M. Lewis (Eds.), *Health behavior and health education: Theory, research, and practice* (3rd ed., pp. 121–143). San Francisco: Jossey-Bass.
Weinstein, N. D., Rothman, A., & Sutton, S. (1998). Stage theories of health behavior. *Health Psychology, 17,* 290–299.
Whaley, B. B. (Ed.). (2000). *Explaining illness: Research, theory, and strategies.* Mahwah: Erlbaum.
Whelan, T., Levine, M., Willan, A., Gafni, A., Sanders, K., Mirsky, D., et al. (2004). Effect of a decision aid on knowledge and treatment decision making for breast cancer surgery. *Journal of the American Medical Association, 292,* 435–441.
Witte, K. (1992a). Putting the fear back into fear appeals: The extended parallel process model. *Communication Monographs, 59,* 329–349.

Witte, K. (1992b). Preventing AIDS through persuasive communications: A framework for constructing effective, culturally-specific, preventive health messages. *International and Intercultural Communication Annual, 16,* 67–86.

Witte, K. (1994). Generating effective risk messages: How scary should your risk communication be? *Communication Yearbook, 18,* 229–254.

Witte, K. (1998). Fear as motivator, fear as inhibitor: Using the extended parallel process model to explain fear appeal successes and failures. In P. A. Andersen & L. K. Guerrero (Eds.), *Communication and emotion: Theory, research, and applications* (pp. 424–451). Burlington: Academic Press.

Witte, K., Peterson, T. R., Vallabhan, S., Stephenson, M. T., Plugge, C. D., Givens, V. K., et al. (1993). Preventing tractor-related injuries and deaths in rural populations: Using a Persuasive Health Message (PHM) framework in formative evaluation research. *International Quarterly of Community Health Education, 13,* 219–251.

Witte, K., Stokols, D., Ituarte, P., & Schneider, M. (1993). Testing the health belief model in a field study to promote bicycle safety helmets. *Communication Research, 20,* 564–586.

Witte, K., Meyer, G., & Martell, D. (2001). *Effective health risk messages.* Thousand Oaks: Sage.

Wright, K. B., Sparks, L., & O'Hair, H. D. (2013). *Health communication in the 21st century* (2nd ed.). Oxford: Blackwell.

Zhao, X., Villagran, M. M., Kreps, G. L., & McHorney, C. (2011). Gain versus loss framing in adherence-promoting communication targeting patients with chronic diseases: The moderating effect of individual time perspective. *Health Communication,* DOI:10.1080/10410236.2011.569002

An Anthropology of Caregiving

Frances K. Barg, Shimrit Keddem, Wendy Shiekman Cohen and Rebecca Henderson

Anthropology is a lens through which we might understand the diversity of issues inherent in the ways that contemporary humans care for one another. The anthropology of caregiving provides an understanding of the range of behaviors, perceptions, and feelings associated with providing care for another person. Culture, a concept central to anthropology, comprises the implicit and explicit set of assumptions, behavioral guidelines, and interconnected beliefs that are shared by members of a society (Helman 2001). Culture shapes both the experience of illness and that of giving care, and informs the ways that these roles are perceived by others. Illness behaviors are often linked to social factors, gender norms, ethnic factors, and politics, as well as differences in philosophies, cultures, and in socioeconomic status (Brown and Barrett 2009). This chapter will explore fundamental concepts from medical anthropology and describe their contributions to our understanding of caregiving.

Humans have been caregivers since prehistoric times. There is archaeological evidence that early modern humans cared for aging and ill members of their groups. Archaeologists have found remains of humans who lived with significant disability during their lifetime, requiring the attention of a caregiving individual to enable them to sustain life (Hublin 2009).

F. K. Barg (✉)
Department of Family Medicine and Community Health,
University of Pennsylvania School of Medicine,
141-2 Anatomy and Chemistry, 3620 Hamilton Walk,
Philadelphia, PA 19104 , USA
e-mail: Fran.Barg@uphs.upenn.edu

S. Keddem
University of Pennsylvania, Philadelphia, USA

W. S. Cohen
Accenture, Philadelphia, USA

R. Henderson
Philadelphia, USA

R. C. Talley, S. S. Travis (eds.), *Multidisciplinary Coordinated Caregiving,*
Caregiving: Research • Practice • Policy, DOI 10.1007/978-1-4614-8973-3_9,

Introduction: Medical Anthropology

Background and Current Status of Medical Anthropology

Medical anthropology is a subdiscipline within anthropology that addresses the interrelationships among health, illness, culture, and the environment (Brown and Barrett 2009). Medical anthropology views illness as socially, culturally, and linguistically constructed, rather than as a strictly biological entity. Illness itself is defined and labeled through language, and these definitions create a culturally mediated "symbolic reality" in which language and cultural symbols structure and shape experience (Kleinman 1973). Further, meanings and experiences of illness are constructed differently in the context of each particular culture, and these meanings are passed from adults to children and through social networks. (Brown and Barrett 2009). The illness experience is shaped by many factors: social realities of illness, gender hierarchies, ethnic relations, politics and philosophy of the culture, and socioeconomic class.

Medical anthropologists question the ways that knowledge about biomedicine is produced, and investigate the ways that power, politics, and economic factors affect and are affected by interaction with biomedicine. The use of anthropologic theory, along with selected items from the anthropologist's toolkit can aid in gaining a more complete, multifaceted, and nuanced understanding of the caregiving process. As Hinton et al. (1999) note, an anthropological approach to caregiving helps to highlight ways that history, macrosocial and microsocial forces interact with family and individual factors to yield an enriched understanding of providing care to aging and/or ill family members.

Major Anthropological Concepts of Health and Illness in the United States

Ethnomedical studies in anthropology look at ways that culture informs beliefs about illness and the delivery of medical care. Culture influences careseeking, symptom recognition, treatment, and perceptions about what constitutes illness and what constitutes an illness problem. Sontag (1989) has written about ways that metaphors used to describe illness, such as the "war on cancer", reveal the underlying ideas that Americans have about illness. In the USA, disease is often referred to in terms of economics, using capitalistic terms such as "spending, consumption, wasting, and squandering vitality." Likewise, through science-fiction metaphors, cancer is perceived as the ultimate mutation, "a disease of the Other." It is alien, possessing a strange kind of fierce energy. Cancer cells are "chaotic" growing ceaselessly out of control (Sontag).

Use of warfare metaphors in relation to disease is also common. In the twentieth century, people began to describe bacteria as "invading" or "infiltrating" the human body. Treatment has often been described as aiming to "bombard," "kill," or "destroy." Americans make reference to the body's "defenses" and their ability or inability to cope with the disease (Sontag 1989). Establishing the National Cancer Act of 1971, Nixon promised to "conquer" cancer. There is also the notion of the "fight" against cancer or the idea that cancer is a "killer" disease. Those who have cancer have been considered "victims" (Payer 1996; Sontag 1989).

Payer asserts that doctors in the USA adhere to the battle notion in their fight against disease. Regardless of the medical condition, doctors in the USA have tended to use aggressive tactics. "Americans not only want to *do* something, they want to do it fast and if they cannot, they often become frustrated" (Payer 1996). While some Americans are reluctant to broaden health concepts beyond those currently recognized by science and technology, others seem to be enveloped by a "biotechnological embrace," in which hope is embodied by an ever-evolving high-technology medicine (DelVeccio Good 2010). Americans look for technical solutions to medical problems. They pursue risky experimental treatment plans and choose life-extending mechanical devices in pursuit of medical "rescue" and increasingly view death as a failure (Chapple 2010). This ethos of aggression can place caregivers and their families in a position where they are tempted to "do everything."

Medical Pluralism

Family perceptions of health and health care often reflect the culture in which they are situated. While the biomedical perspective may seem ubiquitous in Western culture, cultural ideas are not homogenous, and many other perspectives exist within a single society. While many families have health beliefs that are congruent with the dominant biomedical model of health and illness, many other healing traditions have survived in parallel alongside biomedical systems (Baer et al. 2004). This concept, known as medical pluralism, refers to the notion that there are often multiple, sometimes competing, medical systems in operation at one time in any given culture.

Concepts of indigenous and Western medicine are grounded in an interaction between knowledge and belief. While "knowledge" is the understanding of a truth or fact, "belief" is the conviction that this fact is true (Good 1994; O'Connor 1995). In our society, science is considered to have "clarity of viewpoint" and "rigor of method" that transcend cultural values and interest-group bias. For the most part, however, the general public pursues scientific information but does not rely on it as a means of confirming all knowledge (O'Connor 1995). Quite often, they do not have absolute trust in scientific data. Thus, knowledge of health and medicine is "context-dependent" based on social, political, and cultural belief systems.

It is a combination of attitudes toward health and illness and personal theories about the origins and remediation of disease that guide health seeking behavior. Many studies have shown that despite having sufficient access to and knowledge of biomedical services, people continue to utilize alternative healing methods. Helman (2001) discusses this trend of medical pluralism in modern, urbanized societies: "Besides official healthcare systems, which include the medical and nursing professions, there are usually smaller, alternative systems such as homeopathy, herbalism, and spiritual healing in many Western countries." In many instances, one set of highly traditional health beliefs and practices coexist with biomedical beliefs and practices.

There are also several barriers to using biomedicine. In remote locations, where access to services and facilities is limited, people are sometimes forced or persuaded to use nonconventional healing resources. Moreover, financial restriction may restrict health care options (Strathern and Stewart 1999).

Caregiving, Culture, and Identity

What is Caregiving?

What do we mean when we talk about caregiving? While at the surface the answer to this question seems self-evident, caregiving has a number of different meanings in different cultures and contexts. As Grant et al. (2004) point out, there is clearly a difference between "caring for" and "caring about." Questions about the meaning of caregiving include: Who should care for whom? What activities constitute care? Who are ideal caregivers? What role does technology play in care? And the extent to which care is an ethical obligation in society. We can think about care as a product of loving relationships, as a commodity in an industry of service providers, or as a part of social services or a governmental policy. The cultural ideas surrounding caregiving are clearly of primary importance in any society. Biomedical anthropologists tend to emphasize the meaning that care is given by those intimately involved in caregiving. In examining caregiving through the perspectives of those who enact it, anthropologists hope to gain an understanding of the fundamental cultural concepts at work.

Family Concepts of Caregiving

When we talk about caregiving, what are we talking about? There is no universal notion of caregiving. Not all families conceptualize caregiving in the same way. Nor do caregivers all perform the same level or type of duties. When family caregivers begin caregiving, they rarely have a clear idea about the full responsibilities they ultimately assume. They are also rarely prepared for these responsibilities. Frequently, they start by providing some degree of assistance such as transportation, shopping, hygiene, dressing, or nourishment (Montgomery and Kosloski 2009). Gradually, caregivers take on more and more tasks until they have the full responsibility of caring for a loved one. Studies have shown that caregiving entails more than just assistance for functional limitations (Wright 1997).

In the past, caregiving tasks were defined in terms of help with Activities of Daily Living (ADLs). However, evaluation of the necessities associated with ADLs provides only a limited understanding of caregiver demands (Albert 1991). Clearly, caregiving involves far more than the activities that make up the ADLs, and a myriad of other duties have been identified by caregivers. Some examples include "just being with Mother" or "having to encourage her to do things" (Albert 1991). These duties represent activities that are important to the family members who experience caregiving every day, rather than activities that are important from a strictly biomedical perspective. Researchers frequently define caregiving from the viewpoint of service needs rather than the caregiver's perception and their definitions may not mirror the ideas of those who are actually providing care.

In Albert's investigation of caregivers' cognition of various tasks, the most salient tasks were bathing, dressing, cooking, providing medicine, helping to use the toilet, shopping, going to the doctor, and getting elders up (Albert 1991). Caregivers tended to categorize tasks based on type of impairment, location of caregiving, and patient competency. Type of impairment was divided into either physical or cognitive-emotional. Thirty percent of respondents used the description "physical care" while 18 % used the classification "handling a parent's emotional needs." ADL tasks such as bed, toilet, mobility, dress, meals, and look good were differentiated from IADL (Instrumental Activities of Daily living), such as doctor, medication, feeding, simple tasks, and phone (Albert 1991).

Just as caregiving activities differ when described by caregivers instead of medical professionals, so too do family-centered measures of caregiving successes. Schumacher et al. (2000) attempted to gauge qualities of success in family caregiving skill in nine key processes: monitoring, interpreting, making decisions, taking action, making adjustments, providing hands-on care, accessing resources, working together with the ill person, and negotiating the health care system. They found that family caregivers succeeded when they were able to utilize previously developed skills alongside new ones. Family caregivers felt that the most successful care was tailored to the personalities of each individual, and evolved and developed with time and experience (Schumacher et al. 2000). Success in family caregiving goes beyond following medical instructions, and includes domains outside those defined by a hospital or nursing home.

Becoming a Caregiver

Caregiving is a role that many people assume willingly. However, most caregivers are unprepared for the many tasks that await them (Barg et al. 1998). Furthermore, because so much of caregiving takes place in isolation, caregivers have few role models from whom to learn. How do caregivers learn about managing the instrumental tasks, the emotions, the role changes, and the tangible requirements of caregiving? Many caregivers learn about the values related to caregiving from the greater values present in a culture. Several resources are available for lay caregivers for more tangible and explicit types of guidance. They address the impact of caregiving with an aim to educate caregivers about the emotional, physical, professional, financial, and cultural implications of care. Because caregivers must often give up their lifestyle, their job, and their social life in order to care for a loved one, these resources portray caregiving as a life altering task.

The emotional impact a caregiver endures is described as colored by a myriad of feelings. The many changes in caregivers' lives create a paradox of emotions (Cheung and Hocking 2004). A sense of loss is often paired with a feeling of reward, a feeling of restriction is coupled with a sense of authority, and helplessness is contrasted by strength. Health professionals frequently assume that the caregiver is unhappy when in reality there are many positive emotions associated with caregiving.

It is very common for caregivers to experience depression and anxiety (Carretero et al. 2009). Books and websites for caregivers normalize these emotions. Frequently, caregivers feel sadness and anger for the loss of their former life. Sometimes they feel angry and resentful at having to care for someone who may have wronged them in the past. They feel angry at being trapped in a hopeless situation. On the other hand, many caregivers describe the act of caring in terms of a duty that is owed to their loved one. This may produce feelings of guilt and an irrational sense of responsibility. In addition, caregivers are often worried about impending change in a loved one's condition or, even worse, a lack of change.

Some books describe the positive sentiments that caregivers express. They feel a sense of pride and accomplishment for being able to achieve and persevere through some of the onerous tasks of caring. In fact, many caregivers must learn new skills such as administering medication or monitoring feeding tubes. Proficiency in these tasks gives caregivers confidence and a sense of accomplishment. They also feel grateful for having the opportunity to reciprocate care and support to a loved one. This is a rewarding experience that gives many individuals a sense of purpose. For example, many studies of older male caregivers have shown that men take a great deal of satisfaction and pride in their new roles as "capable and competent carers" (Russell 2001). Caregivers who are able to find meaning in their caregiving activities and identities report lower levels of depression and higher self-esteem (Noonan and Tennstedt 1997).

Facing illness, a family member's role is transformed. As caregivers, family members become "advocates, providers, trusted companions, and decision makers" (Levine 1999). They feel that they must speak for the patient especially when the patient is too cognitively impaired to express themselves. As providers, they clean, feed, and medicate loved ones. Family members become even more intimately involved in their loved one's life because they are participating in their illness and sometimes their death. This role transformation is usually not a smooth, continuous process, but may be characterized by periods of stability and dramatic shifts in identity due to changes in the caregiving context (Montgomery and Kosloski 2009).

Not only is the caregiver's role dramatically altered, but their relationship with the patient is also changed. A husband caring for a debilitated spouse may find that he no longer sees her as an intimate partner, but more as a child (Hayes et al. 2009). On the other hand, a child taking care of a parent must transform from the submissive role of a child to the authoritative role of a parent. Changing a parent's identity also affects the identity of the child- "the predictable mother-daughter pattern of interaction, reciprocity, and occupation of the past has been disrupted, as has that aspect of the caregiver's biographical self that was embedded in the shared identity" of daughter and mother (Hasselkus and Murray 2007). Thus, in the context of caregiving, the roles that are so deeply ingrained in family and tradition may become vague and altogether changed.

Communicating with the Doctor

Misinterpretation and miscommunication are common in doctor–patient–family interactions. Physicians may not be aware of patient and family perceptions of illness, and may communicate in different ways with different patients, particularly if they are from different ethnic backgrounds, from an older or younger generation, or a different gender (Bertakis 2009; Ferguson and Candib 2005). Some studies have found that patients from minority groups, especially those that do not speak English, receive less empathy and less information from physicians (Ferguson and Candib 2005). Therefore, health professionals would benefit from situating the patient and family into a broader social and cultural context (Helman 2001). Both doctor and patient are limited by their personal history including "education, social ties, and class aspects of culture" (Strathern and Stewart 1999).

Furthermore, the power differential between patients and their doctors sometimes serves to limit the free flow of information (Ainsworth-Vaughan 1998). For example, physicians communicate differently with patients and caregivers of differing socioeconomic classes, imparting more information and allowing more involvement when patients are of a higher class (Willems et al. 2005). The presence of caregivers also affects the doctor–patient interaction, as doctors can sometimes see a caregiver as a "hidden patient" with separate needs to be considered (Flocke et al. 1998).The caregiver's ability to remember information may also be compromised by stress and memory loss. In a study of the needs of cancer and patients and their main caregivers, Soothill et al. (2001) found that caregivers and patients stressed the importance of having good relationships with health care providers and receiving reliable information.

Culture Informs Ideas of Illness and Caregiving

Cultural values are linked to caregiving in many ways. Culture influences views on illness and aging, and may create profound differences in the ways that families identify illness in loved ones, plan a course of care, and find meaning in caregiving. Individuals from different cultural backgrounds may view the same illness in entirely disparate ways. Culture informs the ways families understand the causes of their loved ones' illness, its severity, and its status in society.

For example, illnesses like dementia and Alzheimer's disease require intensive caregiving from their earliest stages. Loved ones are often the first to recognize the changes in behavior that lead to the need for lifelong care, and a majority of Alzheimer's sufferers receive care at home from family and friends (National Academy on an Aging Society 2000). However, initial symptoms are not always clear-cut, and family members must appraise behaviors and decide on the appropriate course of action to best care for their loved one. This symptom appraisal and care planning is based not only on family's knowledge and access to resources but also on cultural beliefs.

Many Asian cultures view symptoms of Alzheimer's and dementia as normal features of the aging process, and thus as unalarming and not worthy of medical investigation (Yeo et al. 2002) The idea that an aging mind is normally more forgetful, and that this forgetfulness is not necessarily a medical problem, can cause some Chinese families to have higher threshold for concern and thus a later diagnosis of Alzheimer's or dementia (Hsia-Rei Hicks and Sau-Ching Lam 1999). Contrastingly, some studies find that Latino families do not see these illnesses as a normal part of aging, but instead associate the onset of dementia with a sadness, loss, or trauma. The negative emotions of this trauma were seen by caregivers as an important cause of dementia (Hinton and Levkoff 1999; Karlawish et al. 2011).

Cultural explanations can also cause increased stigmatization. Although dementia may be seen as a normal part of aging, in some Chinese and Vietnamese families, chronic mental illness can be associated with a moral failure, either on the part of the individual, or the family, through a failure of filial obligations (Dilworth-Anderson and Gibson 2002; Liu et al. 2008). Several studies have shown that some Chinese and Chinese-American caregivers may attempt to hide dementia symptoms in order to avoid societal stigmatization (Mahoney et al. 2005; Hinton and Levkoff 1999). These findings correlate with studies of Chinese caregivers of individuals with other chronic mental illnesses such as schizophrenia (Ryder et al. 2000). The perception of mental illness as a source of familial shame profoundly changes the experience of caregiving for these family members.

Similarly, in Japan, senility or *boke* is associated with a loss of engagement in mental, physical, and social activities. Continued participation in these activities through personal effort is seen as crucial to remaining mentally alert. The onset of dementia or Alzheimer's disease can thus be seen as resulting in this case from a personal moral failure in which the individual becomes disengaged from both the mental and social worlds. In this way, older individuals are perceived as a societal "burden" engaging in fundamentally antisocial behavior (Henderson and Traphagan 2005).

Yet while these illnesses may be stigmatized in some cultures, one study of American Indians has found that aspects of dementia could come to be categorized positively. For these individuals, the hallucinations associated with dementia provided a "supernormal" connection with the afterlife that should be respected for its ability to provide a "window to the unknown" (Henderson and Henderson 2002).

Cultural definitions can profoundly change the ways that family members and caregivers experience the progression of illness. In their cross-cultural study of dementia and caregiving, Hinton et al. (1999) note that while African-American and

Irish-American caregivers equated dementia with a loss of self or identity, Chinese-American caregivers reported the experience mostly in terms of obligations of care and changing social roles.

Cultural ideas about dementia, aging, and illness clearly shape the experiences of caregivers, impacting their experiences of diagnosis and illness progression by giving dementia meaning. Dementia comes to have a natural or unnatural place in the life course, personal or moral causes, and implications beyond the strictly biomedical—all of which shape the ways that caregivers think about their roles and their loved ones.

Culture and Caregiving Practices

Culture can also help explain differences in caregiving practices such as the willingness to accept help from sources outside the family. For example, white caregivers in the USA are more likely to use personal or nursing care services than African-American or Hispanic caregivers. They are also more likely to place their loved one in a nursing home (National Alliance for Caregiving & AARP 2004). Some have tied this difference to an American emphasis on the values of individualism and independence, as compared to cultures that emphasize family and community unity (Knight and Sayegh 2010).

For example, many Hispanic caregivers see family-based home care as absolutely necessary, and a key part of beliefs about family obligation, reciprocity, and respect for elders (Mahoney et al. 2005). Yet one study found that younger Latinos, and those who had spent more time living in the USA, identified less strongly with these traditional values of "familismo" (Kao and Travis 2005).

Cultural, political, and economic forces can also affect the extent to which caregivers utilize formal services. Reports have shown that African-American caregivers in the USA are more likely to use informal sources of support than white caregivers (Guidry et al. 1997). They may also be less likely to consult with a physician, use prescription medication, or use psychotropic drugs than white caregivers. Some studies have noted African-American caregivers make use of informal social networks which extend beyond the confines of immediate family and include friends and religious communities (Barker et al. 1998). However, Fox et al. (1999) question the extent to which these extended family ties make a concrete difference in the lives of caregivers. Instead, they emphasize that ethnicity or culture must not be allowed to obscure the important and often devastating role that structural factors and large scale sociopolitical forces such as "residential, educational and occupational segregation, racism and economic exploitation" play in creating observed differences in reactions to caregiving.

In Asian culture in general, caregiving is deeply rooted in intergenerational obligations. For example, Burgess et al. (1999) describe ways that Thai families reflect strong Buddhist values of honoring family members through caregiving. Similarly, in Hong Kong, the parent–child relationship has been defined by specific expectations.

A mother cares for her children, and they, in turn, provide for her in old age. This perpetuates the continuity of family ancestry—a cherished value in Chinese society. These values are closely linked to the Confucian sense of self, which is based on *jen,* the notion that "a human must be within the social realm in order to be considered a human" (Holroyd 2001). In caring for their parents, children are occupying the "correct place in an ordered position on earth under heaven," and fulfilling their Confucian duty (Holroyd 2001).

However, shifting from tradition, some members of the younger generation rely on a new model. Hong Kong's contemporary urban culture stresses "youth, modernity, autonomy, spontaneity, and affection" (Holroyd 2001). This transformation is especially evident in the changing societal role of women. Daughters now feel obligated to provide not only for their mothers but also for their husband and children. Further complicating this conflict is the desire to fulfill the needs of their employers and be successful in their careers (Holroyd 2001).

In Korea, beliefs about care over the lifespan are similarly characterized by filial obligation and cyclical reciprocity (Chee and Levkoff 2001). As in Hong Kong, however, changing lifestyles and shifting traditions often prevent this idealized system from becoming reality, causing a discrepancy between ideal attitudes and actual behavior (Shin 1999). Perhaps as a result of this discrepancy, some studies have found that Korean and Korean-American caregivers report higher levels of anxiety, depression, and feelings of burden than white caregivers (Youn et al. 1999).

Similar shifts away from traditionally defined, multigenerational coresidence patterns have begun to be noted in Japanese society by Takagi and Silverstein (2006). Pragmatic concerns such as economics or poor health at times lead older parents to live with unmarried children, contrary to cultural norms. Some researchers believe that after the Second World War, many Japanese were increasingly influenced by American values of individualism and personal productivity, rather than by traditional family values. In addition, a steep decline in birthrates has caused an increase in burden among aging caregivers. However, elders living with their adult children is still far more common in Japan than in the USA (Asahara et al. 1999).

Gender and Caregiving

Across all ethnic groups, caregivers are primarily women—they made up 66 % of caregivers in 2009 (National Alliance for Caregiving & American Association for Retired Persons 2009). Traditionally, care has been perceived as a female occupation. In America, a historical gendered division of labor led to a division of roles in the "breadwinner-caregiver family" (Cancian and Oliker 2000). While aggression, emotional neutrality, and competitiveness became qualities of the masculine provider, the affection and intimacy of caring has come to be linked to qualities associated with femininity. Women are socialized from an early age to take on caring roles through a variety of means, including the kinds of toys they are given, activities and jobs they are encouraged to participate in, and qualities or traits that are praised or discouraged, and ideal roles that are portrayed in mass media (Brewer 2001).

Some feminist scholars argue that the gendered, unpaid, and invisible nature of caregiving leads to its current devalued and diminished status (Cancian and Oliker 2000; Treas and Mazumdar 2004). Further, the unequal division of unpaid care work may also be contributing to higher levels of poverty among older women (Arendell and Estes 1994).The link between perceived gender roles and caregiving also has other important consequences, as in many cultures women undertake this role by default and may judge themselves by their ability to fulfill it. In Hong Kong, for example, while sons are expected to provide monetary support, daughters provide ongoing daily assistance. If they are unable to meet these social obligations, many women feel conflicted and guilty (Holroyd 2001).

Similarly, in the USA, researchers have found differences in the types of caregiving tasks sons and daughters are expected to perform. One study found that Americans tended to assign daughters the intimate tasks of daily caregiving, like showering, cooking, giving medication, making the bed, and doing the laundry, while sons were given more distant, managerial tasks such as organizing finances and services (Lawrence and Goodnow 2002). Men are often seen as having "legitimate excuses" for not participating in care to the same extent as females (Finch and Mason 1993; Campbell and Martin-Matthews 2003). Several studies have shown that female caregivers had higher levels of burden and depression, and lower levels of subjective well-being and physical health (Pinquart and Sorenson 2006). However, increasingly this gendered division of caregiving is changing. In 1987, 75 % of caretakers for the elderly were women, as compared to 73 % in 1997, and 66 % in 2009 (Wagner 1997; National Alliance for Caregiving & American Association for Retired Persons 2009). Male caregivers also struggle with traditional gender roles in which it may be seen as "unmasculine" for men to take time away from the workplace to give care or if they talk about caregiving (Thompson 2002). Men are also more likely to initially resist seeking formal support, preferring to remain "stoic" and to "go it alone" rather than admitting the need for assistance (Thompson). However, many men report high levels of satisfaction and gratification from taking on a caregiving role (Carpenter and Miller 2002; Russell 2001).

Anthropology and Aging

Attitudes about caregiving are linked to ways that Americans conceptualize aging. An anthropology of aging developed in the 1980s, and since then anthropologists have shed light on ways that aging is perceived (Cohen 1994). Aging presents a conflict for Americans, who believe on the one hand in limitless potential of individuals, but also see aging as an inevitable, if unpredictable decline (Solimeo 2009). Further, aging is associated with a loss of independence, autonomy, and productivity, all of which are important cultural ideals for Americans (Kaufman 1994). Americans at once struggle to constantly forestall aging, but also to plan for care in old age. Increasingly, it has become difficult for Americans to distinguish between sickness, chronic conditions, and the "normal" processes of aging (Solimeo 2009).

Americans strongly link aging with appearance and the physical body, including "gray hair, baldness, wrinkles, slowness, bifocals" and possess and consume an increasing range of products designed to conceal and deny these outward signs (Solimeo 2009). Faircloth argues that "the aging mask" or the outward manifestations of aging hide the salient characteristics of the individual (2003). He also suggests that the dominant discourse about aging perpetuates stereotypes of aging individuals.

In one study, older interviewees do not see being old as central to their "experienced self" (Cohen 1994). Often, elders see their bodies as "receptacles" for individuals "true selves" which are hiding inside, so that while bodies are old, personalities are not (Clarke 2001). This idea of the "ageless self" also asserts a continuity of identity over the lifespan (Clarke 2001). Aging Americans may further feel "trapped" in bodies, they may feel "betrayed" by them, becoming more difficult to control. Minds and personalities are seen as separate from bodies, and more important to asserting selfhood (Clarke 2001).

This experience of physical aging— the relationship between the aging body and aging self—may vary across class, cultural, and social differences (Cohen 1994). They also vary by gender, as many have pointed out the "double standard" of aging, in which women's aging appearances are judged more harshly than men's (Clarke 2001).

The disconnections between ideals and reality are also evident in the American tendency to "medicalize" old age (Cohen 1994; Kaufman 1994). In the USA, the life of the elderly is shaped by constant medical interaction. Although aging is a natural part of the life cycle, it has become a stigmatized condition (Brown and Powell-Cope 1991). The elderly are increasingly identified by what has been recorded in their medical chart (Brown and Powell-Cope 1991; Cohen 1994). As Kaufman (1994) notes, "The lived experience of the old person *becomes* the problem list". This medicalization goes both ways, however, as the elderly also often desire biomedicine to "fix" their problems and believe "in the power of the American health care system to restore, manage, and order" (Kaufman 1994).

Culture, Caregiving, and Food

Food is a significant and symbolic cultural concept, central to societal organization and world view. As food and food preparation are essential tasks for caregivers, it is important to understand the many ways that food and its meaning can be interpreted. Traditional "comfort foods" are often used by caregivers to demonstrate caring and nurturing to their loved ones (Locher et al. 2005). Locher et al. (2005) note that comfort foods were consumed when individuals were "feeling down and needed comfort, or when they needed an extra boost to get them through some task". Traditional foods can also be an important means of asserting individual and group identities, and have important emotional implications. For example, one study of Chinese cancer patients and their caregivers noted that the ability to eat traditional Chinese foods was central to patients' feelings of well-being, despite often contradicting the instructions of nutritionists and doctors (Bell et al. 2009).

Foods are also used to communicate emotion, social status, and celebration. Food can be categorized as "sacred," permitted by religious beliefs, or "profane," prohibited by religious beliefs (Helman 2001). Cross culturally, food is prohibited during certain traditional religious events. Yom Kippur, a Jewish holiday, is a 25-hour fast, and Ramadan, a Muslim fast, requires avoidance of food and drink from dawn to sunset during the 9th month of the lunar calendar (Helman 2001).

In many cultures, food is grouped into "hot" and "cold" categories. This classification is not solely based on temperature, but is derived according to the physical properties of the food. (Helman 2001). Often, medicine, food, and illness are interconnected. "Hot" and "cold" categories are not only used to classify foods but also to define illness. This notion is followed by the idea that "hot" illnesses should be treated with "cold" food and vice versa. In some cases, particular diets are assigned for treatment of certain illnesses or psychological disturbances. (Helman 2001).

Food is also a public symbol characterizing relationships, social status, gender, and group identity. Frequently, communal meals are controlled by the norms of a culture or group. Ritual is inherent in the preparation, service, and clean-up of meals. Food itself is culturally unique—every cuisine has distinct size, color, smell, and taste. Different types of meals can reveal the relationships and values of those sharing the food. A barbeque, for example, is much less formal and intimate than a private dinner party. Across all cultures, special meals and drinks mark important landmarks in the human life cycle and other festive occasions (Helman 2001).

Future Needs and New Directions for an Anthropology of Caregiving

Several subdisciplines within anthropology (medical anthropology, anthropology of aging, and anthropology of disability) have begun to explore caregiver issues. As issues and technologies continue to evolve, a number of areas stand out as essential to our increased understanding of issues of caregiving. End of life research, including research into the ways that caregivers make decisions about end of life care are increasingly important in an age of "rescue" oriented technology (Chapple 2010). Further, the meaning of these new medical technologies, and their relevance to the ways that we care for others, are just beginning to be explored.

As individuals around the world continue to live longer, the anthropology of aging also takes on a renewed importance. Several authors have pointed to the experiences of the aging "baby boomer" population as an important avenue of research (Leibing and Cohen 2006). Aging research has important implications for addressing ideas identity and personhood, as well as the stigmatization of age and the ethics of aging well. The relationship between aging identities and caregivers is an especially vital avenue of exploration.

Finally, anthropology has much to offer to caregiver research in the way of methodology. Anthropology's tradition of inductive research has much to offer the growing body of qualitative and mixed methods research on caregiving (Poirier and Ayres 2002). Weitzman and Levkoff (2000) have explored ways that anthropological field methods in combination with quantitative survey methods enriched the methodological rigor of studies of minority elders caring for family members with dementia. Albert (1990) has used cultural consensus analysis (Borgatti 1999; Handwerker and Borgatti 1998; Weller and Romney 1988) along with ethnographic field methods to examine shared, and therefore, cultural notions about caregiving related to dependency and obligation. Karlawish et al. (2011) used similar techniques to understand cultural concepts of dementia among Latina and white family caregivers. Mixed methods approaches to understanding patient and family notions about depression and depression management have been useful in identifying cultural features that affect mental health helpseeking and treatment adherence (Barg et al. 2006; Gallo et al. 2005).

References

Ainsworth-Vaughan, N. (1998). *Claiming power in doctor-patient talk.* Berkeley: University of California Press.

Albert, S. M. (1990). Caregiving as a cultural system: Conceptions of filial obligation and parental dependency in urban America. *American Anthropologist, 92*(2), 319–331.

Albert, S. M. (1991). Cognition of caregiving tasks: Multidimensional scaling of the caregiver task domain. *Gerontologist, 31*(6), 726–734.

Arendell, T., & Estes, C. (1994). Older women in the post-regan era. In: E. Fee & N. Krieger (Eds.), *Women's health, politics, and power* (pp. 333–349). Amityville: Baywood.

Armelagos, G. J., Ryan, M., & Leatherman, T. (1990). Evolution of infectious disease: A biocultural analysis of AIDS. *American Journal of Human Biology, 2*(9), 353–363.

Ashara, K., Konishi, E., Soyano, A., & Davis, A. (1999). Long-term care for the elderly in Japan. *Geriatric Nursing, 20,* 23–7.

Baer, H., Singer, M., & Susser, I. (2004). *Medical anthropology and the world system.* Westport: Praeger.

Barg, F. K., Pasacreta, J. V., Nuamah, I. F., Robinson, K. D., Angeletti, K., Yasko, J. M., et al (1998). A description of a psychoeducational intervention for family caregivers of cancer patients. *Journal of Family Nursing, 4*(4), 394–413.

Barg, F. K., Huss-Ashmore, R., Wittink, M. N., Murray, G. F., Bogner, H. R., & Gallo, J. J. (2006). A mixed methods approach to understand loneliness and depression in older adults. *Journals of Gerontology: Social Sciences, 61B*(6), S329–S339.

Barker, J., Morrow, J., & Mitteness, L. (1998). Gender, informal social support networks, and Elderly Urban African Americans. *Journal of Aging Studies, 12*(2), 199–222.

Bell, K., Lee, J., Ristovski-Slijepcevic, S. (2009). Perceptions of food and eating among chinese patients with cancer: Findings of an ethnographic study. *Cancer Nursing, 32*(2), 188–126.

Bertakis, K. D. (2009). The influence of gender on the doctor-patient interaction. *Patient Education Counseling, 76*(3), 356–60.

Boddy, J., Cameron, C., & Moss, P. (2006). *Carework, present and future.* New York: Routledge.

Borgatti, S. (1999). Cultural consensus theory. In J. Schensul & M. Weeks (Eds.), *The ethnographic toolkit* (pp. 115–151). Newbury Park: Sage.

Brewer, L. (2001). Gender socialization and the cultural construction of elder caregivers. *Journal of Aging Studies, 15,* 217–235.

Brown, M. A., & Powell-Cope, G. M. (1991). AIDS family caregiving: Transitions through uncertainty. *Nursing Research, 40*(6), 338–345.

Brown, P. J., & Barrett, R. (2009). *Understanding and applying medical anthropology*. Toronto: Mayfield Publishing Company.

Burgess, M., Stephenson, P., Ratanakul, P., & K. Suwonnakaote, K. (1999). End of life decisions: Clinical decisions about dying and perspectives on life and death. In H. Coward & P. Ratanakul (Eds.), *Cross-cultural dialogue on health care ethics* (pp. 190–206). Waterloo: Wilfrid Laurier University Press.

Campbell, L., Martin-Matthews, A. (2003) The gendered nature of men's filial care. *Journal of Gerontology, 58B*(6), S350–S358.

Cancian, F., & Oliker, S. (2000). *Caring and gender*. Walnut Creek: AltaMira.

Carpenter, E., & Miller, B. (2002). Psychosocial challenges and rewards experienced by caregiving men: A review of the literature and an empirical case example. In B. Kramer & E. Thompson (Eds.), *Men as caregivers*. Amherst: Prometheus Books.

Carretero, S., Garces, J., Rodenas, F., & Sanjose, V. The informal caregiver's burden of dependent people: Theory and empirical review. *Archives of Gerontology and Geriatrics, 49*(1), 74–79.

Chapple, H. (2010). *No place for dying: Hospitals and the ideology of rescue*. Walnut Creek: Left Coast.

Chee, Y. K., Levkoff, S. E. (2001). Culture and dementia: Accounts by family caregivers and health professionals for dementia-affected elders in South Korea. *Journal of Cross-Cultural Gerontology, 16,* 111–125.

Cheung, J., & Hocking, P. (2004). The experience of spousal carers of people with multiple sclerosis. *Qualitative Health Research, 14*(2), 153–166.

Clarke, L. (2001). Older women's bodies and the self: The construction of identity in later life. *Canadian Review of Sociology and Anthropology, 38*(4), 441–464.

Cohen, L. (1994). Old age: Cultural and critical perspective. *Annual Review of Anthropology, 23,* 137–158.

DelVecchio Good, M. (2010). The medical imaginary and the biotechnical embrace: Subjective experiences of clinical scientists and patients. In B. Good, M. Fischer, S. Willen, & M. DelVecchio Good (Eds.), *A Reader in Medical Anthropology*. Blackwell.

Dilworth-Anderson, P., & Gibson, B. (2002). The cultural influence of values, norms, meanings, and perceptions in understanding dementia in ethnic minorities. *Alzheimer's Disease and Associated Disorders, 16,* S56–S63.

Evercare & National Alliance for Caregiving (2008) Hispanic family caregiving in the US: Findings from a National Study.

Faircloth, C. A. (2003). Different bodies and the paradox of aging: Locating aging bodies in images and everyday experience. In C. A. Faircloth (Ed.), *Aging bodies: Images and everyday experience* (pp. 1–26). Walnut Creek: AltaMira.

Ferguson, W. J., & Candib, L. M. (2002). Culture, language, and the doctor-patient relationship. *Family Medicine, 34*(5), 353–361. Review. http://www.ncbi.nlm.nih.gov/pubmed/12038717 (May).

Finch, J., & Mason, J. (1993). *Negotiating family responsibilities*. London: Routledge.

Flocke, S. A., Goodwin, M. A., & Strange, K. G. (1998). The effects of a secondary patient in the family practice visit. *Journal of Family Practice, 46,* 429–439.

Fox, K., Hinton, W. L., & Levkoff, S. (1999). Take up the caregiver's burden: Stories of care for urban African American elders with dementia. *Culture Medicine and Psychiatry, 23* (4), 501 (Dec).

Gallo, J. J., Bogner, H. R., Morales, K. H., & Ford, D. E. (2005). Patient ethnicity and the identification and active management of depression in late life. *Archives of Internal Medicine, 165*(17), 1962–1968.

Good, B. J. (1994). *Medicine, rationality and experience: An anthropological perspective*. Cambridge: Oxford University Press.
Grant, K., Amaratunga, C., Armstrong, P., Boscoe, M., Pederson, A., & Willson, K. (2004). *Caring for/caring about: Women, home care, and unpaid caregiving*. Aurora: Garamond.
Guidry, J. J., Aday, L. A., Zhang, D., & Winn, R. J. (1997). The role of informal and formal support networks for patients with cancer. *Cancer Practice, 5*(4), 241–246.
Handwerker, W. P., & Borgatti, S. P. (1998). Reasoning with numbers. In H. R. Bernard (Ed.), *Handbook of methods in cultural anthropology* (pp. 549–587). Walnut Creek: AltaMira.
Hasselkus, B., & Murray, B. (2007). Everyday occupation, well-being, and identity: The experience of caregivers in families with dementia. *The American Journal of Occupational Therapy, 61*(1), 9–20.
Hayes, J., Boylestein, C., & Zimmerman, M. (2009). Living and loving with dementia: Negotiating spousal and caregiver identity through narrative. *Journal of Aging Studies, 23*(10), 48–59.
Helman, C. G. (2001). *Culture, health and illness*. Oxford: Butterworth-Heinemann Ltd.
Henderson, J. N., & Henderson, L. C. (2002). Cultural construction of disease: A "supernormal" construct of dementia in an American Indian tribe. *Journal of Cross-Cultural Gerontology, 17*, 197–212.
Henderson, J. N., & Traphagan, J. W. (2005). Cultural factors in dementia: Perspectives from the anthropology of aging. *Alzheimer Disease and Associated Disorders, 19*(4), 272–274.
Hinton, W. L., Fox, K., & Levkoff, S. (1999). Introduction: Exploring the relationships among aging, ethnicity and family dementia caregiving. *Culture, Medicine and Psychiatry, 23*, 403–413.
Holroyd, E. (2001). Hong Kong Chinese daughters' intergenerational caregiving obligations: A cultural model approach. *Social Science & Medicine, 53*, 1125–1134.
Hsiao-Rei Hicks, M., & Sau-Ching Lam, M. (1999). Decision-making within the social course of dementia: accounts by Chinese-American caregivers. *Culture, Medicine and Psychiatry, 23*, 415–452.
Hublin, J. (2009). The prehistory of compassion. *Proceedings of the Academy of Sciences of the United States of America, 106*(16), 6429–6430.
Hudson, P. (2004). Positive aspects and challenges associated with caring for a dying relative at home. *International Journal of Palliative Nursing, 10*(2), 58–65.
Johnson, R. W. (2007). Choosing between paid elder care and unpaid help from adult children: The role of relative prices in the care decision. In M. E. Szinovacz & A. Davery (Ed.), *Caregiving contexts: Cultural, familial and societal implications* (pp. 35–70). New York: Springer.
Kao, H., & Travis, S. (2005). Effects of acculturation and social exchange on the expectations of filial piety among Hispanic/Latino parents of adult children. *Nursing and Health Sciences, 7*, 226–234.
Karlawish, J., Barg, F. K., Augsburger, D., Beaver, J., Ferguson, A., & Nunez, J. (2011 March). What Latino Puerto Ricans and non-Latinos say when they talk about Alzheimer's disease. *Alzheimer's and Dementia, 7*(2), 161–170.
Kaufman, S. (1994). Old age, disease, and the discourse on risk: Geriatric assessment in US healthcare. *Medical Anthropology Quarterly, 8*(4), 430–447.
Kleinman, A. (1973). Medicine's symbolic reality. *Inquiry: An Interdisciplinary Journal of Philosophy, 16*(1–4), 206–213.
Knight, B., & Sayegh, P. (2010) Cultural values and caregiving: The Updated sociocultural stress and coping model. *Journal of Gerontology Series B Psychological Sciences and Social Sciences, 65B*(1), 5–13.
Lawrence, J. A., Goodnow, J. J., Woods, K., & Karantzas, G. (2002). Distributions of caregiving tasks among family members: The place of gender and availability. *Journal of Family Psychology, 16*(4), 493–509.
Leibing, A., & Cohen, L. (2006). *Thinking about dementia: Culture, loss, and the anthropology of senility*. New Brunwick: Rutgurs University Press.
Levine, C. (1999). The loneliness of the long-term caregiver. *New England Journal of Medicine, 340*, 1587–1590.

Liu, D., Hinton, L., Tran, C., Hinton, D., & Barker, J. (2008). Reexamining the relationships among dementia, stigma, and aging in immigrant Chinese and Vietnamese family caregivers. *Journal of Cross-Cultural Gerontology, 23,* 283–299.

Locher, J., Yoels, W., Maurer, D., & van Ells J. (2005). Comfort foods: An exploratory journey into the social and emotional significance of food. *Food and Foodways: Explorations in the History and Culture of Human Nourishment, 13*(4), 273–297.

Mahoney, D. F., Cloutterbuck, J., Neary, S., & Zhan, L. (2005). African American, Chinese, and Latino family caregivers' impression of the onset and diagnosis of dementia: cross cultural similarities and differences. *The Gerontologist, 45*(6), 783–792.

Montgomery, R., & Kosloski, K. (2009). Caregiving as a process of changing identity: Implications for caregiver support. *Journal of the American Society on Aging., 33*(1), 47–52.

National Academy on an Aging Society. (2000). Alzheimer's disease and dementia: A growing challenge. *Challenges for the 21st Century: Chronic Conditons.* 11.

National Alliance for Caregiving & American Association for Retired Persons (NAC/AARP). (2004). *Caregiving in the U.S.* Washington: Authors.

National Alliance for Caregiving & American Association for Retired Persons (NAC/AARP). (2009). *Caregiving in the U.S.* Washington: Authors.

Noonan, A., & Tennstedt, L. (1997). Meaning in caregiving and its contribution to caregiving well-being. *The Gerontologist, 37,* 785–794.

O'Connor, B. B. (1995). *Healing traditions: Alternative medicine and the health professions.* Philadelphia: University of Pennsylvania Press.

Payer, L. (1996). *Medicine & culture.* New York: Owl Books.

Pinquart, M., & Sorensen, S. (2005). Ethnic differences in stressors, resources, and psychological outcomes of family caregiving: A meta-analysis. *Gerontologist, 45*(1), 90–106.

Pinquart, M., & Sörensen, S. (2006). Gender differences in caregiver stressors, social resources, and health: An updated meta-analysis. *The Journals of Gerontology. Series B, Psychological Sciences and Social Sciences, 61*(1), p33–45 (Jan). http://www.ncbi.nlm.nih.gov/pubmed/16399940\t_blank.

Poirier, S., & Ayres, L. (2002). *Stories of family caregiving: Reconsideration of theory, literature, and life.* Indianapolis: Center Nursing Publishing.

Russell, R. (2001). In sickness and in health: A qualitative study of elderly men who care for wives with dementia. *Journal of Aging Studies, 15*(4), 351–367.

Ryder, A., Bean, G., Dion, K. (2000). Caregiver responses to symptoms of first-onset psychosis: A comparative study of Chinese- and Euro-Canadian families. *Transcultural Psychiatry, 37*(2), 255–265.

Schumacher, K., Stewart, B., Archbold, P., Dodd, M., & Dibble, S. (2000). Family caregiving skill: Development of the concept. *Research in Nursing and Health, 23,* 191–203.

Shin, S. (1999). Social transformation of Korean familism. *Korean Association of Family Relations, 4,* 165–192.

Sokolovsky J. (Ed.). (1997). *The cultural context of aging: Worldwide perspectives* (2nd ed.). CT: Bergin & Garvey.

Solimeo, S. (2009). *With shaking hands: Aging with Parkinson's disease in America's Heartland.* Hartford: Rutgers University Press.

Sontag, S. (1989). *Illness as metaphor and AIDS and its metaphors.* New York: Anchor Books.

Soothill, K., Morris, S. M., Harman, J. C., Francis, B., Thomas, C., & McIllmurray, M. B. (2001). Informal carers of cancer patients: What are their unmet psychosocial needs? *Health and Social Care in the Community, 9*(6), 464–475.

Strathern, A., & Stewart, P. J. (1999). *Curing and healing: Medical anthropology in global perspective.* Durham: Carolina Academic Press.

Takagi, E., & Silverstein, M. (2006). Intergenerational coresidence of the Japanese elderly: Are cultural norms proactive or reactive? *Research on Aging, 28*(4), 473–492.

Thompson, E. (2002). *What's unique about men's caregiving?* In Kramer, B. & Thompson, E. (Eds.), *Men as caregivers.* Amherst: Prometheus.

Treas, J., & Mazumdar, S. (2004). Kinkeeping and caregiving: Contributions of older people in immigrant families. *Journal of Comparative Family Studies, 35*(1), 105–122.
Turner, H. A., & Catania, J. A. (1994). The prevalence of informal caregiving to persons with AIDS in the United States: Caregiver characteristics and their implications. *Social Science and Medicine, 38,* 1543–1552.
Wagner, D. (1997). Comparative analysis of caregiver data for caregivers to the Elderly, 1987 and 1997. *National Alliance for Caregiving Report.*
Weiss, M. L., & Mann, A. E. (1990). *Human biology and behavior: An anthropological perspective* (5th ed.). Glenview: Scott, Foresman/Little, Brown.
Weitzman, P. F., & Levkoff. S. E. (2000). Combining qualitative and quantitative methods in health research with minority elders: Lessons from a study of dementia caregiving. *Field Methods, 12*(3), 195–208.
Weller, S. C., & Romney, A. K. (1988). *Systematic data collection.* Newbury Park: Sage.
Willems, S., De Maesschalck, S., Deveugele, M., Derese, A., & De Maeseneer, J. (2005). Socio-economic status of the patient and doctor–patient communication: does it make a difference? *Patient Education and Counseling, 56,* 139–146.
Wright, L. K. (1997). Health behavior of caregivers. In D. S. Gochman (Ed.), *Handbook of health behavior research III: Demography, development, and diversity III* (pp. 267–284). Walnut Creek: AltaMira.
Yeo, G., Tran, J., Hikoyeda, N., & Hinton, L. (2002). Conceptions of dementia among Vietnamese American caregivers. *Journal of Gerontological Social Work, 36*(1–2), 131–152.
Youn, G., Knight, B. G., Jeong, H. S., & Benton, D. (1999). Differences in familism values and caregiving outcomes among Korean, Korean American, and white American dementia caregivers. *Psychology and Aging, 14,* 355–364.

Caregiving in Late Life: A Life Span Human Development Perspective

Karen A. Roberto and Shannon E. Jarrott

As a discipline, human development embraces a philosophical stance that incorporates biopsychosocial frameworks to guide the study of individuals, families, and communities across the lifespan. Historically, scholars trained in this integrative, multidisciplinary tradition have relied on theories and models developed in the behavioral and social sciences to inform and advance their work. As early as the 1920s, academic scholars forged alliances with traditional disciplines, such as psychology and sociology, to examine issues related to the needs and abilities of children (Grant 1997). Drawing on the work of behavioralists, such as John B. Watson, and developmentalists, including John Dewey and G. Stanley Hall, researchers and practitioners advanced society's understanding of the principles of development and how to best raise children. As the USA began to experience significant shifts in its demographic makeup, the focus on families with young children and adolescents expanded to the interdisciplinary study of development across the life span. Within this broader life span focus, the study of aging in general, and families in late life in particular, caregiving emerged as a significant area of research with far-reaching implications for practice and policy initiatives.

In this chapter, we present the primary tenets of five theoretical frameworks commonly used by scholars in human development to study family caregiving in late life: (a) life span perspective; (b) life course perspective; (c) stress and coping; (d) exchange theory; and (e) formal service use. We provide examples from the literature illustrating the utility of each of these frameworks for studying the effects of caregiving on spouses, adult children, and other family members providing care for

K. A. Roberto (✉)
Center for Gerontology and the Institute for Society, Culture and Environment,
Virginia Polytechnic Institute and State University, Blacksburg, VA 24061, USA
e-mail: kroberto@vt.edu

S. Jarrott
Department of Human Development, Virginia Polytechnic Institute and State University,
Blacksburg, VA 24061, USA
e-mail: sjarrott@vt.edu

R. C. Talley, S. S. Travis (eds.), *Multidisciplinary Coordinated Caregiving,*
Caregiving: Research • Practice • Policy, DOI 10.1007/978-1-4614-8973-3_10,

their older relatives. We conclude the chapter with suggestions for the explicit use of individual- and contextual-level theories to advance future caregiving research, practice, and policy.

A Life Span Perspective

The life span perspective proposed by Baltes (1987) entails five key tenets that together specify a coherent meta-theoretical view on the nature of human development. Incorporating concepts and constructs from multiple disciplines (e.g., biology, psychology, and sociology), acknowledging the influence of internal mechanisms and external forces, and recognizing the diverse experiences of individuals as they proceed through the life course, this perspective provides a framework for the study of consistency and change in caregiving behavior and response (Roberto and Jarrott 2008).

According to the life span perspective, individual development is a *lifelong process* influenced by the life tasks facing individuals, which are typically associated with various chronological ages and influenced by historical or nonnormative events. Second, development is *multidimensional* and *multidirectional* including both growth and decline across multiple domains (e.g., physical, cognitive, emotional). Baltes (1987, p. 616) also suggests that "any developmental progression displays at the same time new adaptive capacity as well as the loss of previously existing capacity." Throughout their lives, individuals encounter *historical* and *societal forces* that shape the course of their development. As suggested by this third tenet, individual development is influenced by the multiple social contexts in which one engages, including family, neighborhoods, work, church, and community. The fourth tenet of the life span perspective, *plasticity*, refers to intraindividual variability. It suggests a capacity for differential behavior in response to different situations because of development or intervention. Finally, the course of development can best be understood as the outcome of interactions among three systems of developmental influences : *age-graded*, *history-graded*, and *nonnormative*. Age-graded changes are biologically or culturally influenced changes with strong ties to chronological age. History-graded influences affect an individual's development and may explain the attitudinal and behavioral differences among cohorts. Few people experience nonnormative events or events that occur off time for a particular stage of life.

Although few researchers explicitly name or address the specific tenets of the life span perspective in their research (Roberto and Jarrott 2008; Shifren 2009), investigations grounded in life span principles have generated important knowledge about individual issues surrounding family caregiving. Collectively, the literature acknowledges the multiple dimensions of caregiving and their influence on individual caregivers' physical health, psychological well-being, personal relationships, employment, and so forth. As researchers identified and solidified outcomes across life domains, more integrated and comprehensive investigations of caregiving have emerged. For example, supporting and giving greater confidence to the earlier causal assertions from cross-sectional studies of caregivers' physical and mental health outcomes, findings from a recent 10-year study of informal caregivers of persons with dementia showed that caregivers with elevated depressive symptoms at multiple measurement points reported poorer and worsening physical health over time (O'Rourke et al. 2007). Although the mechanisms behind this relationship have yet to be identified, the findings suggest the need for treating depression in caregivers to prevent health declines and premature institutionalization of their family members. Interventions such as skill building to become better at the caregiving tasks may help increase caregivers' level of personal mastery, and indirectly increase positive affect (Chen et al. 2010; Hepburn et al. 2003).

Despite the pervasive focus on negative outcomes or loss in the caregiving literature, family members also experience positive outcomes or gains including greater positive affect (Riberio and Paúl 2008; Robertson et al. 2007), higher self-esteem (Lopez et al. 2005; Noonan and Tennstedt 1997) and self-efficacy (Semiatin and O'Connor 2012), and improved psychological and social well-being (Hilgeman et al. 2007; Lévesque et al. 1995). Another positive aspect of family caregiving is the opportunity for growth in personal competencies. Stephens and Franks (1995) found that such personal growth was frequently reported by caregiving daughters and was positively associated with higher levels of positive affect among study participants.

The differences in caregiving outcomes may be attributed to moderating variables that enhance caregivers' ability to endure the care demands while maintaining other roles. Consistent with the primary tenets of the life span human development perspective, caregivers' potential for positive as well as negative development may be, at least, partly dependent on their personal coping styles (Wilcox et al. 2001), norms of filial responsibility (Gans and Silverstein 2006; Stein et al. 1998), and relationships among family members (Ingersoll-Dayton et al. 2003; Riberio and Paúl 2008).

A Life Course Perspective

According to Elder (1977; 1998), the life course can be viewed as a multilevel phenomenon shaped by historical time and prevalent social structures. Embedded within this broader context, individuals experience an intertwining of events, transitions, and turning points in their roles and relations that influence the course of their lives. Central themes of the life course perspective include the interplay of human lives and historical times, the social meaning of age, age norms, and age-graded roles and events, the timing, sequencing, and duration of life events, the linking and interdependence of lives, and human agency in choice making.

According to a life course perspective, the experiences and expectations of family caregivers will vary depending on the historical time and place in which they live. For example, contemporary policies that promote and sustain family care in the USA may contribute to a more positive caregiving experience for aging families compared to several decades ago, when few services and programs were available to support older adults and their caregivers (Wacker and Roberto 2014). With the passage of time, succeeding cohorts also face changes in social norms and roles and the evolution of cultural values that inform family caregiving decisions. Consider first- and second-generation American families coming from diverse ethnic backgrounds as an example. Due to the long tradition of filial piety, elderly immigrants from Asian and Latin American countries typically expect care exclusively from family members. However, family caregivers who demonstrated higher levels of acculturation also demonstrated fewer positive views of caregiving and were quicker than their Latina counterparts, who had more positive views of caregiving, to institutionalize their elderly relative (Mausbach et al. 2004). Younger generations modified their belief in *familismo*, which places the value of family above all else, as they faced competing influences and challenges of their new cultural environments.

Age norms, based on a system of age-grading, assign people to various roles and obligations according to their biological age and family expectations and events that surround each age interval. Although the traditional family caregiver is most often identified as a middle-aged or older female (Wolff and Kasper 2006), what constitutes the appropriate age to assume the caregiving role for an aging relative depends on individual and family circumstances. As suggested by the life course perspective, people construct their lives with the constraints of their social and physical worlds. For example, Burton's (1996) study of three generations of African-American women found that the role of a family caregiver in the lives of these women was shaped by culturally and contextually defined family timetables and differed by class and geographic residence. As a result of changing family demographics and women's increasing participation in the workforce, a growing number of men (Calastani and King 2007; Kramer and Thompson 2005) and young family members (Dellmann-Jenkins et al. 2000; Hamill 2012; Shifren 2001) are assuming responsibility for elder care. Regardless of gender, caring for an older relative while shouldering parental and work responsibilities is often associated with role conflict and strain (Fredriksen-Goldsen and Scharlach 2006).

A life course perspective also posits the principle of "linked lives," which refers to the interactions that emerge from the social roles and events of one life intersecting with those of another. The lives of family caregivers are embedded in and interconnected with the lives of their elderly care recipient, other kin, friends, and colleagues. Adult children with spouses or dependent children may experience both benefits and challenges of their linked lives while caring for a parent. For example, a spouse may be a source of support but can also be a demand on the caregiver's time that detracts from care work and contributes to tension experienced by the caregiver (Stephens and Franks 1995). When considering a person caring for an elderly while simultaneously caring for a child, the demands of caregiving can affect the child indirectly, via the strain placed on the caregiver (MaloneBeach et al. 1998), and directly, as the child shares care responsibilities (Fruhauf and Orel 2008) and deals with changes in the relationship with his or her grandparent (Celdrán et al. 2012).

Caregiving demands also constrict caregivers' ability to maintain social relationships. Spouses frequently manage their caregiving responsibilities by limiting interactions outside of the family (Blieszner et al. 2007). Even if a caregiver wants to maintain non-kin relationships, the amount of contact often declines. For example, adult children providing elder care reported that their relationships with friends (as well as with other family members) deteriorated due to their lack of sensitivity to the responsibilities and emotions involved in caring for a parent with dementia (Suitor and Pillemer 1993).

In addition to family and friend connections, researchers consistently document strain created by competing workplace demands and family expectations of being an available, responsible caregiver. Gender differences present themselves in studies of employed caregivers with women experiencing greater stress from balancing work with caregiving (Fredriksen-Goldsen and Scharlach 2006). While occupying multiple roles inherently presents the potential for relationship conflict, some researchers identified positive "spillover" benefits across relationships. For example, married adult daughters caring for an elderly relative reported that perceived competence in the caregiving role gave an enhanced sense of well-being in their spousal roles (Stephens and Franks 1995). Caregivers who are also parenting may provide a powerful role model of care for their children (Piercy and Chapman 2001). As did their parents before them, grandchildren in caregiving households grasped the family rule, whether spoken or unspoken, that younger generations care for the oldest as the oldest once cared for them.

Stress and Coping Models

Stress and coping paradigms guide much of the research on the influences of caregiving on physical and emotional well being. One frequently used model, put forth by Pearlin et al. (1990), highlights four aspects of the stress process. In this model, initial attention is given to the background and context variables, which focus on the key characteristics of caregivers (e.g., ascribed statuses and attainments), the caregiving history, the relationship between the caregiver and care receiver, social network composition and interaction, and the caregiver's access to and use of resources and community programs. Considered next are the primary stressors, including objective indicators, such as the care receiver's cognitive status, problematic behaviors, and limitations in performing activities of daily living as well as subjective indicators, which include the caregiver's role overload and relational deprivation. The third element of the model, secondary stressors, includes both role strains associated with family or job conflict or economic problems and intrapsychic strains manifested as low self-esteem and mastery, feeling captive in the caregiving role, and experiencing loss of the sense of self. Finally, the outcome or consequence of caregiving may include depression, anxiety, disturbances to cognitive functioning or physical health, and premature yielding of the caregiver role. Primary and secondary stressors and outcomes can be mediated by coping strategies and social support.

As suggested by the *stress process model* and confirmed in the collective literature using this model, distress among caregivers has multiple pathways. Caregivers' cultural beliefs and values, psychosocial health, and mastery or competence in providing care (Dilworth-Anderson et al. 2004) as well as their commitment to the care process

(Goodman et al. 1997) influence the caregivers' ability to handle stress successfully. As time passes, if caregiving responsibilities increase or behaviors associated with cognitive impairment become more erratic, levels of distress and depression increase (Gaugler et al. 2000; Hooker et al. 2002). Relationship type and gender also influence the caregiving experiences and outcomes. Spouse caregivers typically report a different, greater stress and burden than adult child caregivers (Pinquart and Sörensen 2011). Female caregivers tend to experience more stressors and to have access to fewer social resources than their male counterparts, and they have lower levels of psychological and physical health (Pinquart and Sörensen 2006).

In one of the first studies to use the model as a conceptual framework for examining stress of male caregivers (Lévesque et al. 2008), 323 husband caregivers of functionally or cognitively impaired spouses were interviewed twice over a 1-year period. Husband caregivers were divided into quartiles by their baseline psychological distress score. Results showed considerable stability in distress (high–high or low–low) over time. Caregivers who consistently reported symptoms of distress experienced more role overload and role captivity than caregivers who were consistently asymptomatic. None of the subjective stressors distinguished between the two groups. According to Pearlin's model, objective stressors should have elicited subjective stressors. The authors speculated that the low frequency of the wives' behavior problems may have contributed to the lack of findings in this area.

Theories of Social Exchange

The basic premise underlying theories of social exchange (Blau 1964; Homans 1961; Thibaut and Kelley 1986) is that people engage in relationships that maximize rewards and minimize costs. By comparing themselves to similar others or larger social norms, individuals evaluate the balance and extent of the rewards and costs in their relationships. When the costs of the relationship are high and continually outweigh the rewards, the person or persons involved are likely to disband the relationship. In interdependent family relationships, such as marriage and parent–child relations, costs and rewards occur in the context of reciprocal exchanges that take place over the course of the relationship. That is, reciprocity, when defined by familial norms, is a generalized process that does not require that exchanges occur at the same point in time and do not necessarily involve giving and receiving the same things (Ingersoll-Dayton and Antonucci 1988).

When applied to the study of family caregiving in late life, exchange theories highlight three important aspects of caregiving relationship. First, caregiving involves a mutual exchange between the caregiver and care recipient. Diminished capacity to maintain reciprocity affects both caregivers and care receivers. For example, loss of reciprocity can add strain to the caregiver, who may feel guilty or flustered by the incompetent attempts made by the care receiver at being helpful (Ingersoll-Dayton et al. 2001). Newsom and Schulz (1998) explored the negative reactions of care receivers to assistance received. Those with low self-esteem in particular responded negatively (i.e., experienced emotional strain) to the receipt of assistance. The authors related this reaction to the care receivers' perceived inadequacy and inability to reciprocate support. In contrast to the costs associated with the care receiver's inability to provide instrumental support, Ingersoll-Dayton et al. (2001) described the positive value of emotional support provided by elders to their family caregivers. Adult children perceived their affective relationship with their parents as mutually dependent and satisfying. If this capacity for emotional exchange is lost, relational deprivation may occur, which has been associated with more reports of loneliness and depression among daughter caregivers and greater anger among mother care recipients (Walker et al. 1992). Such findings mirror other investigations that found less satisfying relationships with care receivers associated with higher levels of depression and role captivity among family caregivers (Lawrence et al. 1998).

A second assertion of social exchange theories is that caregiving may provide an avenue for achieving balance in family relationships. Asymmetry in exchange typically characterizes the caregiving relationship "in the moment" with family caregivers bearing greater burden in the relationship while care receivers disproportionate benefit from the relationship. The duty to provide care may be tied to beliefs associated with the marital vow or filial piety, but it can also be explained by a long view of reciprocity. Caregivers explained that their commitment to caregiving stemmed from earlier periods in their relationship with the older care recipients (Harris et al. 1998; Raschik and Ingersoll-Dayton 2004). Spouses and adult children viewed their time as caregivers as a chance to "repay" their older family members for the care and support received from them throughout their lives.

Third, exchange theories suggest that family members experience both costs and rewards as a result of their care responsibilities. Although the caregiving literature tends to emphasize the negative aspects of caregiving, there are several identifiable positive outcomes associated with caring for older family members, including enhanced feelings of competence (Peacock et al. 2010) and overall life satisfaction (Raschick and Ingersoll-Dayton 2004). The positive, benefits resulting from engaging in family care have been associated with caregivers' enhanced capacity to cope with care stressors and the ability to maintain the caregiving role (Mausbach et al. 2004).

Model of Service Use

Despite the availability of formal services in most communities, relatively few caregivers look beyond themselves or close family members for help and support (Jarrott et al. 2005). According to Anderson's *Behavioral Model of Health Service Use*, reliance on services is a function of an individual's predisposition to use the service, enabling factors that either facilitate or impede use of a service and the need for the service (Anderson 1995; Anderson and Newman 1973). Certain individuals are more inclined than others to use services because of personal characteristics that are present before the need for a service arises. These predisposing characteristics include the demographic factors of age and gender. They also include social structure characteristics, such as marital status, education, occupation, and ethnicity, as well as coping skills and abilities and the availability of informal and formal resources to provide assistance. General beliefs or attitudes about support services also predict service use.

Individuals predisposed to using services will not do so unless they can access those services. The enabling characteristics that facilitate the use of services include personal and family characteristics of income level, insurance coverage, access to transportation, and awareness of services. At the community level, the enabling characteristics include availability of the service and the distance to the service. Finally, service need can either be an individual's subjective assessment of need or an evaluated need provided by a professional. Need alone does not predict service use unless the person is predisposed to use the service and then has the necessary enabling resources.

Applied to the study of family caregiving, researchers have suggested that predisposing factors, such as gender, age, and ethnicity, living arrangement, family relationships, and enabling factors, such as rural–urban location, availability of transportation, and medical insurance, may be as important, if not more important, predictors of service utilization when compared with need variables (Kosloski et al. 2002; Scharlach et al. 2008). The type of services examined may account for study findings. For example, although an investigation of human and health service used by a person with Alzheimer's disease and the family caregiver (Toseland et al. 2002) revealed that enabling variables explained more variance in the use of health and human services than that by need or predisposing variables, analyses based on service type showed that the model predicted more variance in the use of human services than in the use of health services. Specifically, experiencing objective burden, caring for a person who wandered, the availability of public and private transportation, being a spouse, living separately from the care recipient, and having a higher educational level predicted the use of human services but not health services.

Although Anderson's model identifies predisposing, enabling, and need factors as determinants of service use, it does not fully explore how these three domains, or their measures, are interrelated. Bradley et al. (2002) argued that because the model combines race and ethnicity with other demographic characteristics included as predisposing factors, the omission of the interrelationships among these variables may oversimplify the role of race and ethnicity in service use. Their study, which included 96 elderly African-American and White focus group participants, revealed that psychosocial variables may mediate the effect of race and ethnicity on long-term care service use. Compared with White participants, African-American participants perceived poorer access to needed information, reported stronger norms of family caregiving, and had more concerns about potential loss of privacy and self-determination in long-term care settings. The findings suggest the need for more sophisticated modeling of race and ethnicity for understanding the propensity of using long-term services by older adults and their caregivers.

Advancing Future Research, Practice, and Policy

The strength of human development as a multidisciplinary field of study is its propensity toward the integration of knowledge. The focus on individual development with the context of a larger society guides the work of human development researchers and practitioners who seek to understand and improve the lives of late life family caregivers. The complexities inherent to the study of human development present several challenges to this community of scholars as they strive to advance this field of study and practice.

To fully capture and understand the issues of family caregiving in late life, the use of longitudinal designs and advanced statistical methods is required. Although these approaches pose conceptual and resource challenges, they will advance the study of caregiving by allowing researchers to consider age-related and age-graded changes in caregiving structures, the influence of personal and societal history (i.e., cohorts' effects) on caregivers' actions, diversity in the ways families accept and address their caregiving responsibilities, and the effectiveness of community services designed to support caregivers' growth and development.

We encourage academic scholars to acknowledge explicitly the influence of theory on their research efforts. Without well-articulated theories, the processes and dynamics of family caregiving and the influence that giving and receiving care has on the daily lives of individuals and families cannot be explained precisely (Roberto et al. 2006). Only by grounding research in theoretical principles of human nature and behavior will scholars be able to achieve a full understanding of what the empirical findings reveal about the diversity and complexity of late life caregiving families and apply this information widely (Krauss 2006).

While theories are powerful tools in understanding and predicting antecedents and consequences of family caregiving in late life, an important contribution of theorized research is its potential for informing educational programs, professional practice, and policy development through a dynamic interchange among professionals (Roberto et al. 2006). For example, Fredricksen-Goldsen and Scharlach (2006) lamented that working caregivers report more strain from balancing multiple roles now than ever before. According to the authors, "most workplace family friendly programs and policies have served to increase employees' availability for work without attending to the overall issue of work demands v. family needs" (Fredricksen-Goldsen and Scharlach 2006, p. 450). Attention to state and federal policies and not just employer policies that allow workers to consider how to meet family care needs at the same time that they consider how to meet work responsibilities will better address the heart of the caregiving matter. To ensure that future policy initiatives consider the multiple ways that aging families respond to the multiple demands associated with elder care, it is incumbent upon scholars to produce theoretically sound, evidence-based information. They must actively engage community practitioners and policy makers in discussions about demographic trends and their impact on family structure that will continue to affect families' abilities to provide quality elder care (Feldman et al. 2001).

When information is shared across professions, it can enhance future academic scholarship and further understanding of the patterns and behaviors of family caregivers that practitioners see in their daily practices. As policy is inextricably linked to the creation and fiscal backing of local and national programs for caregivers, the exchange of information among researchers, practitioners, and policy makers is critical to garnering support for the development and implementation of new services and interventions that will support the physical, social, and psychological well being of family caregivers in the twenty-first century and beyond.

References

Anderson, R. (1995). Revisiting the behavioral model and access to medical care: Does it matter? *Journal of Health and Social Behavior, 36,* 1–10. doi:10.2307/2137284.

Anderson, R., & Newman, J. (1973). Societal and individual determinants of medical care utilization in the United States. *Milbank Memorial Fund Quarterly, 51,* 95–124. doi:10.1111/j.1468-0009.2005.00428.x.

Baltes, P. B. (1987). Theoretical propositions of life-span developmental psychology: On the dynamics between growth and decline. *Developmental Psychology, 23,* 611–626. doi:10.1037/0012-1649.23.5.611.

Blau, P. (1964). *Exchanges and power in social life*. New York: Wiley.

Blieszner, R., Roberto, K. A., Wilcox, K. L., Barham, E. J., & Winston, B. L. (2007). Dimensions of ambiguous loss in couples coping with mild cognitive impairment. *Family Relations, 56,* 195–208. doi:10.1111/j.1741-3729.2007.00452.x.

Bradley, E. H., McGraw, S. A., Curry, L., Buckser, A., King, K. L., Kasl, S. V., & Andersen, R. (2002). Expanding the Andersen model: The role of psychosocial factors in long-term care use. *Health Services Research, 37,* 1221–1242. doi:10.1111/1475-6773.01053.

Burton, L. M. (1996). Age norms, the timing of family role transitions, and intergenerational caregiving among aging African American women. *The Gerontologist, 36,* 199–208. doi:10.1093/geront/36.2.199.

Calasanti, T., & King, N. (2007). Taking 'women's work' 'like a man': Husbands' experiences of care work. *The Gerontologist, 47,* 516–527. doi:10.1093/geront/47.4.516.

Celdrán, M., Villar, F., & Triadó, C. (2012). When grandparents have dementia: Effects on their grandchildren's family relationships. *Journal of Family Issues, 33,* 1218–1239. doi:10.1177/0192513X12443051.

Chen, Y. M., Henrick, S. C., & Young, H. M. (2010). A pilot evaluation of the Family Caregiver Support Program. *Evaluation and Program Planning, 33*(2), 113–119. doi:10.1016/j.evalprogplan.2009.08.002.

Dellmann-Jenkins, M., Blankemeyer, M., & Pinkard, O. (2000). Young adult children and grandchildren in primary caregiver roles to older relatives and their service needs. *Family Relations, 49,* 177–186. doi:10.1111/j.1741-3729.2000.00177.x.

Dilworth-Anderson, P., Goodwin, P. Y., & Williams, S. W. (2004). Can culture help explain the physical health effects of caregiving over time among African American caregivers? *Journals of Gerontology: Social Sciences*, *59*, S138–S145. doi:10.1093/geronb/59.3.S138.

Elder, G. (1977). Family history and the life course. *Journal of Family History, 2,* 279–304. doi:10.1177/036319907700200402.

Elder, G. (1998). The life course and human development. In R. M. Lerner (Ed.), *Handbook of child psychology: Vol: 1. Theoretical models of human development* (5th ed, pp. 939–991). New York: Wiley.

Feldman, P. H., Nadash, P., & Gursen, M. (2001). Improving communication between researchers and policy makers in long-term care: Or, researchers are from mars; policy makers are from venus. *The Gerontologist, 41,* 312–321. doi:10.1093/geront/41.3.312.

Fredriksen-Goldsen, K. I., & Scharlach, A. E. (2006). An interactive model of informal adult care and employment. *Community, Work & Family, 9,* 441–455. doi:10.1080/13668800600925084.

Fruhauf, C. A., & Orel, N. A. (2008). Developmental issues of grandchildren who provide care to grandparents. *The International Journal of Aging and Human Development, 67,* 209–230. doi:10.2190/AG.67.3.b.

Gans, D., & Silverstein, M. (2006). Norms of filial responsibility for aging parents across time and generations. *Journal of Marriage and Family, 68,* 961–976. doi:10.1111/j.1741-3737.2006.00307.x.

Gaugler, J. E., Pearlin, L. I., Davey, A., & Zarit, S. H. (2000). Modeling caregiver adaptation over time: The longitudinal impact of behavior problems. *Psychology and Aging, 15,* 437–450. doi:10,103 7//0882-7974.15.3.437.

Goodman, C. R., Zarit, S., & Steiner, V. L. (1997). Personal orientation as a predictor of caregiver strain. *Aging and Mental Health, 1,* 149–157. doi:10.1080/13607869757245.

Grant, J. (1997). Modernizing mothers: Home economics and the parent education movement, 1920–1945. In S. Stage, & V. B. Vincenti (Eds.), *Rethinking home economics: Women and the history of a profession* (pp. 55–74). Ithaca: Cornell University Press.

Hamill, S. B. (2012). Caring for grandparents with Alzheimer's disease: Help from the "Forgotten" generation. *Journal of Family Issues, 33,* 1195–1217. doi:10.1177/0192513X12444858.

Harris, P. B., Long, S. O., & Fuji, M. (1998). Men and elder care in Japan: A ripple of change? *Journal of Cross-Cultural Gerontology, 13,* 177–198. doi:10.1023/A:1006571508069.

Hepburn, K. W., Lewis, M., Sherman, C. W., & Tornatore, J. (2003). The Savvy Caregiver Program: Developing and testing a transportable dementia family caregiver training program. *The Gerontologist, 43,* 908–915. doi:10.1093/geront/43.6.908.

Hilgeman, M. M., Allen, R. S., DeCoster, J., & Burgio, L. D. (2007). Positive aspects of caregiving as a moderator of treatment outcome over 12 months. *Psychology and Aging, 22,* 361–371. doi:10.1037/0882-7974.22.2.361.

Homans, G. (1961). *Social behavior: Its elementary forms*. New York: Harcourt Brace & World.

Hooker, K., Bowman, S. R., Coehlo, D. P., Lim, S. R., Kaye, J., Guariglia, R., & Li, F. (2002). Behavioral change in persons with dementia: Relationships with mental and physical health of caregivers. *Journal of Gerontology: Psychological Sciences, 57,* P453–P460. doi:10.1093/geronb/57.5.P453.

Ingersoll-Dayton, B., & Antonucci, T. C. (1988). Reciprocal and nonreciprocal social supports: Contrasting sides of intimate relationships. *Journal of Gerontology: Social Sciences, 43,* S65–S73. doi:10.1093/geronj/43.3.S65.

Ingersoll-Dayton, B., Neal, M. B., & Hammer, L. B. (2001). Aging parents helping adult children: The experience of the sandwiched generation. *Family Relations, 50,* 262–271. doi:10.1111/j.1741-3729.2001.00262.x.

Ingersoll-Dayton, B, Neal, M. B., Ha, J., & Hammer, L. B. (2003). Redressing inequity in parent care among siblings. *Journal of Marriage and the Family, 65,* 201–212. doi:10.1111/j.1741-3737.2003.00201.x.

Jarrott, S. E., Zarit, S. H., Stephens, M. A. P., Townsend, A., & Greene, R. (2005). Instrumental help and caregivers' distress: Effects of change in informal and formal help. *American Journal of Alzheimer's Disease and Related Dementias, 20,* 181–190. doi:10.1177/153331750502000308.

Kosloski, K., Schaefer, J., Allwardt, D., Montgomery, R., & Karner, T. (2002). The role of cultural factors on clients' attitudes toward caregiving, perception of service delivery, and service utilization. *Home Health Care Services Quarterly, 21,* 65–88. doi:10.1300/J027v21n03_04.

Kramer, B. J., & Thompson, E. H. (2005). *Men as caregivers*. Amherst: Prometheus Books.

Krauss, N. (2006). Social relationships in late life. In R. H. Binstock, & L. K. George (Eds.), *Handbook of aging and the social sciences* (pp. 182–201). San Diego: Academic Press.

Lawrence, R. H., Tennstedt, S. L., & Assmann, S. F. (1998). Quality of the caregiver–care recipient relationship: Does it offset negative consequences of caregiving for family caregivers? *Psychology and Aging, 13,* 150–158. doi:10.1037/0882-7974.13.1.150.

Lévesque, L., Cossette, S., & Laurin, L. (1995). A multidimensional examination of the psychological and social well-being of caregivers of a demented relative. *Research on Aging, 17,* 332–360. doi:10.1177/0164027595173005.

Lévesque, L., Ducharme, F., Zarit, S. H., Lachance, L., & Giroux, F. (2008). Predicting longitudinal patterns of psychological distress in older husband caregivers: Further analysis of existing data. *Aging & Mental Health, 12,* 333–342. doi:10.1080/13607860801933414.

Lopez, J., Lopez-Arrieta, J., & Crespo, M. (2005). Factors associated with the positive impact of caring for elderly and dependent relatives. *Archives of Gerontology and Geriatrics, 41,* 81–94. doi:10.1016/j.archger.2004.12.001.

MaloneBeach, E. E., DeGenova, M., & Otani, H. (1998). Conflict, well-being, and depression: Young adults in intergenerational caregiving and noncaregiving families. *Korean Journal of Research in Gerontology, 8,* 5–16.

Mausbach, B. T., Coone, D. W., Depp, C., Rabinowitz, Y. G., Wilson-Arias, E., Kraemer, H. C., et al. (2004). Ethnicity and time to institutionalization of dementia patients: A comparison of Latina and Caucasian female family caregivers. *Journal of the American Geriatric Society, 52,* 1077–1084. doi:10.1111/j.1532-5415.2004.52306.x.

Newsom, J. T., & Schulz, R. (1998). Caregiving from the recipient's perspective: Negative reactions to being helped. *Health Psychology, 17,* 152–162. doi:10.1037/0278-6133.17.2.172.

Noonan, A. E., & Tennstedt, S. L. (1997). Meaning in caregiving and its contribution to caregiver well-being. *The Gerontologist, 37,* 785–794. doi:10.1093/geront/37.6.785.

O'Rourke, N., Cappeliez, R., & Neufeld, E. (2007). Recurrent depressive symptomatology and physical health: A 10-year study of informal caregivers of persons with dementia. *La Revue Canadienne de Psychiatrie, 52,* 434–441.

Peacock, S., Forbes, D., Markle-Reid, M., Hawranik, P., Morgan, D., Jansen, L., Leipert, B. D., & Henderson, S. R. (2010). The positive aspects of the caregiving journey with dementia: Using a strengths-based perspective to reveal opportunities. *Journal of Applied Gerontology, 29,* 640–659. doi:10.1177/0733464809341471.

Pearlin, L. I., Mullan, J. T., Semple, S. J., & Skaff, M. M. (1990). Caregiving and the stress process: An overview of concepts and their measures. *The Gerontologist, 30,* 583–594. doi:10.1093/geront/30.5.583.

Piercy, K. W., & Chapman, J. G. (2001). Adopting the caregiver role: A family legacy. *Family Relations, 50,* 386–393. doi:10.1111/j.1741-3729.2001.00386.x.

Pinquart, M., & Sörensen, S. (2006). Gender differences in care-giving stressors, social resources, and health: An updated meta-analysis. *Journal of Gerontology: Psychological Sciences, 61,* P33–45.

Pinquart, M., & Sörensen, S. (2011). Spouses, adult children, and children-in-laws as caregivers of older adults: A meta-analytic comparison. *Psychology and Aging, 26,* 1–14. doi:10.1037/a0021863.

Raschick, M., & Ingersoll-Dayton, B. (2004). Costs and rewards of caregiving among aging spouses and adult children. *Family Relations, 53,* 317–325. doi:10.1111/j.0022-2445.2004.0008.x.

Ribeiro, O., & Paúl, C. (2008). Older male carers and the positive aspects of care. *Ageing & Society, 28,* 165–183. doi:10.1017/S0144686X07006460.

Roberto, K. A., & Jarrott, S. E. (2008). Caregiving in late life: A life-span human development perspective. *Family Relations, 57,* 100–111. doi:10.1111/j.1741-3729.2007.00486.x.

Roberto, K. A., Blieszner, R., & Allen, K. R. (2006). Theorizing in family gerontology: New opportunities for research and practice. *Family Relations, 55,* 513–525. doi:10.1111/j.1741-3729.2006.00422.x.

Robertson, S. M., Zarit, S. H., Duncan, L. G., Rovine, M. J., & Femia, E. E. (2007). Family caregivers' patterns of positive and negative affect. *Family Relations, 56,* 12–23. doi:10.1111/j.1741-3729.2007.00436.x.

Scharlach, A. E., Giunta, N., Chow, J. C., & Lehning, A. (2008). Racial and ethnic variations in caregiver service use. *Journal of Aging and Health, 20,* 326–346. doi:10.1177/0898264308315426.

Semiatin, A. M., & O'Connor, M. K. (2012). The relationship between self-efficacy and positive aspects of caregiving in Alzheimer's disease caregivers. *Aging & Mental Health.* doi:10.1080/13607863.2011.651437.

Shifren, K. (2001). Early caregiving and adult depression: Good news for young caregivers. *The Gerontologist, 41,* 188–190. doi:10.1093/geront/41.2.188.

Shifren, K. (2009). Introduction: A life span perspective on caregivers. In K. Shifren (Ed.), *How caregiving affects development: Psychological implications for child, adolescent, and adult caregivers* (pp. 3–35). Washington, DC: American Psychological Association.

Stein, C. H., Wemmerus, V. A., Ward, M., Gaines, M. E., Freeberg, A. L., & Jewell, T. C. (1998). Because they're my parents: An intergenerational study of felt obligation and parental caregiving. *Journal of Marriage and the Family, 60,* 611–622. doi:10.2307/353532.

Stephens, M. A. P., & Franks, M. M. (1995). Spillover between daughters' roles as caregiver and wife: Interference or enhancement? *Journal of Gerontology: Psychological Sciences, 50,* P9–P17. doi:10.1093/geronb/50B.1.P9.

Suitor, J. J., & Pillemer, K. (1993). Support and interpersonal stress in the social networks of married daughters caring for parents with dementia. *Journal of Gerontology: Social Sciences, 48,* S1–S8. doi:10.1093/geronj/48.1.S1.

Thibaut, J. W., & Kelley, H. H. (1986). *The social psychology of groups.* New York: Wiley.

Toseland, R. W., McCallion, P., Gerber, R., & Bank, S. (2002). Predictors of health and human services use by persons with dementia and their family caregivers. *Social Science & Medicine,* 55, 1255–1266. doi:10.1016/S0277-9536(01)00240-4.

Wacker, R. R., & Roberto, K. A. (2014). *Community resources for older adults: Programs and services in an era of change* (4th ed.). Thousand Oaks: Sage.

Walker, A., Martin, S. S. K., & Jones, L. L. (1992). The benefits and costs of caregiving and care receiving for daughters and mothers. *Journal of Gerontology: Social Sciences, 47,* S130–S139. doi:10.1093/geronj/47.3.S130.

Wilcox, S., O'Sullivan, P., & King, A. C. (2001). Caregiver coping strategies: Wives versus daughters. *Clinical Gerontologist, 23,* 81–97. doi:10.1300/J018v23n01_08.

Wolff, J. L., & Kasper, J. D. (2006). Caregivers of frail elders: Updating a national profile. *The Gerontologist, 46,* 344–356. doi:10.1093/geront/46.3.344.

Contributions of Public Health to Caregiving

Ronda C. Talley, John E. Crews, Donald Lollar, Diane Elmore, Martha R. Crowther and Janet Valluzzi

The findings and conclusions in this chapter are those of the authors and do not necessarily represent the views of the Centers for Disease Control and Prevention.

R. C. Talley (✉)
Department of Psychology, College of Education and Behavioral Sciences,
Western Kentucky University, 1906 College Heights Boulevard,
GRH 3023, Bowling Green, KY 42101, USA
e-mail: Ronda.Talley@wku.edu

R. C. Talley · J. E. Crews · D. Lollar · J. Valluzzi
Division of Human Development and Disability,
National Center on Birth Defects and Developmental Disabilities,
Centers for Disease Control and Prevention,
1600 Clifton Road, Atlanta, GA 30299, USA
e-mail: jcrews@cdc.gov

D. Lollar
Oregon Institute on Disability and Development,
Oregon Health and Science University,
Child Development and Rehabilitation Center,
707 SW Gaines Road, 97239 Portland, OR, USA
e-mail: lollar@ohsu.edu

D. Elmore
American Psychological Association, 750 First Street,
Washington, DC, NE 20002, USA
e-mail: delmore@apa.org

Policy Program Director, National Center for Child Traumatic Stress,
Duke University Medical Center, 27701 Durham, NC, USA
e-mail: diane.elmore@duke.edu

M. R. Crowther
Department of Psychology, University of Alabama,
PO Box 870348, Tuscaloosa, AL 35487, USA
e-mail: mrcrowther@as.ua.edu

J. Valluzzi
2151 Jamison Avenue #609, Alexandria, VA 22314, USA
e-mail: Janet.Valluzzi@cms.hhs.gov

R. C. Talley, S. S. Travis (eds.), *Multidisciplinary Coordinated Caregiving*,
Caregiving: Research • Practice • Policy, DOI 10.1007/978-1-4614-8973-3_11,

Contributions of Public Health to Caregiving

Health is a concern of every American. As a large portion of the US population ages (Giguere 2007; Kausler and Kausler 2001), the avoidance of illness and disease is increasingly viewed as both desirable and obtainable for the majority of the population. Middle and old age, viewed through the lenses of a generation of aging individuals who consider all things to be possible, have been psychologically transformed from the stereotypical view as a time to wind down and prepare for life's end to a time of enrichment and opportunity for new experiences and adventures. As life spans lengthen for most individuals (U.S Census Bureau 2005, 2006a, b), concerns about the quality of life become paramount. A public health model supports this shift by calling for not only disease prevention, but also health promotion (CDC 2007a).

Much public attention is now focused on the remarkable health advances available to the elderly. However, a public health approach that addresses the needs of individuals throughout the life span is essential if we are to enhance the public's health, prevent disease, and extend life's quality as well as its quantity. A public health perspective calls for society to embrace new modes of conceptualizing health, moving from the treatment of diseases and injuries to their prevention, then forward to a perspective that regards health not only as the absence of illness, but also as the presence of positive physical and mental well-being (Fredrickson and Losada 2005; Keyes 2007). Within this model, care for the individual, as a member of society, begins with preventive action, such as the administration of folic acid to young adult women, which reduces the chance of spina bifida in the newborn. A public health approach is a societal process that begins prior to birth and extends through end of life.

Only recently has caregiving been regarded as a public health issue. Historically, care needs have been framed from psychological or medical models without emphasis on the environmental contexts of care (Clark and Weist 2000; Hacker and Darcy 2006; Knight and Maines 2001; Rozensky 1994; Wallace 1998; Winslow 1920). Talley and Crews articulated the importance of caregiving as a public health issue (Talley et al. 2004; Talley and Crews 2007), arguing that within a public health model, caregiving is an essential function. They assert that caregiving occurs between not only the family caregiver—care recipient dyad, but also with a third group of individuals—professional caregivers. Within this collaborative partnership, multiple family and professional caregivers may serve the care recipient in varying durations and with diverse functions throughout the disability or disease course. For example, a mother or father may be the newborn's first caregiver, with a pediatrician, pediatric nurse, or other specialist serving as the first professional caregivers involved in the child's life. However, the care triad will change as the child develops, with other family caregivers, such as grandparents, aunts, uncles, older siblings, or neighbors, serving as additional layers of care providers. As the child grows to adulthood, other givers of care, such as teachers, coaches, club leaders, and religious elders, will model and instruct the child through pathways of care.

In this chapter, we explore the foundations of public health, its history, and its leadership within the USA. We examine how these concepts provide a context for considering current issues in public health. Specifically, we highlight the current status of public health practice, the education and training of public health professionals, surveillance and research in public health, and policy and advocacy in the field. Importantly, we relate this information to a critical public health issue: the care of family and friends during times of illness and disability. As an emerging public health issue, caregiving has captured the nation's attention.

Public Health Caregiving

The Committee for the Study of the Future of Public Health (Institute of Medicine [IOM] 1988) defines public health as "what we, as a society, do collectively to assure the conditions in which people can be healthy" (p. 1). Both public and private groups are involved in the public health system, which is responsible for preventing epidemics and disease spread, protecting against environmental hazards, eliminating injuries, promoting healthy behavior, assisting communities to recover from disasters, and enhancing the quality and accessibility of health services (*Healthy People 2010,* 2000).

Public health agencies are charged with the core functions of assessment, policy development, and assurance (IOM 1988, 2002b; see Fig. 1). The assessment function involves monitoring and evaluating health information while diagnosing public health issues. Policy development addresses comprehensive public health issues and the mobilization of community resources (Veazie et al. 2001). The assurance function is directed to enforcing laws, evaluating progress, and ensuring a competent public health workforce. These functions have been translated into 10 essential public health services (Table 1) and applied to diverse settings (Adelman and Taylor 2006; Lollar 2002; Weist 2005).

Public Health Caregiving Defined

As discussed in the introductory chapter, caregiving refers to assistance by a family member or friend to an individual who is ill or disabled (see Chap. 1). Table 2 presents caregiving by the public health dimensions of assessment, health promotion, and disease prevention with sample caregiving questions, activity types, and potential outcomes. In addition, caregiving is colored by the individual's discipline-specific orientation. For instance, as outlined in Table 3, the application of public health, psychological, or medical models may lead to differing societal outcomes.

In this chapter, we use the term *public health caregiving* to refer to the nexus between public health and caregiving. While there is considerable overlap between the two areas on dimensions of population-based assessment, needs, and interventions, there are some caregiving needs outside of the public health domain and many areas of public health that encompass caregiving, but are not restricted to it. For instance, in caregiving, both population-based public health strategies, as well as individually-based interventions may be needed. However, in addition to caregiving, a public health framework is used for health promotion and disease prevention in physical and mental health, addressing issues, such as diseases like cancer, diabetes, Alzheimer's disease, and depression (Thompson 2003). Thus, public health caregiving is a specialized area of concern involving the application of public health theory,

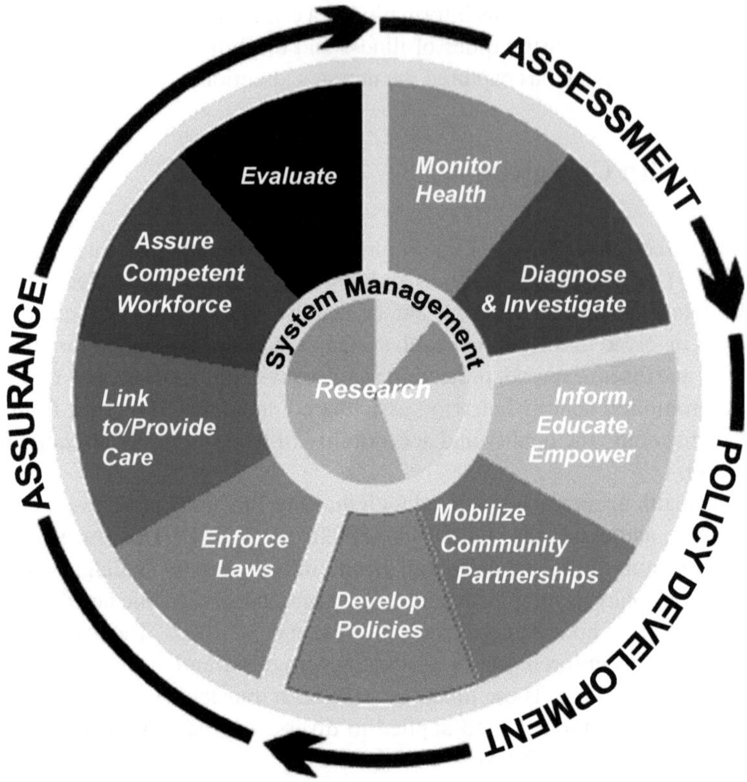

Fig. 1 Public health functions. (Adopted: Fall 1994, Source: Public Health Functions Steering Committee, Members (July 1995): American Public Health Association, Association of Schools of Public Health, Association of State and Territorial Health Officials, Environmental Council of the States, National Association of County and City Health Officials, National Association of State Alcohol and Drug Abuse Directors, National Association of State Mental Health Program Directors, Public Health Foundation, U.S. Public Health Service, Agency for Health Care Policy and Research, Centers for Disease Control and Prevention, Food and Drug Administration, Health Resources and Services Administration, Indian Health Service, National Institutes of Health, Office of the Assistant Secretary for Health, Substance Abuse and Mental Health Services Administration.)

research, education, support, and practice, which are derived from public health principles, to supporting those who provide care to another in need.

Public Health Leadership on Caregiving

A variety of federal and state agencies and departments, as well as scientific organizations and professional associations have engaged the issue of public health caregiving (Turnock 2004). At the national level, these include the President, who convenes the White House Conference on Aging and the President's Council on Bioethics; federal departments, such as the US Department of Health and Human Services (HHS), and offices within the department, such as the Surgeon General's Office, the Admin-

Table 1 Competencies for providing essential public health services. (From *Essential Public Health Services*. Adopted Fall 1994 by the Public Health Functions Steering Committee.)

1	Monitor health status to identify community health problems
2	Diagnose and investigate health problems and health hazards in the community
3	Inform, educate, and empower people about health issues
4	Mobilize community partnerships to identify and solve health problems
5	Develop policies and plans that support individual and community health efforts
6	Enforce laws and regulations that protect health and ensure safety
7	Link people to needed personal health services and assure the provision of health care when otherwise unavailable
8	Assure a competent public health and personal health care workforce
9	Evaluate effectiveness, accessibility, and quality of personal and population-based health services
10	Research for new insights and innovative solutions to health problems

istration on Aging (AoA), the Centers for Disease Control and Prevention (CDC), and the National Institutes of Health (NIH); and the Department of Veterans Affairs (VA). Other relevant organizations include the Institute of Medicine (IOM) and the American Public Health Association (APHA), both because of their history, as well as their potential to advance a caregiving agenda. National leadership is essential to public health caregiving since it provides recognition of caregivers and their needs, promulgates legislation and policies to address these needs, and allocates resources for caregiving initiatives.

National Leadership

Presidential Leadership

White House Conferences on Aging

Since their inception, White House conferences on aging have rallied leadership and focus on the health care needs of older Americans (White House Conference on Aging 2005a). Begun in 1961, the first White House Conference on Aging focused on health care. It was followed a decade later with a conference on income maintenance; in 1981 with a conference on social security; and in 1995, with a focus on support for existing "safety net" programs, such as Medicaid, Medicare, and the Older American's Act (White House Conference on Aging 2005b). Held from December 11 to 14, 2005, the fifth White House Conference on Aging was attended by over 3,000 people. Delegates voted for the top 50 of 73 resolutions that were presented based on a multi-year input process (White House Conference on Aging 2005a). Key resolutions pertaining to caregiving are presented in Table 4. These resolutions contain ones that are directly related to caregiving, such as the adoption of long-term care strategies and the delivery of high quality services, as well as those indirectly related, but which make the caregiver's tasks easier, such as the design of accessible buildings and innovative technology. Of the 25 proposed resolutions that contain caregiving concepts, 21 were passed by the delegation (White House Conference on

Table 2 Public health caregiving

Public health dimensions	Sample caregiving questions	Sample caregiving activity types	Potential caregiving outcomes
Assessment/ surveillance	How many caregivers are there?	BRFSS optional caregiver module administered by each state	State-level, population-based documentation of the caregiver incidence and prevalence over time
	What are their caregiving responsibilities?	Telephone surveys administered by various groups (AARP, Metlife, NAC, FCA, AD Association)	Information on caregiver experience in relation to designated disease or issue criteria (e.g., AD caregiving or intergenerational caregiving)
	How much time do they spend caregiving?		
	What are the most prevalent disabilities, diseases, and injuries do they experience?		
Health promotion	What variables impact caregiver health?	Design, implementation, and evaluation of caregiver intervention programs addressing ways to prevent caregiver disability, disease, or injury before it occurs	Increased caregiver resilience and physical/mental health at the start of and throughout the caregiving experience
		Design, implementation, and evaluation of individual and group caregiver-directed interventions to maintain health and well-being of caregivers throughout their caregiving careers	Increased understanding of and ability to deal with disability, illness, or injury of care recipient
Disease prevention	What may be done to "inoculate" caregivers against disability, disease, and injury?	Research on caregiver disease risks	Increased understanding of risk factors for caregivers and ways to decrease risk of caregiver disability, disease, or injury

Table 2 (continued)

Public health dimensions	Sample caregiving questions	Sample caregiving activity types	Potential caregiving outcomes
	What existing interventions are evidence-based and effective?	Development, implementation, and evaluation of caregiver-directed inventions before, during, and after death of the care recipient	Community mobilization, cross-agency collaborations, and formation of caregiving coalitions to address caregivers' needs
	What community supports are needed to promote caregiver wellness and quality of life?	Individual and group activities for caregivers designed to	
	What is the level of "community caregiving capacity?"	Development, initiation, and evaluation of community-level and community-wide supports to decrease caregiver stress and burden	

Aging 2005c), although no action has occurred on them to date. Thus, while White House conferences can help set an agenda (White House Conference on Aging 2005d) and are important in their own right, action-oriented recommendations, such as those in Table 4 pertaining to public health and caregiving, must be carried forth by groups with implementation power.

President's Council on Bioethics

Established on November 28, 2001, by Presidential Executive Order 13237, the President's Council on Bioethics advises the President on bioethical issues brought to light by biomedical science and technology advances. The Council was renewed on September 23, 2003, by Executive Order 13316, and again on September 29, 2005, by Executive Order 13385. As an advisory group, the Council's mission is to:

> (1) undertake fundamental inquiry into the human and moral significance of developments in biomedical and behavioral science and technology; (2) to explore specific ethical and policy questions related to these developments; (3) provide a forum for a national discussion of bioethical issues; (4) facilitate a greater understanding of bioethical issues; and (5) explore possibilities for useful international collaboration on bioethical issues. (Presidential Executive Order 13237 2001).

Table 3 Comparison of three care models

	Public health model	Psychological model	Medical model
Definition	Population-focused on all aspects of health	Individually-focused on mental health	Individually-focused on physical health
Emergence			
Philosophy			
Mission	Disease prevention Health promotion Fulfillment of society's interest in assuring the conditions in which people can be healthy (IOM 1988)		
Substance	Organized community efforts aimed at the prevention of disease and the promotion of health (IOM 1988)		
Organizational framework	Activities undertaken within the formal structure of government and the associated efforts of private and voluntary organizations and individuals (IOM 1988)		
Consumers	Communities Health care services Individuals		
Surveillance			
Assurance			
Prevention			
Health promotion			
Practice/intervention			
Care standards			
Education standards			
Continuing education	Required dependent on specific health profession	Required for all practicing health psychologists	Required for all professional medical staff
Evaluation standards			
Policy/advocacy			
Reimbursement/financing			
Insurance			

Table 4 Caregiving-related resolutions considered by the 2005 White House conference on aging. (From *Index of Resolutions* 2005a, White House conference on aging)

Resolution area number	Resolution area	Priority number (consecutively numbered across resolution areas)	Resolution
I	Planning along the lifespan	5[a]	Foster innovations in financing long-term care services to increase options available to consumers
II	Workplace of the future	13	Promote assistive technology in the workplace to help older workers remain in the workforce
III	Our community	14[a]	Expand opportunities for developing innovative housing designs for seniors' needs
		16	Encourage advancement of intergenerational strategies
		17[a]	Encourage community designs to promote livable communities that enable aging in place
		26[a]	Support older adult caregivers raising their relatives' children
		27	Expand integrated aging and disability resource centers nationwide
IV	Health and long-term living	30[a]	Develop a coordinated, comprehensive long-term care strategy by supporting public and private section initiatives that address financing, choice, quality, service delivery, and the paid and unpaid workforce
		31[a]	Apply evidence based research to the delivery of health and social services where appropriate
		32[a]	Evaluate payment and coordination policies in the geriatric healthcare continuum to ensure continuity of care
		34[a]	Improve the health and quality of life of older Americans through disease management and chronic care coordination
		40[a]	Attain adequate numbers of healthcare personnel in all professions who are skilled, culturally competent, and specialized in geriatrics
		41[a]	Support geriatric education and training for all healthcare professionals, paraprofessionals, health profession students, and direct care workers
		42[a]	Promote innovative models of non-institutional long-term care
		43[a]	Ensure appropriate care for seniors with disabilities

Table 4 (continued)

Resolution area number	Resolution area	Priority number (consecutively numbered across resolution areas)	Resolution
		44[a]	Reduce healthcare disparities among minorities by developing strategies to prevent disease, promote health, and deliver appropriate care and wellness
		46[a]	Promote innovative evidence-based and practice-based medical and aging research
		48[a]	Ensure appropriate recognition and care for veterans across all healthcare settings
		53[a]	Improve access to care for older adults living in rural areas
		55[a]	Improve patient advocacy to assist patients in and across all care settings
V	Civic and social engagement		None
VI	Technology and innovation in the marketplace	61[a]	Promote the integration of health and aging services to improve access and quality of care for older Americans
		65	Promote an accessible nation by expanding the availability and utilization of assistive and universally designed technologies through private-public incentives
	Cross cutting	67[a]	Support a broad strategy for supporting informal caregivers of seniors to enable adequate quality and supply of services
		71[a]	Improve state and local based integrated delivery systems to meet twenty-first century need of seniors
		72[a]	Review alignment of government programs that delivery services to older Americans

[a]Resolution passed

Activities of the Presidential Council on Bioethics are addressed here because of their recent interest in caregiving. *Taking Care: Ethical Caregiving in Our Aging Society* (2005a) was produced by the Council "to gain attention for a burgeoning social problem and to offer ethical guidance regarding the care of our elders who can no longer care for themselves" (Presidential Council on Bioethics 2005a, p. 5). Among other recommendations, the report called for a Presidential Commission on Aging, Dementia, and Long-Term Care to focus the nation's attention on caregiving. The report went largely unrecognized by the caregiving community (cited only eight times in PubMed articles since it issuance) even though it did recognize the crisis in caregiving that is emerging as baby boomers age. As reasons for this general disregard, Eckenwiler (2006) suggests that the report's focus was too narrow and supports a conservative political agenda, covers ground addressed in other reports, and perpetuates the stigma between death and old age. Thus, even though the report indicates presidential attention to the issue of caregiving, the resources and professional time represented by the report suggests another missed opportunity to provide support to caregivers and to advance the direction of the field.

Departmental Leadership

US Department of Health and Human Services

The US Department of Health and Human Services serves as the federal governmental organization dealing with public health. Within the department's broad framework, four entities have, or have the potential to have, substantive foci on issues pertaining to caregiving: the Administration on Aging, the Centers for Disease Control and Prevention, the Surgeon General's office, and the National Institutes of Health.

Administration on Aging

The Administration on Aging is charged with implementation of premiere legislation to provide caregiver support: the National Family Caregiver Support Program (NFCSP) of the Older Americans Act Amendments of 2000. Currently funded at US$ 162 million, the NFCSP authorizes state divisions on aging to work with area agencies on aging throughout the state and local community-service providers to provide a range of services. These include: (a) information to caregivers about available services; (b) assistance to caregivers in gaining access to services; (c) individual counseling, organization of support groups, and training to assist the caregivers in making decisions and solving problems relating to their caregiving roles; (d) respite care to enable caregivers to be temporarily relieved from their caregiving responsibilities; and (e) limited supplemental services to complement the care provided by caregivers (AoA 2007).

Since its inception, more than 750,000 family caregivers nationwide have received services through the NFCSP. There are four eligible groups: (1) family caregivers of older adults, age 60 years or older; (2) caregivers of a person with Alzheimer's disease or a related disorder, regardless of age; (3) grandparents and relative caregivers, 55 years of age or older, of children no older than 18 years of age; relative caregivers, age 55 years or older, of an adult child aged 19–59 with a disability (not including natural or adoptive parents). In addition, the program requires states to give priority to older individuals who provide care to children or adults with severe disabilities.

In 2001, the first year of the National Family Caregiver Support Program, the AoA administered 3-year caregiver innovation grants to state and area agencies on aging, nonprofit community service providers, institutions of higher education, and national organizations (AoA 2004). An additional, US$ 5 million in grants were awarded to tribal organizations to provide caregiver support services for Native American and Native Hawaiian elders with an additional US$ 6.3 million to Native Americans in fiscal year 2007.

Two other AoA caregiver initiatives are noteworthy. First, AoA works closely with the National Aging Services Network of federal, state, and local organizations to plan, coordinate, and provide home- and community-based services to older persons and their caregivers. Second, AoA supports a nationwide, toll free information and assistance directory and website called the Eldercare Locator (800-677-1116, www.eldercare.gov), which connects older persons and their caregivers with the National Aging Services Network. Using this resource, older individuals and their caregivers can find needed services.

Centers for Disease Control and Prevention

As one of 13 major operating entities of the US Department of Health and Human Services (CDC 2007a), the Centers for Disease Control and Prevention's mission is "to promote health and quality of life by preventing and controlling disease, injury, and disability" (CDC 2006a). To accomplish its mission, the CDC works with organizations throughout the USA and the world to perform eight core functions: (1) monitor health, (2) detect and investigate health problems, (3) conduct research to enhance prevention, (4) develop and advocate sound public health policies, (5) implement prevention strategies, (6) promote healthy behaviors, (7) foster safe and healthful environments, and (8) provide leadership and training (CDC n.d.). Founded in 1946 with a US$ 10 million budget and 400 employees, the CDC has expanded considerably beyond its original charge of controlling malaria to address a broad range of public health issues, including pandemic influenza terrorism, obesity, chronic diseases, cancer, and disabilities (Lumpkin 2005). With 9,300 employees, the CDC's FY'08 budget request is US$ 8.8 billion for program support (CDC 2007b, c).

CDC's health impact goals are relevant to the caregiving community. They address: (a) healthy people in every stage of life across the entire life span; (b) healthy people in healthy places, including homes, schools, workplaces, communities, and healthcare settings; (c) people prepared for emerging health threats, such as hurricanes, tornadoes, floods, or terrorism; and (d) healthy people in a healthy world, including health protection, promotion, and diplomacy (CDC 2007b).

Within the CDC, as noted by the work of the Disability and Health Team of the National Center on Birth Defects and Developmental Disabilities (NCBDDD) and the Healthy Aging Program of the National Center for Chronic Disease Prevention and Health Promotion, caregiving has emerged very rapidly as a public health concern and the initiative has enjoyed considerable support.

National Center on Birth Defects and Developmental Disabilities, Disability and Health Team Within the NCBDDD, the Disability and Health Team addresses the health and prevention of secondary conditions in people with disabilities, including the health of their caregivers. The team's mission is "to improve the health and well-being of people with disabilities" (CDC 2006b, (1). Caregiving program goals are founded on the assumption that the better the health of caregivers, the longer and more successfully they can remain in caregiving roles, and as a consequence, care recipients will enjoy greater health and an improved quality of life than they would if the caregiver could not function. The pathway of improved health and quality of life for people with disabilities, in this initiative, is through family caregivers. To achieve its mission, the Disability and Health Team develops strategies to create, implement, and evaluate a broad national program intended to bring a pronounced CDC emphasis on public health and public health policy to this large population. The scientific and programmatic imperatives of the Disability and Health Team are driven by the conceptual framework created by the World Health Organization's (WHO) *International Classification of Functioning, Disability and Health* (ICF; WHO 2001).

While caregiving has been promoted at CDC for a number of years, caregiver research sponsored the Disability and Health Team, began in 2004 when grant awards made to Dr. Karen Kuhlthau at Harvard-Massachusetts General Hospital and Dr. Elena Andresen at the University of Florida. With grant funds, Dr. Kuhlthau analyzed data from the State and Local Area Integrated Telephone Survey (SLAITS) on the health effects of caregiving upon parents of young children with disabilities. She found that parents of young children with disabilities did not access routine health care as regularly as parents who did not have children with disabilities. Dr. Andresen and her colleagues developed a caregiver module for the Behavioral Risk Factors Surveillance System (BRFSS), which was piloted in North Carolina (Neugaard et al. 2007). In addition, Andresen examined two caregiver questions from the 2000 to 2001 BRFSS core to estimate the prevalence of caregiving for older people.

Continued advancement of the caregiving agenda occurred in late 2005 when the CDC director, Dr. Julie Gerberding, made US$ 1 million available to the CDC Coordinating Center on Health Promotion, in which NCBDDD and the Health and Disability team reside. The purpose of the competitive funds was to support innovative programming ideals. The caregiving program applied for and was awarded a third of the director's discretionary funds, receiving the largest grant made. Funded activities provided for the expansion of current program activities and the addition of several exciting initiatives.

One component of the award funded continuing development of the BRFSS caregiving module. To further module development, three cash awards of US$ 5,000 were made to states that successfully competed to become field-test sites for the module: Hawaii, Kansas, and. In addition to the cash awards, states also received technical assistance and outcome reports from the University of Florida team that initially developed and tested the module in North Carolina. Concurrently, the Disability and Health Team worked collaboratively with the BRFSS staff at CDC to continue the approval process for the module to be made an official optional module of the BRFSS, with the goal of having an approved BRFSS caregiving module for use by all states in 2009. Administration of the caregiving module by the states will allow national-level, population-based data on caregiving to be tabulated for the first time.

A second component of the director's discretionary award funded the development of a searchable database on caregiver research with specific attention to both government and nongovernmental instruments that contain caregiver-related variables or that can inform caregiver health and behavior if used in combination. In addition, a funded meta-analysis on caregiver health effects provided a synthesis of research on this topic.

The final component of the director's discretionary award funded an expert panel to advise on the latter two activities in combination with previously initiated and on-going caregiving work, and to produce a report on recommendations for future action of the Disability and Health Team to support caregivers.

Drawing on this and other research, the caregiver initiative has evolved into a well integrated area of research and programmatic efforts. In addition, writing on caregiving issues by Disability and Health science team members includes a 2007 *American Journal of Public Health* peer reviewed article, *Framing the Public Health of Caregiving* (Talley and Crews 2007), which conceptualizes caregiving as a public health issue. This was followed by a June 2007 article in the *Mortality and Morbidity Weekly Report* that examines the results of the initial field-testing of the caregiving module in North Carolina (Neugaard et al. 2007). Lastly, *The Multiple Dimensions of Caregiving and Disability* (Talley and Crews 2007), which is edited by members of the Disability and Health team, is in production.

In the future, the Disability and Health Team will provide national leadership in collaboration with other national agencies and groups to advance the field of caregiving and the health of caregivers and care recipients.

National Center for Chronic Disease Prevention and Health Promotion Healthy Aging Program Housed with the National Center for Chronic Disease Prevention and Health Promotion (NCCDPHP), the CDC Healthy Aging Program has five primary objectives: (1) to link public health and aging services networks at the national, state, and local levels; (2) to provide high-quality health information to public health and aging professionals and to the general public; (3) to partner with the healthcare system to enhance communication and promote the broader use of clinical preventive services; (4) to monitor health trends of older Americans to guide program efforts; and (5) to work with communities to translate effective prevention research findings into community-based programs.

The Healthy Aging Program is examining existing data to better understand the characteristics of caregivers and the caregiving situation for people caring for an older adult who has a cognitive impairment. More specifically, they have a special focus on understanding caregiving among American Indian and Alaskan Natives, with an emphasis on tribal-based elders receiving supportive care. Finally, the Health Aging Program is committed to identifying and putting into practice effective programs. To this end, they explore avenues to move evidence-based interventions into practice, thus resulting in improved health and well-being of caregivers.

The Disability and Health team in the NCBDDD and Healthy Aging Program in the NCCDPHP have worked collaboratively since 2003 to promote caregiving as an important issue within CDC. One example of this is the caregiving symposium of the programs co-sponsored at the 2007 Behavioral Risk Factor Surveillance System (BRFSS) conference.

Surgeon General

The Surgeon General of the US Public Health Service in the Department of Health and Human Services provides national leadership to the country's public health system. Appointed in 1871, the first person to hold this role was John M. Woodworth, a founder of the American Public Health Association and Supervising Surgeon of the Marine Hospital Service, the precursor to the US Public Health Service. Interestingly, Dr. Woodworth also designed the seal of the US Public Health Service, which with modification, remains to this day. In 1873, the position title was changed to Supervising Surgeon General and, in 1902, it was revised again to the title currently used, Surgeon General. There have been 17 Surgeon Generals since the position's inception; however, the official Office of the Surgeon General was established in abolished in 1968, then re-established in 1987 (U.S. Department of Health and Human Services [HHS] 1981).

The Surgeon General has numerous duties and forums to offer public health leadership. Duties include serving as an advisor to the President and the Secretary of Health and Human Services on public health, health policy, and health prevention. The Surgeon General also supervises the Commissioned Corps of the US Public Health Service, informs the nation about critical public health issues, and offers a visible public presence on these issues by delivering speeches, sponsoring conferences, and giving interviews (HHS 1981). Three additional responsibilities of the Surgeon General will be discussed next: developing Public Health Reports of the Surgeon General, issuing Calls to Action on public health issues, and setting national public health goals.

Public Health Reports The first Public Health Report was released in 1964 by Surgeon General Luther L. Terry, MD, the 9th Surgeon General. The impetus for the report was the Public Health Cigarette Smoking Act of 1969, which required the Surgeon General to produce an annual report reviewing the latest scientific findings on the effects of smoking on health. As a result of this Act, over half of all public health reports during the past 43 years have had smoking as a central issue. Recent reports have addressed the health consequences of involuntary exposure to tobacco smoke (2006) and smoking (2004b) as well as smoking and women (2001a), bone health and osteoporosis (2004a), and youth violence (2001b).

Each Surgeon General has championed specific issues and the Public Health Reports reflect that interest. For example, in 1979, Surgeon General Julius B. Richmond issued *Healthy People: The Surgeon General's Report on Health Promotion and Disease Prevention,* which focused on exercise, nutrition, environmental factors, and occupational safety. Surgeon General C. Everett Koop, who served from 1981 to 1989, released the *Surgeon General's Report on Acquired Immune Deficiency Syndrome* (1986). In 1999, Surgeon General David Satcher issued *Mental Health A Report of the Surgeon General*, marking an expansion of the Surgeon General's concerns beyond a predominant focus on diseases of the body

National Public Health Priorities Announced in 2006, the Surgeon General's public health priorities (HHS 2006b) are: (a) preventing disease, with attention to the issues of decreasing the number of Americans who are overweight or obese, born with birth defects, or become ill due to HIV/AIDS or tobacco use and increasing the numbers of persons who engage in physical activity; (b) eliminating health disparities, specifically addressing the greater burden of death and disease from breast cancer, prostate cancer, cervical cancer, cardiovascular disease, diabetes, and other illnesses in minority populations; (c) strengthening public health preparedness, with a focus on planning to deal with terrorism, emerging infections, and natural disasters, as well as mental health and resilience; (d) improving health literacy for the more than 90 million Americans who cannot adequately understand basic health information; and (e) increasing organ donations to respond to the 95,557 individuals who are on the waiting list as of March 23, 2007 (Office of Organ Procurement and Transportation [OPTN] 2007b), with 300 added to the waiting list each month and approximately 77 individuals added to the list each day (Health Resources and Services Administration 2007a).

US Department of Veterans Affairs

The precursor to the Department of Veterans Affairs (VA), the Veterans Administration was created by Executive Order 5398, signed by President Herbert Hoover on July 21, 1930. The second largest cabinet department, the VA is responsible for providing federal benefits to veterans and their families, including health care, financial assistance, and burial benefits (U.S. Department of Veteran's Affairs 2006). Currently, approximately 63 million veterans, family members, or survivors of veterans are potentially eligible for VA benefits and services. Benefits or pensions can cover multiple generations: currently, five children of Civil War veterans and 440 children and widows of Spanish–American War veterans still draw benefits or pensions.

When the system began, there were 31,600 employees working in 54 hospitals to serve 4.7 million living veterans. Currently, the Department of Veterans Affairs has 235,974 employees in 113 ambulatory care and community-based outpatient clinics, nursing homes, residential rehabilitation treatment programs, veterans centers, and comprehensive home-care programs serving 5.3 million veterans, with an additional 2.4 million veterans enrolled (VA 2006). In 2005, the VA spent US$ 1.55 billion on research from federal (US$ 731 million) and nonfederal (US$ 819 million) sources. With more than half of the physicians practicing in the nation receiving some education at the VA, it is the operator of the country's largest medical education and health professions training program, matriculating 83,000 health professionals each year. For FY'08, the VA has requested a budget of US$ 1.724 billion dollars (VA 2007d).

Based on a 2002 needs assessment (VA 2002), in 2003, the VA started a care coordination program that utilizes information technology to enhance or extend care and case management (VA 2007a). They developed this model based on a 2000 pilot program, which was expanded in 2002, 2003, and 2004. National adoption of the care coordination model was completed in 2005. Understanding the needs of the caregiver in the home and finding ways to link them with local support sources is a vital element of the program (VA 2007b).

Beginning in 2005, the VA's care coordination program incorporated concepts of patient self-management and shared decision-making. At that time, the care coordination program had three foci : (1) care coordination home telehealth; (2) care coordination general telehealth; and (3) care coordination involving store-and-forwards telehealth (VA 2007a, c). In the first model, home telehealth technologies provide in-home support while in the second model, videoconferencing technologies, including telemental health and telesurgery, are shared among VA facilities. The store- and forwards telehealth model was developed by the VA in collaboration with the Department of Defense and the Joslin Vision Network in Boston. Based on a primary care paradigm, under the third model, diabetic veterans are screened for retinopathy using a nonmydriatic teleretinal imaging program and referred for needed treatment.

National Association Leadership

American Public Health Association

The American Public Health Association (APHA), the nation's leading advocacy organization for public health professionals, was founded in 1872 (APHA 2007b). As an organizational leader in the field of public health (APHA 2007a), the support of APHA for caregiving issues is paramount. A search of the APHA website revealed no association policies expressly about caregiving, but three caregiving-related policies: women's issues, expanded family and medical leave, and end-of-life care. In the latter document, APHA specifically addresses caregivers' needs in this context: "families and caregivers of persons with chronic terminal illnesses often experience increased morbidity or premature mortality resulting from the stress and strains associated with a loved one's terminal decline" (APHA 2005, p. 1). A search of the association's newsletter, *The Nation's Health*, yielded 37 hits using "caregiving" as the search term, while a similar search of the association's journal, the *American Journal of Public Health*, yielded four articles with "caregiving" in the title, 114 additional articles with caregiving in the text, and 11 articles with caregiver in the title. While a foundation for public health caregiving advocacy has been laid, clearly, a great deal of additional work is needed by APHA members in order to rally the association's considerable influence to the benefit of America's caregivers.

National Scientific Leadership

National Academies: The Institute of Medicine

Under a charter approved by President Abraham Lincoln in 1863, the National Academies were created as independent sources for the scientific review of important public issues. The non-governmental National Academies consist of four organizations: the Institute of Medicine, the National Academy of Sciences, the National Academy of Engineering, and the National Research Council. The National Academy of Sciences was established in the same year as the charter, with the other three groups organized at later dates. The creation of the Institute of Medicine in 1970 marked the last of the four organizations established under the original charter (The National Academies 2007).

As a private organization with no direct ties to the federal government, the Institute of Medicine was established to fill the need for an independent, nonpartisan entity to provide scientific advice on health matters. While the IOM is not directly funded by the federal government, the majority of studies it conducts is for government agencies and is paid for with their appropriations. Experts appointed to IOM panels serve free of charge, a requirement of the original charter. Expert panel meetings may be public or private, and each IOM report must be evidence-based and undergo a rigorous peer review process before release to the public (IOM 2006a).

Recent IOM reports of critical importance to the public health caregiving community include *Disability in America: Toward a National Agenda for Prevention* (2002a), *Health Insurance is a Family Matter* (2002c), *Workshop on Disability in America: A New Look—Summary and Background Papers* (2006c), and, most recently, *The Future of Disability in America* (2007a). A new IOM project of currency to the public health caregiving constituency is *The Future Health Care Workforce for Older Americans* (2006b). With a looming shortage of health personnel trained in geriatric care (Giguere 2007), the workforce report, due in 2008, will illuminate a subject of growing public concern: caring for the aging population, including those aging with disabilities. Since most Americans wish to remain in their home while receiving care (Larsson et al. 2004), *Psychosocial Services to Cancer Patients and Families in a Community Setting* (IOM 2007b) is another projected IOM report that will also provide leadership on how we can better support family caregivers who provide home-based care. Lastly, the IOM currently supports an expert panel on *Adolescent Health Care Services and Models of Care for Treatment, Prevention, and Healthy Development,* which will release its report in April 2008. While always an important area of concern, the care of adolescents, both as caregivers and care receivers, has received little attention in the national caregiving literature (see *Intergenerational Caregiving,* this series). The IOM report will direct much needed focus on adolescents' care needs.

State Leadership

State public health leadership is important to increase awareness of caregivers' needs, promote caregiver health, and fund caregiving-related services.

State Departments of Public Health

State departments of public health coordinate state-wide efforts in this area. Departments have great variability in their structures (IOM 1988). For example, in some states, mental health is addressed within the department of public health while other states have this as a separate department or a part of some larger state entity. Likewise, some states have the elder abuse program in the department of public health while others do not. Thus, state departments of public health exhibit great heterogeneity in structure and focus (Hodge et al. 2006).

A state's emphasis on caregiving is reflected in its placement within state government. In a majority of states, caregiving issues are addressed within departments or divisions on aging. This placement ignores both the life span and the nature of caregiving, which affects children, youth, and other non-seniors, and its public health dimensions. Currently, most states' primary caregiver support activities are dictated by the National Family Caregiver Support Program, which, as previously discussed, is administered by the Administration on Aging in the US Department of Health and Human Services. Since funding comes to states from this source, it is logical that state leadership on caregiving currently is housed within aging units. Perhaps in the future, as caregiving is increasingly recognized for the life span topic it is, the issue will be jointly owned by several departments, including aging, children and youth services, mental health, and public health. However, the assurance function of public health caregiving must rest in public health.

Importance of Public Health Caregiving

Current Issues in Public Health Caregiving

Issues in public health caregiving are myriad. In this section, we discuss applications of public health practice to family and professional caregivers with particular emphasis on the role of public health officials. The education and training of public health caregivers is explored and issues in surveillance and research are surveyed. Lastly, advances in public health caregiving policy and advocacy are noted.

Public Health Practice: Family and Professional Caregivers

Public Health Officials Public health officials, many of whom are government employees, communicate scientific information to the general public and media (Regidor et al. 2007). Public health workers also promote public health practice within the government bureaucracy where they are employed and, outside of their government employment, may serve as advocates for advances in public health practice. Examples of employment settings for public health officials include both public and private settings, such as local and state health departments, health-related agencies of the federal government, the military, academia, and medical care facilities. Communication by public health officials generally are meant to inform or persuade. Examples of persuasive communications include health advisories on prenatal care and long-term care planning. Informational communication includes the dissemination of information on outbreaks, such as influenza or tuberculosis; emergency preparedness procedures for handicapped individuals and their caregivers to increase readiness for disasters, such as hurricanes, earthquakes, and floods; and environmental risk analysis for mobility, which is needed for physically impaired persons, or for disease, such as cancer or Alzheimer's disease (Brookmeyer et al. 1998).

When addressing caregiving issues, public health officials face a new challenge in communicating with the family and professional caregivers, care recipients, the general public, and the media. Historically, public health officials have not been concerned with caregiving issues, but as the population ages, increasing attention must be given to providing these officials with information and intervention knowledge that will prepare them to fulfill their responsibilities to this group.

Education and Training of Public Health Providers Public health service providers, including those who work in both public agencies and private settings, such as hospitals, schools, faith-based entities, managed care organizations, non-profit organizations, and businesses, form the backbone of the nation's public health infrastructure. In terms of education and training, public health officials at the local, county, state, and national levels are responsible for delivering services that range from monitoring health status to conducting research (Table 1). In order to deliver these services, public health officials must have a number of competencies. Using an eight-domain structure, the Council on Linkages Between Academia and Public Health Practice (2001) defined these as: (1) analytic/assessment, (2) policy development/program planning, (3) communication, (4) cultural competency, (5) community dimensions of practice, (6) basic public health sciences, (7) financial planning and management, and (8) leadership and systems thinking.

Surveillance and Research in Public Health Caregiving

While a number of important studies have drawn the attention of the public and policymakers to the needs of caregivers (Family Caregiver Alliance 2004; Feinberg et al. 2006; National Alliance for Caregiving [NAC]/AARP 2004), none to date has been conducted with the population-based focus of public health.

In order to address this need, in 2004 CDC began work with the University of Florida to develop an optional caregiver module to the BRFSS. Currently, the CDC Disability and Health Team is working collaboratively with the CDC BRFSS staff to conduct cognitive testing of individual items and to prepare the module for official approval. The goal is to have an approved BRFSS caregiving module for use by all states in 2009. This achievement will allow national-level, population-based data on caregiving to be tabulated for the first time. When a majority of states have administered the module, a report will be issued providing national and state-by-state data. The document will be useful as states define their caregiving populations and provide needed interventions.

Another CDC effort involves the development of a searchable database on caregiver research with specific attention to both government and nongovernmental instruments that contain caregiver-related variables or that can inform caregiver health and behavior if used in combination. Mathematica is currently completing this project with the goal of having the database posted on the CDC website by early 2008. In addition, to inform the program's caregiving agenda, a meta-analysis on caregiver health effects has been commissioned.

Public Health Caregiving Policy and Advocacy

Policy can serve as a potent agitator of change (Cassady et al. 2006; Hemenway 2005; Hoagwood and Johnson 2003).

Along with the 2001 reauthorization of the Older Americans Act to include the National Family Support Program, the long-awaited National Respite Care Act was the second major piece of legislation passed by Congress within the past decade. Designed to amend the Public Health Service Act to establish a program to assist family caregivers in accessing affordable and high-quality respite care, it became Public Law 109–442, the Lifespan Respite Care Act of 2006.

Future Directions in Public Health Caregiving

Public Health Caregiving Practice

1. Community-based caregiving coalitions should be formed in partnership with local and county health departments to assess their locale's caregiver health and support needs; develop collaborative cross-agency, cross-sector plans to support caregivers; fund interventions from blended funding streams; implement caregiver programs and other supports; and regularly evaluate these efforts.
2. Professional and family caregivers.
3. Evidence-based caregiving interventions—find, document, and disseminate to public health departments at all levels.

4. Since the VA has responsibility not only just for veterans, but also for their spouses, survivors, and dependents, we need to utilize its tremendous reach to implement evidence-based intergenerational caregiving interventions that span multiple generations. With support and commitment, the VA may be used as a caregiving practice model for the country.

Education and Training of Public Health Providers

1. Encourage public and private schools—primary grades through college—to teach caregiving in classes designed to prepare future providers and inoculate caregivers-to-be to the negative health effects of caregiving.
2. Enlist university schools of public health, community colleges, technical schools, and private schools to provide education on caregiving and preparation for the caregiver role. Utilize training programs to develop credentials for new levels of health care workers to provide professional caregiving services and to support family caregivers.
3. Since the VA manages the largest medical education and health professions training program in the USA, public health professionals should collaborate with VA facilities to ensure that health providers are informed about and are sensitive to the needs of caregivers and their care recipients. Since VA facilities are affiliated with 107 medical schools, 55 dental schools, and more than 1,200 other schools across the country; and train about 83,000 health professionals each year; and has provided professional education to more than half of the practicing US physicians, it is a key organization in educating professional caregivers about communicating with family caregivers and assessing caregivers' mental and physical health needs. It is also organizations that can quick-start, then model, a major training shift in professional caregiver education.

Surveillance and Research in Public Health Caregiving

In 1870, when the first U. S. was conducted of individuals 65 years of age or older, an estimated 1.2 million people were considered "old" (3 % of the total population of 40 million; Kausler and Kausler 2001). For past 160 years, optimal life expectancy has increased by a quarter of a year every year (Oeppen and Vaupel 2002). With a burgeoning group of 77 million Baby Boomers (Said 2005), we have come a long way since that first census. However, we have not come far enough. To promote surveillance and research in public health caregiving, we recommend:

1. National surveillance of caregiver-care recipient characteristics and current forms of support is urgently needed. The BRFSS optional Caregiver Module, which is being developed by the CDC for use in 2009, is one means by which this profile may emerge. A population-based report card on caregiving, nationally, by state, and by metropolitan district, should be developed based on these data.

2. State BRFSS departments should be encouraged to adopt and administer the optional BRFSS Caregiver Module in its entirety at the first available opportunity, ideally in 2009.
3. An optional Disability Module should be developed for the BRFSS. An analysis of data from the Caregiver Module and the Disability Module will provide a much-needed picture of the state of caregiving in America from the perspectives of both the caregiver and the care recipient.
4. To gather additional information about caregiver health, other national surveillance measures, such as the National Health Interview Survey, should insert caregiving questions in their core. For example, collecting information on whether the respondent is a caregiver, activity limitations, and environment would allow analyses of datasets that are currently not possible.
5. Build on the Agency on Health Research Quality- and CDC-funded Mathematica studies and the CDC searchable database on caregiver health to include additional dimensions of caregiving knowledge. Expand the database to be an essential research and practice information source for professional and family caregivers, as well as for caregiving researchers and policy analysts.
6. Increase federally funded research on caregiver physical and mental health and on evidence-based interventions to support caregivers. Fund dissemination of results and knowledge translation to states and local communities.
7. External and internal researchers should work within the VA to implement and evaluate family caregiver interventions and to replicate and disseminate information about successful projects.

Caregiving-Oriented Public Health Policy and Advocacy

1. Caregiving as a critical public health issue should be recognized by all pertinent agencies of the federal government. Cross-agency collaborations should be established to promote federal leadership on this issue, fund research and other forms of knowledge development, provide necessary surveillance, and disseminate information to state governments; appropriate organizations, such as national professional associations that represent public health professionals, as well as disease-specific entities; university schools of public health; and the general public.
2. Caregiving and caregiver health should be more directly included in the nation's health goals and objectives. As a cross-cutting issue that is dealt with on a daily basis by individuals of all illnesses, diseases, and disabilities and their families, caregiving health effects should be monitored, goals for caregiver health should be established, and federal agencies should be assigned specific responsibilities for promoting the health of caregivers across the life span.
3. National public health organizations, such as the American Public Health Association, should recognize caregiving as a critical public health issue. Associations representing a caregiving workforce or advocating for family care should develop policy statements about caregiving, determine ways to highlight the health

effects of caregiving, distribute informational materials, and participate in alliances that encourage the dissemination of information about caregiver health and evidence-based interventions.

4. Interested organizations should advocate with the Surgeon General's office to the issue of caregiving as a public health issue. *A Call to Action* or *Surgeon General's Report on Caregiving* would provide high visibility to caregiver health as a national public health issue.
5. The Institute of Medicine should be commissioned to study caregiving as a public health issue, to summarize what is known about caregiving in the USA, and to make recommendations for needed future action. This action was proposed in 2001 and should be championed and funded by a coalition of organizations, agencies, associations, businesses, and foundations with caregiving interest.
6. State-affiliates of national organizations, such as the American Public Health Association, should adopt a caregiving policy statement that recognizes caregiving as an issue faced by a growing number of its citizens. They should disseminate information on caregiving as a public health issue to their constituents.
7. Amend the National Family Caregiver Support Program to provide services to all family caregivers, regardless of age. To underscore a life span perspective, engage the Administration on Children and Youth to co-administer the program with the Administration on Aging.
8. To better address children's needs, amend the Individuals with Disabilities Education Act to acknowledge the caregiving burden faced by parents and siblings of children with disabilities, and provide directed funds to support and respite care to family members who care for a school-aged child with disabilities. Through the Act, provide targeted funds to schools to teach specialized caregiving curricula for teachers, counselors, and school psychologists.
9. Regidor et al. (2007) suggest that future communication in public health be characterized by a range of mediums. Therefore, we recommend the implementation of a national awareness campaign on caregiving and caregiver health that emphasizes prevention, health promotion, early intervention, and the need for community support using all available media. Major businesses should fund paid-time advertising while the Ad Council, a major producer of public service announcements, provides expertise in a multi-year effort.

Conclusions

In *The Future of the Public's Health* (IOM 1988), the authors note:

> The history of public health has been one of identifying health problems, developing knowledge and expertise to solve problems, and rallying political and social support around the solutions. (p. 70)

Caregiving has emerged as a critical public health concern. Following the historical tradition of public health, its constituents—in both the public and private sectors—should act as key leaders in identifying caregiving issues, funding science, generating policy, and advocating for increased caregiver support. The issue now highlighted is one of care—one of the most basic gifts one person can give to another—and public health must fulfill its historic destiny by recognizing the health problems associated with caregiving, providing surveillance and research, and communicating the science with which leaders may make informed decisions about care relationships that involve millions of lives.

In this chapter, we have addressed the public health of caregiving. By exploring its dimensions, we have illustrated how a public health framework applies to care issues. Public health has much to contribute to caregiving in our nation. Public health officials, at national, state, and local levels, bear a scientific responsibility to have the knowledge and an ethical responsibility to have the commitment to address this critical issue. Caregivers need and deserve the attention of a public health system that mobilizes its considerable resources to improve their health and well-being—and thus, their care recipient's life. The time for public health caregiving has come.

References

Adelman, H. S., & Taylor, L. (2006). Mental health in schools and public health. *Public Health Reports, 121*(3), 294–298.

Administration on Aging. (2004). Promising practice in the field of caregiving: 28 national innovations program and 11 projects of national significance. http://www.aoa.gov/prof/aoaprog/caregiver/careprof/nfcsp_projects/PromisingPractices.pdf.

Administraton on Aging. (2007). *The national family caregiver support program*. Washington, DC: U.S. Department of Health and Human Services.

American Public Health Association. (2005). Supporting public health's role in addressing unmet needs at the end-of-life. http://www.apha.org/NR/rdonlyres/223F989B-AFCC-4F85-AEAA-724EFF156BCF/0/GROUPC32005.pdf.

American Public Health Association. (2007a). Building a healthier future: Annual report, fiscal year 2006. http://www.apha.org/NR/rdonlyres/A435EE47-5EF4-4475-B68C-15F03827A452/0/Anreportforweb.pdf.

American Public Health Association. (2007b). Home page. http://www.apha.org/.

Brookmeyer, R., Gray, S., & Kawas, C. (1998). Projections of Alzheimer's disease in the United States and the public health impact of delaying disease onset. *American Journal of Public Health, 88,* 1337–1342.

Cassady, D., Vogt, R., Oto-Kent, D., Mosley, R., & Lincoln, R. (2006). The power of policy: A case study of healthy eating among children. *American Journal of Public Health, 96,* 1570–1571.

Centers for Disease Control and Prevention. (2006a). About CDC: Vision, mission, core values, and pledge. http://www.cdc.gov/about/mission.htm.

Centers for Disease Control and Prevention. (2006b). Disability and health. http://www.cdc.gov/ncbddd/dh/default.htm.

Centers for Disease Control and Prevention. (2007a). About CDC: Our story. http://www.cdc.gov/about/ourstory.htm.

Centers for Disease Control and Prevention. (2007b). Health protection goals and objectives. http://www.cdc.gov/osi/goals/Objectives0307.pdf.

Centers for Disease Control and Prevention. (2007c). State of CDC. http://www.cdc.gov/about/stateofcdc/cdrom/SOCDC/SOCDC2006.pdf.

Centers for Disease Control and Prevention. (2007d). Who's the "public" in public health? http://blogs.inside.cdc.gov/ConnectingConversations/?author=8.

Centers for Disease Control and Prevention. (n.d.). Strategic imperatives and health protection goals: Portable guide. http://www.cdc.gov/osi/goals/SIHPGPostcard.pdf.
Clark, N. M., & Weist, E. (2000). Mastering the new public health. *American Journal of Public Health, 90*(8), 1208–1211.
Council on Linkages Between Academia and Public Health Practice. (2001). Core competencies for public health professionals. http://www.phf.org/competencies.htm.
Crews, J. E., & Talley, R. C. (Vol. Eds., in production). *Introduction: The multiple dimensions of caregiving and disability*. R. C. Talley (Series Ed.). New York: Oxford University Press.
Eckenwiler, L. A. (2006). A missed opportunity: The President's Council on Bioethics report on ethical caregiving. *American Journal of Bioethics, 6*(2), W20–23.
Family Caregiver Alliance. (2004). *The state of the states in family caregiver support: A 50-state study*. San Francisco: Family Caregiver Alliance, National Center on Caregiving. http://www.caregiver.org/caregiver/jsp/content_node.jsp?nodeid=1220.
Family caregiving and public policy: Principles for change. (2003). http://www.caregiving.org/data/principles04.pdf.
Feinberg, L. F., Wolkwitz, K., &, Goldstein, C. (2006, March). Ahead of the curve: Emerging trends and practices in family caregiver support (Research report). Washington, DC: AARP Public Policy Institute. http://www.aarp.org/research/longtermcare/resources/Articles/2006_09_caregiver.html.
Fredrickson, B. L., & Losada, M. F. (2005). Positive affect and the complex dynamics of human flourishing. *American Psychologist, 60*(7), 678–686.
Giguere, N. (2007, January 22). Graying of America drives work force needs. Minneapolis-St. Paul Star Tribune. http://www.startribune.com/1758/v-print/story/951746.html.
Hacker, K., & Darcy, K. (2006). Putting "child mental health" into public health. Public Health Reports, 121(3), 292–293.
Hemenway, D. (2005). A public health approach to firearms policy. In D. Mechanic, L. B. Rogut, D. C. Colby, & J. R. Knickman (Eds.), *Policy challenges in modern health care*. Piscataway: Rutgers University Press. http://www.rwjf.org/files/research/085-Part%202-Chapter%206.pdf.
Hoagwood, K., & Johnson, J. (2003). School psychology: A public health framework: From evidence-based practices to evidence-based policies. *Journal of School Psychology, 41*(1), 3–21.
Hodge, J. G., Gostin, L. O., Gebbie, K., & Erickson, D. L. (2006). Transforming public health law: The turning point model state public health act. *Journal of Law, Medicine & Ethics, 34*(1), 77–84.
Index of resolutions. (2005). http://www.whcoa.gov/about/resolutions/whcoa_voting_results%2050.pdf.
Individuals with Disabilities Education Improvement Act of 2004, P.L. 108–446, H.R. 1350. 20 U.S.C. § 1400.
Institute of Medicine, Committee for the Study of the Future of Public Health. (1988). *The future of the public's health*. Washington, DC: National Academies Press.
Institute of Medicine. (2002a). *Disability in America: Toward a national agenda for prevention*. Washington, DC: National Academies Press.
Institute of Medicine. (2002b). *The future of the public's health in the 21st century*. Washington, DC: National Academies Press.
Institute of Medicine. (2002c). *Health insurance is a family matter*. Washington, DC: National Academies Press.
Institute of Medicine. (2002d). *Who will keep the public healthy? Educating public health professionals for the 21st century*. Washington, DC: National Academies Press.
Institute of Medicine. (2003). *Who will keep the public healthy? Workshop summary*. Washington, DC: National Academies Press.
Institute of Medicine. (2006a). *Frequently asked questions*. Washington, DC: Institute of Medicine of the National Academies. http://www.iom.edu/?id=5774.
Institute of Medicine. (2006b). *Projects: The future health care workforce for older Americans*. Washington, DC: Institute of Medicine of the National Academies. http://www.iom.edu/CMS/3809/40113.aspx.

Institute of Medicine. (2006c). *Workshop on disability in America: A new look—Summary and background papers*. Washington, DC: National Academies Press.
Institute of Medicine. (2007d). *Challenges in adolescent health care: Workshop report*. Washington, DC: Author.
Institute of Medicine. (2007a). *The future of disability in America*. Washington, DC: National Academies Press.
Institute of Medicine. (2007b). *Psychosocial services to cancer patients and families in a community setting*. Washington, DC: National Academies Press.
Institute of Medicine. (2007c). *Training physicians for public health careers*. Washington, DC: National Academies Press.
Kausler, D. H., & Kausler, B. C. (2001). *The graying of America: An encyclopedia of aging, health, mind, and behavior* (2nd ed.). Champaign:University of Illinois Press.
Kellehear, A. (2005). *Compassionate cities: Public health and end-of-life care*. New York: Routledge.
Kellehear, A. (2006). Third-wave public health? Compassion, community, and end-of-life care. *International Journal of Applied Psychoanalytic Studies, 1*(4), 313–323.
Keyes, C. L. M. (2007). Promoting and protecting mental health as flourishing: A complementary strategy for improving national mental health. *American Psychologist, 62*(2), 95–108.
Knight, B. G., & Maines, M. (2001). Mental disorders and mental health services in late life: Issues for public health and public policy.In G. L. Caravaglia (Ed.), *Aging and public health*. Springfield, IL: Charles C. Thomas, Ltd.
Larsson, B. W., Larsson, G., & Carlson, S. R. (2004). Advanced home care: Patients' opinions on quality compared with those of family members. *Journal of Clinical Nursing*, 13(2), 226–233.
Levine, C. (Ed.). (2004). *Always on call: When illness turns families into caregivers (updated & expanded)*. Nashville: Vanderbilt University Press.
Lifespan Respite Care Act of 2006, P.L. 109–442. (H.R. 3248 [109th]). http://www.govtrack.us/congress/bill.xpd?bill=h109-3248.
Lollar, D. J. (2002). Framing and using measures of chronic conditions in childhood: A public health perspective. *Ambulatory Pediatrics, 2*(1), 24–25.
Lumpkin, J. R. (2005, December). Public health's historic achievements: Leading the way to visionary change. Keynote presentation at the annual meeting of the American Public Health Association. Philadelphia, PA. http://www.rwjf.org/newsroom/featureDetail.jsp?featureID=1246&pageNum=1&type=4.
National Alliance on Caregiving & AARP. (2004). *Caregiving in the U.S.* Washington, DC: Authors.
Neugaard, B., Andresen, E. M., DeFries, E. L., Talley, R. C., & Crews, J. E. (2007). Characteristics and health of caregivers and care recipients—North Carolina, 2005. *Mortality and Morbidity Weekly, 56*(21), 529–532.
Oeppen, J., & Vaupel, J. W. (2002). Demography: Enhanced: Broken limits to life expectancy. *Science, 296*(5570), 1029–1031.
President's Council on Bioethics. (2005a). Taking care: Ethical caregiving in our aging society. http://www.bioethics.gov/reports/taking_care/index.html.
President's Council on Bioethics. (2005b). Taking care: Ethical caregiving in our aging society: Letter of transmittal. http://www.bioethics.gov/reports/taking_care/transmittal.html.
Presidential Executive Order 13237. (2001). Creation of the President's council on bioethics. http://www.bioethics.gov/about/executive.html.
Presidential Executive Order 13316. (2003). Continuance of certain federal advisory committees (including the President's Council on Bioethics). http://www.bioethics.gov/about/executive2.html.
Presidential Executive Order 13385. (2005). Continuance of certain federal advisory committees (including the President's Council on Bioethics). http://www.bioethics.gov/about/executive2005.htm.
Public Health Cigarette Smoking Act of 1969, 15 U.S.C. § 1331, 91st Congress, 1st Session.
Public Health Functions Steering Committee Members. (1995, July). Essential public health services. http://www.health.gov/phfunctions/public.htm.

Public Health in America Project. (1999). Public health in America. http://www.health.gov/phfunctions/public.htm.
Regidor, E., de la Fuente, L., Gutierrez-Fisac, J. L., de Mateo, S., Pascual, C., Sanchez-Paya, J., et al. (2007). The role of the public health official in communicating public health information. *American Journal of Public Health, 97*(Suppl. 1), S93–97.
Rozensky, R. H. (1994). Clinical psychology in medical settings: Psychology's role in health care. *Journal of Clinical Psychology in Medical Settings, 1*(1). 1–5.
Said, C. (2005, March 11). Entrepreneurs getting hip to the graying of America: Marketing machine out to mine gold in Boomers' wallets. San Francisco Chronicle, C1. http://www.sfgate.com/cgi-bin/article.cgi?file=/c/a/2005/03/11/BUGG8BNDTG18.DTL&type=printable.
Talley, R. C. (2004, July). Caregiving as an emerging public health issue. In R. C. Talley (Chair), Caregiving in America as an emerging public health issue: Surveillance and response by the nation's public health system. Symposium presented at the 2nd National Center on Birth Defects and Developmental Disabilities Conference, Washington, DC.
Talley, R. C., & Crews, J. E. (2007). Framing the public health of caregiving. *American Journal of Public Health, 97*(2), 224–228.
The National Academies. (2007). http://www.nationalacademies.org/about/faq1.html.
Thompson, K. (2003). Stigma and public health policy for schizophrenia. *Psychiatric Clinics of North America, 26*(1), 273–294.
Turnock, B. (2004). *Public health: What it is and how it works* (3rd ed.). Sudbury: Jones & Bartlett Publishers.
U.S. Census Bureau. (2005). *65 + in the United States: 2005* (pp. 23–209). Washington, DC: U.S. Government Printing House. http://www.census.gov/prod/2006pubs/p23-209.pdf.
U.S. Census Bureau. (2006a). Census bureau estimates number of adults, older people and school-age children in states. http://www.census.gov/Press-Release/www/releases/archives/population/001703.html.
U.S. Census Bureau. (2006b). Facts for features: Older Americans month: May 2006. http://www.census.gov/Press-Release/www/releases/archives/facts_for_features_special_editions/006537.html.
U.S. Department of Health and Human Services, Health Resources and Services Administration. (2007a). Organdonor.gov. http://www.organdonor.gov.
U.S. Department of Health and Human Services, Health Resources and Services Administration. (2007b). Organ procurement and transportation network (OPTN). http://www.optn.org and www.organdonor.gov.
U.S. Department of Health and Human Services. (1979).Healthy people: The surgeon general's report on health promotion and disease prevention. http://profiles.nlm.nih.gov/NN/B/B/G/K/_/nnbbgk.pdf.
U.S. Department of Health and Human Services. (1986). The surgeon general's report on acquired immune deficiency syndrome. Rockville, MD: Public Health Service. http://profiles.nlm.nih.gov/NN/B/B/V/N/_/nnbbvn.pdf.
U.S. Department of Health and Human Services. (1999). *Mental health: A report of the surgeon general: Executive summary*. Rockville: Substance Abuse and Mental Health Services Administration, Center for Mental Health Services, National Institute of Mental Health, National Institutes of Health.
U.S. Department of Health and Human Services. (2000a). *Healthy people 2010, chapter 23, public health infrastructure* (Vol. 2). Washington, DC: Government Printing Office.
U.S. Department of Health and Human Services. (2000b). Healthy people 2010: With understanding and improving health and objectives for improving health (2nd ed., Vol. 2, Chpt. 23: Public health infrastructure). Washington, DC: Author. http://www.healthypeople.gov/Document/HTML/Volume2/23PHI.htm.
U.S. Department of Health and Human Services. (2001a). Women and smoking: A report of the surgeon general. http://www.cdc.gov/tobacco/data_statistics/sgr/sgr_2001/index.htm.

U.S. Department of Health and Human Services. (2001b). *Youth violence: A report of the Surgeon General*. Rockville: Public Health Services. http://www.surgeongeneral.gov/library/youthviolence/sgsummary/summary.htm.
U.S. Department of Health and Human Services. (2004a). Bone health and osteoporosis: A report of the Surgeon General. Rockville, MD: Public Health Service. http://www.surgeongeneral.gov/library/bonehealth/content.html.
U.S. Department of Health and Human Services. (2004b). The health consequences of smoking: A report of the Surgeon General. http://www.surgeongeneral.gov/library/smokingconsequences/.
U.S. Department of Health and Human Services. (2006a). Office of the Surgeon General: Public health priorities. http://www.surgeongeneral.gov/publichealthpriorities.html.
U.S. Department of Health and Human Services. (2006b). *The health consequences of involuntary exposure to tobacco smoke: A report of the Surgeon General*. Rockville: Centers for Disease Control and Prevention, National Center for Chronic Disease Prevention and Health Promotion, Office on Smoking and Health.
U.S. Department of Health and Human Services, U.S. Public Health Service. (1981). The Surgeon General of the U.S. Public Health Service: Functions and legal responsibilities. http://profiles.nlm.nih.gov/QQ/B/C/H/N/_/qqbchn.pdf.
U.S. Department of Veterans Affairs. (2002). The development and expansion of home tele-health in VHA: A paper summarizing the discussions and recommendations generated from a two day VHA meeting on home tele-health in April 2002. http://www.va.gov/occ/Docs/Recommendations_06-20-2002_v-4.pdf.
U.S. Department of Veterans Affairs. (2006). Fact sheet: Facts about the Department of Veterans Affairs. http://www1.va.gov/opa/fact/vafacts.asp.
U.S. Department of Veterans Affairs. (2007a). Care coordination in VA. http://www.va.gov/occ/CCinVA.asp.
U.S. Department of Veterans Affairs. (2007b). Caregiver issues and support for caregivers in VA: Who are care givers and why are they so important? http://www.va.gov/occ/CGIssues.asp.
U.S. Department of Veterans Affairs. (2007c). History and rationale for care coordination in VA. http://www.va.gov/occ/history.asp.
U.S. Department of Veterans Affairs. (2007d). Fiscal year 2008 budget submission: Summary volume (Vol. 5). http://www.va.gov/budget/summary/VolumeIVSummaryVolume.pdf.
Veazie, M. A., Teufel-Shone, N. I., Silverman, G. S., Connolly, A. M., Warne, S., King, B. F., Lebowitz, M. D., & Meister, J. S. (2001). Building community capacity in public health: The role of action-oriented partnerships. *Journal of Public Health Management and Practice, 7*(2), 21–32.
Wallace, R. B. (1998). Public health & preventative medicine: Trends and guideposts. In R. B. Wallace (Ed.), *Public health and preventative medicine* (14th ed.). Stamford: Appleton and Lange.
Weist, M. D. (2005). Fulfilling the promise of school-based mental health: Moving toward a public mental health promotion approach. *Journal of Abnormal Child Psychology, 33*(6), 735–741.
White House Conference on Aging. (2005a). 50 resolutions as voted by the 2005 White House Conference on Aging delegates (Monday, December 12, 2005 [unranked]). http://www.whcoa.gov/about/resolutions/whcoa_voting_results.pdf.
White House Conference on Aging. (2005b). History: The White House conferences on aging. http://www.whcoa.gov/about/history.asp.
White House Conference on Aging. (2005c). Index of resolutions. http://www.whcoa.gov/about/resolutions/Resolutions.pdf.
White House Conference on Aging. (2005d). Report to the president and the Congress. http://www.whcoa.gov/about/about.asp#report.
Winslow, C. E. A. (1920). The untilled field of public health. *Modern Medicine,* 2183–2191.
World Health Organization (WHO). (2001). *International Classification of Functioning, Disability, and Health: ICF*. Geneva: Author.

Public Policy and Caregiving

Nora Super

Public Policy and Caregiving

Public policymakers are always faced with the challenge of designing and evaluating social programs that take into consideration the budgetary implications, political realities, and ethical dilemmas of a wide spectrum of stakeholders. It is from this perspective of multiple competing priorities that public policy makers consider caregiving and what is known and what is needed.

Population Trends and Implications for Caregiving

Policymakers have been hearing about the impending retirement of the baby boom generation for decades. As the largest number of baby boomers approach age 65 in 2010, the day of reckoning is just around the corner. As we near that date, it seems important to consider what these demographic trends will mean for public health programs today and in the future.

Policymakers understand that people are living longer. The number of Americans aged 65 and older grew rapidly throughout the twentieth century, nearly tripling, between 1950 and 2000 (Friedland and Summer 2005). Improvements in life expectancy have increased the proportion of individuals who are aged 85 and older. This population will double to nearly 10 million by the year 2030 (U.S. Census Bureau 2004).

Since 1960, family structure has changed considerably. Men and women marry later, on average, and divorce rates have risen (U.S. Census Bureau 2004). A higher

N. Super(✉)
George Washington University, Washington, USA

U.S. Department of Health & Human Services,
200 Independence Ave SW, Washington, DC, USA
e-mail: Nora.Super@hhs.gov

R. C. Talley, S. S. Travis (eds.), *Multidisciplinary Coordinated Caregiving*,
Caregiving: Research • Practice • Policy, DOI 10.1007/978-1-4614-8973-3_12,

share of children are born to unmarried mothers. Successive generations have fewer children, but longer life expectancies.

An older population will mean more people with health and personal care needs and greater use of health and long-term care services. As individuals age, their need for assistance with activities of daily living (ADLs) such as walking and dressing, and instrumental activities of daily living (IADLs) such as grocery shopping and money management increases. More than 40 % of people over age 70 have at least one ADL or IADL limitation (Shirey and Summer 2000). Such demands are expected to grow significantly as the number of elderly increases.

Yet at the very time the demand for this help is increasing, the traditional supply of both paid caregivers and unpaid caregivers is shrinking. Demographic data show a widening gap between the number of people likely to need care and the number of people who are most likely to provide care. Women between the ages of 25–64 have typically provided the majority of both paid and unpaid care in the USA (Super 2002). However, while the population aged 85 and older is the fastest growing age group in the USA, the number of women aged 25–54 is expected to remain relatively unchanged from 2000 to 2030.

Sociodemographic factors have also affected the supply of formal and informal caregivers. Due to greater opportunities for education and workforce participation by women over the past four decades, fewer new workers are entering the long-term care workforce. These new opportunities also make them less available to care for family members in need of assistance. Marriage and reproductive trends, such as increased number of childless couples, smaller family sizes, and higher divorce raters, have also decreased the pool of potential caregivers. According to the National Family Caregivers Association (NFCA n.d.), the number of potential family caregivers for each person needing care will decrease from 11 in 1990 to an estimated 4 in 2050.

As we enter this brave new world with a much higher proportion of older Americans, it is difficult to predict exactly what these trends will mean for political and policy priorities.

The population aged 65–75 today is healthier, wealthier, and better educated than persons in this age group in past generations (Friedland and Summer 2005). Thus, these older persons may still be engaged in the labor markets long after age 65 and their savings are a necessary component of financial markets.

Nonetheless, certain segments of this population remain vulnerable. For example, older single women have particularly low average incomes. Moreover, large health and long-term health expenses can wipe out the resources of those who previously felt financially secure.

As people live longer, they are more likely to require hands-on assistance from others. Among people aged 65 or over, 20 % have limitations in IADLs. At age 85, over 19 % have limitations in IADLs and another 19 % have limitations in one or more ADLs (see Fig. 1).

On the other hand, disability rates among the elderly could be improving. Among the population aged 65 and older, disability rates remained relatively constant during the 1970s. However, between 1982 and 1999, the proportion of older people with a disability declined from 26 to 20 % (Manton and Gu 2001). This change could

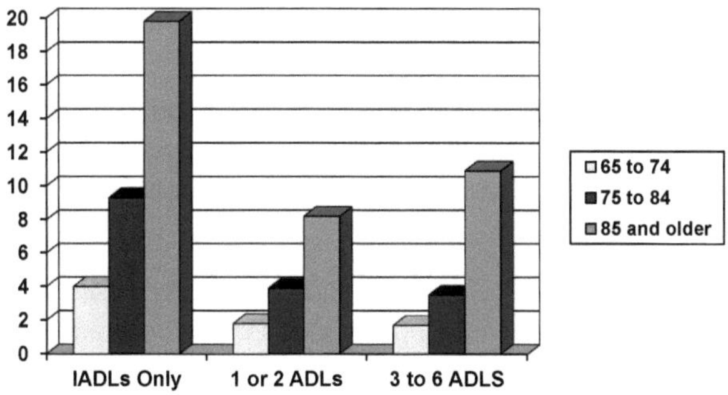

Fig. 1 Percentage of older people with functional limitations who need help from another person. Those with IADLs only said "yes" to needing help with IADLs from another person and "no" to ADL question. Those with ADLs may or may not have an IADL. Those with one or two ADLs responded "yes" to needing help with ADLs and "yes" to fewer than three specific activity questions. Those with 3–6 ADLs responded "yes" to at least three of the follow-up questions about specific activities. (Source: Center on an Aging Society analysis of data from National Health Interview Survey, 2000)

indicate that disability rates may decline in the future for older adults and the number of years free of disability could be increasing; however, it is likely to become more difficult to avoid some level of disability prior to death (Friedland and Summer 2005).

Rising obesity rates among older adults suggest that disability could be more of a burden on family caregivers in the future. People who have difficulty with ADLs and require assistance of another person rely primarily on family and friends. Those who are obese are somewhat more likely to receive help from spouses, children, or grandchildren—77 % compared with 72 % for nonobese adults (Shirey and Summer 2003).

These population trends ensure that in the future there will be a larger proportion of people aged 65 and older. By exactly how much is not known because future mortality, fertility, and life expectancy is uncertain. Also, it is not known exactly what kind of fundamental changes these improvements in life expectancy will have on how education, family formation, living arrangements, and labor force participation are organized over time.

However, it seems likely that these population shifts will in turn require shifts in focus from children to older persons, because certain needs, such as child care and education, will not be in as high demand, while other needs, such as health care and long-term care needs will likely dominate the political agenda.

Although much of the legislative action to assist caregivers occurs on the state level, the federal government also plays a key role in developing policies to support caregivers, both directly and indirectly. The federal government today spends over US$ 600 billion a year for both the Medicare and Medicaid programs combined. As a result, policymakers have begun to look at ways to more effectively manage costs within both of these programs, which will have implications for both Medicare and Medicaid beneficiaries as well as the people who care for them.

Current Status of Caregiving and Public Policy

Public policymakers and those who try to impact public policy have influenced caregiving in the USA both by their lack of early activity and, more recently, by their interest in and action on caregiving policy efforts. (You could name a range of them here).

- improvement of the Medicaid home-and-community-based services (HCBS) option by broadening the Money Follows the Person program;
- Establishment of the Community Living Assistance Services and Supports (CLASS) program, a self-funded and voluntary long-term care insurance choice that helps people with disabilities remain in their homes, communities, and jobs through cash benefits to pay for community support services;
- Provision of support to Medicaid beneficiaries with daily activities and health-related tasks through the ACA Community First Choice Option, which covers community-based attendant services and supports;
- Development of preventative care standards for medical diagnostic equipment;
- Bars discrimination on the basis of pre-existing condition and caps on lifetime benefits; and
- Prohibits insurance companies from discrimination on the basis of medical history or genetic information (starting in 2014). (The White House, 2013).

Due to the broad potential focus of this chapter, with the unfolding ACA as backdrop, we will focus on one primary policy initiative, the Medicare program, its influence by health policy makers and influencers, and how its provision effects caregiving at the levels of practice, education and training, research, and advocacy.

Medicare as Public Policy for Caregivers

Since Medicare began in 1965, the number of people covered by the program has more than doubled; nearly 42 million Americans now receive their health insurance through the Medicare program. In 2004, 35.4 million beneficiaries aged 65 and older participated in Medicare and 6.3 billion beneficiaries qualified for Medicare due to a disability. Total Medicare spending is expected to a total of US$ 325 billion in 2005, according to the Congressional Budget Office (CBO).

A significant share of people with Medicare, and in particular non-elderly people with disabilities and those aged 85 or older, have functional and/or cognitive limitations (Cubanski et al. 2005). One-third of all beneficiaries are limited in their ability to handle basic ADLs, such as bathing and eating, and a quarter of all beneficiaries have a cognitive or mental impairment. Nearly six in ten non-elderly beneficiaries with disabilities have a cognitive or mental impairment.

Public Policy in Practice

Despite these statistics, Medicare's role in financing long-term care is limited. It covers primarily medical care costs, but it also pays for some care provided by nursing homes and other suppliers of long-term care services. These services are generally received over a short period of time and are related to an acute episode. For example, the Medicare coverage of nursing home services is limited to short-term post-acute stay of up to 100 days of illness after hospitalization. Medicare's home health benefit, the closest the program comes to paying for long-term care, does provide up to 35 h per week of in-home services to some persons with chronic conditions as long as they are homebound and also need skilled care. Medicare's expenditures for these types of services are projected to increase from an estimated US$ 34 billion in 2004 to a projected US$ 51 billion in 2020 (CBO 2004).

Despite these high costs, the Medicare program does not cover most types of long-term assistance given by family caregivers at home, such as helping incapacitated relatives shop, eat, bathe, and dress. Medicare also does not cover most types of training to help caregivers learn how to best look after their families.

Yet as the population ages, the trend is to enable older adults to receive care in the least restrictive setting possible. These trends are reflected in the housing choices adopted by Medicare beneficiaries. The vast majority of Medicare beneficiaries live in their own homes or other community-based settings. The rate of nursing home residence has declined among older adults as other types of settings have become more common (Harrow 2005). In 2003, 93 % of Medicare enrollees aged 65 years and over lived in traditional community settings, 2.5 % resided in community settings with services, and 4.4 % resided in long-term care facilities. As might be expected, the settings with greater service availability house the residents with the greatest level of disability. However, 9 % of those residing in a traditional community setting reported having three or more ADLs. Thus, it is likely that a fair amount of care is being delivered informally by family or friends or being paid for out-of-pocket for formal care, which is not well documented.

Medicare Beneficiaries, Chronic Conditions, and Care Needs

Chronic conditions cut across all age groups, although they are especially prevalent among the elderly, who typically are most in need of caregiving services. Because of statutory limitations, Medicare has typically left long-term care coverage to the Medicaid program; however, policymakers have recently become more aware of the growing number of Medicare beneficiaries who have chronic conditions and need care, and their link to higher costs to the program. Beneficiaries with chronic conditions are more likely to experience problems with care coordination because they often receive care from a variety of physicians and specialists. These beneficiaries are also at greater risk of being admitted to the hospital or of visiting emergency rooms for preventable conditions or complications (Super 2004).

More than 80 % of Medicare beneficiaries have at least one chronic condition, therefore, need care coordination. While the prevalence of many conditions increases with age, other conditions, such as emphysema, diabetes, and cognitive/mental impairments are somewhat more prevalent among non-elderly Medicare beneficiaries with disabilities (Cubanski et al. 2005). The prevalence of chronic conditions, which typically require ongoing care and treatment to maintain health and functional status and to slow down the progression of the disease, has been strongly linked to high expenditures and the use of medical resources. More than 75 % of high cost Medicare beneficiaries were diagnosed with one or more of seven major chronic conditions (e.g., chronic obstructive pulmonary disease, congestive heart disease, diabetes; US Congressional Budget Office 2005). Twenty-three percent of beneficiaries with five or more chronic conditions account for 68 % of the program's spending (Anderson 2005). Nearly 20 % of high-cost Medicare beneficiaries were aged 85 or older, compared with 10 % of other beneficiaries (US Congressional Budget Office 2005).

However, under our current payment system, health care providers are not adequately compensated for the extra time needed to properly assess and coordinate care for patients with multiple chronic conditions. According to a study by Duke University Medical Center, the amount of time spent with a patient discussing preventive services can increase threefold if one or more chronic conditions are uncontrolled at the time of the patient's visit (Yarnall 2005). Under the current payment incentive structure, physicians are encouraged to avoid these patients rather than to embrace them (Super 2005), thus potentially resulting in poor care and little or no care coordination.

Private Section Responses

Several private sector initiatives are underway to try to change the incentive structures. In the private sector, many "disease management" firms have sprung up in an effort to assist patients with chronic conditions to adhere to care plans. Disease management has sometimes been used interchangeably with "care coordination" or "case management," although there can be important distinctions (Sprague 2003).

Another popular private sector effort aim that has gained nationwide attention has been to pay for health care services based on performance. "Pay-for-performance" seeks to reward physicians and other care providers for delivering health care services that meet specified standards or achieve defined levels of quality. These payment methods have been adopted across the country by public and private purchasers with some demonstrated success; however, they face important impediments and challenges, too.

Palliative Care

Finally, there has been growth of palliative care programs in US hospitals in response to abundant evidence of poorly treated pain and other symptoms. Overall, the number of programs increased linearly from 632 (15 % of hospitals) in 2000 to 1,027 (25 % of hospitals) in 2003 (Morrison et al. 2005). Palliative care aims to relieve suffering and improve quality of life for patients with multiple chronic conditions and advanced illnesses. It is offered simultaneously with all other appropriate medical treatments and is not limited to the care of the terminally ill. Studies demonstrate that palliative care is effective at reducing suffering of all causes, and patients and families are more satisfied when they receive it (Teno et al. 2004). In practice, palliative care involves expert pain and symptom assessment and management, communication among the patient, family and providers about the goals of care, and coordination of care across multiple settings (Morrison and Meier 2004).

At present, however, Medicare's payment systems not only fail to reward high quality palliative care programs, but also encourage just the opposite—more costly procedures, the most specialists visits, and the most hospital stays for the patients least likely to benefit from them (Super 2005). Data from the Center for Evaluative Clinical Sciences at Dartmouth Medical School suggest that the higher utilization of results from current Medicare payment incentives is not only not associated with improved quality of care for seriously ill Medicare beneficiaries, but counter to the prevailing assumption, more services are actually associated with *higher* (not lower) mortality (Fisher et al. 2003). In contrast, a health care system that provided comprehensive palliative care as the default approach, rather than the exception, would result in more satisfied patients and families, a lower burden of pain and suffering, equivalent or better survival rates, and markedly lower, but appropriate use of complex high-cost procedures and care settings (Morrison and Meier 2004).

Public Policy Advocacy and Legislation

Among its many far-reaching provisions, the Medicare Prescription, Drug, Improvement, and Modernization Act (MMA) of 2003 established many new programs and demonstrations to improve chronic care. Chronic care improvement seems to be one issue that Republicans and Democrats can agree upon in this Congress. CMS has established several new demonstration and pilot programs aimed at improving Medicare's management of chronic conditions. Perhaps most significantly, roughly 180,000 fee-for-service beneficiaries in nine states and the District of Columbia are offered the opportunity to sign up for a pilot program—Medicare Health Support—modeled on private sector disease management program. Potential participants—those diagnosed with diabetes or congestive heart failure, with or without comorbid conditions—were identified through claims data.

In addition, CMS announced on July 1, 2005, the Care Management for High Cost Beneficiaries (CMHCB) demonstration, which tests the ability of direct-care provider models to coordinate care for high-cost/high-risk beneficiaries by providing such beneficiaries with clinical support beyond traditional settings to manage their conditions (Department of Health and Human Services (HHS) 2005). Under the demonstration, provider groups receive a monthly fee to cover their administrative and care management costs for each beneficiary participating in the program.

However, organizations are required to assume financial risk if they do not meet established performance standards for achieving savings to Medicare.

CMS also has several pilot and demonstration projects underway that are designed to link payment to quality. Pay-for-performance (P4P) initiatives are also supported by the Medicare Payment Advisory Commission (MedPAC), whose members support incentives that will improve the quality of care while simultaneously reducing the inappropriate use of physician services (Miller 2005).

Top congressional leaders have introduced legislation that would tie Medicare reimbursement to reporting data on quality measures. Senators Grassley (R-IA), Baucus (D-MT), Enzi (R-WY), and Kennedy (D-MA) introduced the "Medicare Value Purchasing Act of 2005" on June 30, 2005, that would require the Secretary of Health and Human Services to develop and implement value-based purchasing programs under Medicare for acute-care hospitals, physicians and practitioners, Medicare Advantage plans, home health agencies, and skilled nursing facilities. In the first stage, Medicare reimbursement updates will be tied to reporting data on quality measures. The Secretary will be expected to include measures relevant to the frail elderly and those with complex chronic conditions.

In the House, Rep. Nancy Johnson (R-CT), chair of the House Ways and Means Subcommittee on Health, introduced the Medicare Value-Based Purchasing for Physician Services Act of 2005 (H.R. 3617), which would provide a differential payment update to practitioners meeting preestablished thresholds of quality or preestablished levels of improvement.

Roles and Preparation of Caregiving Advocates

To impact legislative and policy initiatives that support both family caregivers and professional caregivers such as physicians, nurses, social workers, psychologists, chaplains, and other members of a care team.

Public Policy to Support Caregiving Practitioner Needs

Despite older Americans' huge demand for health services and resources, most health care professionals are unprepared to provide health care for the aging population either as a specialist in geriatrics or as a generalist with basic geriatric education and training. The current shortage of geriatricians is expected to worsen. Experts estimate that the nation will need approximately 36,000 geriatricians by 2030 (Alliance for Aging Research 2002). Today there are approximately 6,600 certified geriatricians, indicating that the current training output is insufficient to reach. The decision to choose a career focused on the care of older adults remains financially unattractive for young physicians with increasingly large educational debt each year (Association of American Medical Colleges 2003).

Studies of doctor–patient communications have found that clinicians typically fail to discuss patients' values, goals of care, and preferences regarding treatment (Tulsky 2003). Not only are these skills rarely taught in medical school, but any physician who tries to provide these services will soon be forced out of practice due to under-reimbursement. Physicians in practice quickly learn what they have to do to pay their overhead and themselves—see more patients faster and spend most time doing the highest-paid procedures. Talking to patients and families, managing complex symptoms, coordination and communication of care across settings—the kind of care patients and families say they want and what most of us would agree we would want for ourselves and our loved ones—is a sure path to bankruptcy under the current physician payment system (Singer et al. 1999). The Medicare system of the future should assure access to well trained primary care physicians, nurses, and allied professionals who are as well compensated for their time and effort as colleagues doing high technology interventions.

Similar shortages exist in the fields of nursing and social work. Less than 1 % of nurses are certified in geriatrics and only 3 % of advance practice nurses specialize in care of an older adult. Less than one-third of 1 % of physical therapists are certified in geriatrics and of the more than 200,000 pharmacists, only 720 have a geriatric certification. Social workers have no national certification for geriatric work, and registered dieticians and dietetic technicians have no formal program in geriatric nutrition.

Research in Caregiving Public Policy

As Medicare moves in the direction of paying for performance and chronic care management, some important research questions have been raised. Fewer clinical guidelines exist for treatment of beneficiaries with multiple chronic conditions, making identification of the "evidence-based" case more difficult.

Patient self-management is a key component of most commercial disease management programs. Medicare beneficiaries are more likely to be poor, frail, and cognitively impaired than enrollees of commercial plans. Geriatricians have argued that self-management and patient education techniques simply do not work for persons with Alzheimer's disease or related dementia. Similarly, research needs to be done about the applicability of P4P for patients with multiple chronic conditions. Most of the P4P measures under consideration by CMS and Congress are performance-based, but are unproven benefit for vulnerable persons, especially those 75 years and older. Clinicians and advocates have raised concerns that P4P initiatives could create adverse incentives for physicians seeking to deliver high-quality care to patients with multiple chronic conditions and advance complex illness (Boyd et al. 2005). If P4P is to be truly relevant to the costliest Medicare beneficiaries, it will have to utilize measures truly correlated with quality care in this patient population (Super 2005). Quality of care should take into account patient and family preference, as well as the relevance of some indicators for certain patients with advance illnesses. More research should be done to study the effectiveness of these clinical practice guidelines on vulnerable populations before they are applied to the Medicare program at large.

Finally, health care for people in their last year of life accounts for approximately 27 % of Medicare spending—an average of US$ 26,000 per decedent (Last Acts Partnership 2005). Yet we lack the most basic details about how people spend their final months and days—whether they are cared for according to their wishes, whether they are in pain—and the means to measure whether things are moving in a positive direction. In its report, *Describing Death in America*, the Institute of Medicine highlighted how little we know about the "quality, appropriateness, or costs of care dying individuals receive, or the burden on caregivers and survivors" (Foley et al. 2003). One of the central recommendations of the report was to revitalize the National Mortality Followback Survey, a national survey that has not been conducted since 1993.

Future Directions in of Caregiving Public Policy

As Medicare provides no coverage for many services and products typically needed by beneficiaries, people with substantial long-term care needs and limited ability to pay often turn to Medicaid, the single largest source of financing for all long-term services. Estimates of long-term care spending for different age groups are hard to come by, but the CBO estimates that Medicaid paid for about a third of the long-term care spending on the elderly in 2004, including a third of all nursing home costs (O'Brien 2005). The CBO also reports that Medicaid paid a much larger share, an estimated 60 %, of the long-term care spending of non-elderly persons with disabilities. The program exclusively finances the increasingly popular personal care services and care provided to individuals at home or in the community through home- and community-based services (HCBS) waivers.

People who need long-term care services are diverse. They include the elderly with physical and cognitive impairments as well as children and non-elderly adults. People with disabilities in Medicaid include children and adults with mental retardation and developmental disabilities; the severely mentally ill; people with traumatic brain injuries and spinal cord injuries; adults with debilitating illness, such as Parkinson's disease, and multiple sclerosis; people with AIDS; and children born with severe physical and cognitive impairments.

It important to note that most people use their own resources to pay for formal long-term care services when they are needed. Estimates of the sources of payment for nursing home care over the lifetime use of the elderly (that is, all nursing home services used by people from age 65 and above) suggest that a substantial proportion of the elderly with any nursing home use (44 %) paid their own way. In total, in 2003, people with long-term care needs and their families paid US$ 37.5 billion out-of-pocket on long-term care in 2003, accounting for roughly 21 % of all long-term care spending (O'Brien 2005).

Nevertheless, just 17 % of people with long-term care needs receive those services in institutional settings (Smith et al. 2005). The disabled elderly are more likely than non-elderly persons with disabilities to reside in nursing homes; nevertheless, a large number of people with substantial needs are living in their own homes or receiving care in other community settings. What separates the nursing home from the community population is not so much level of impairment, but the presence of family or social supports. Nursing home residents generally lack family or social supports, or have families who have provided substantial care to a disabled person at home, but are no longer able to provide the amount and kind of care needed without assistance.

Public Policy Advocacy and Legislative Needs

There has been substantial growth in Medicaid spending on community-based long-term care services over the past decade, and a significant shift in the distribution of Medicaid long-term care resources from institutional to home- and community-based services (O'Brien 2005). Between 1994 and 2004, spending on home and community-based services increased from US$ 8.4 to $ 31.6 billion, rising from 19 to 36 % of Medicaid long-term care spending. This shift was primarily due to the rapid growth of HCBS waiver spending, which, today accounts for nearly two-thirds of Medicaid long-term care spending in the community.

However, it is important to note that states vary widely in the resources they devote to long-term care. For example, in 2001, Medicaid spending on home and personal care ranged from a high of US$ 7,145 per disabled enrolled in Connecticut to less than US$ 250 in the District of Columbia, Hawaii, and Mississippi (O'Brien 2005). These inequities can have profound impacts on the health and well-being of the frail elderly and non-elderly people with disabilities. Waiting lists for home- and community-based services prevent financially eligible individuals from receiving services, leading to inappropriate institutionalization and unmet needs. One recent study of frail elderly applicants for a Medicaid HCBS waiver in Connecticut found that the elderly applicants who did not participate in the waiver program "appear to get by in the community" through a combination of informal care, use of Medicare home care, and going through without needed services (Long et al. 2005). Their ability to manage in the community, however, was limited. The elderly who applied for but did not receive waiver services were far more likely than those who received HCBS to enter a nursing home within six months following their assessment for waiver services.

Advocacy for consumer direction in long-term care began in the USA during the 1970s with the Independent Living Movement for younger adults with disabilities. Advocates believe that people with disabilities have the ability and the right to make decisions about the services that affects their lives. More recently, many federal and state policymakers have embraced the philosophy of consumer-directed care and applied it to services for elderly populations as well. Consumer-directed programs have also been put forward as a solution to the growing shortage of direct-care workers. In most consumer-directed models, consumers take on all worker management tasks, with the exception of paying the worker.

Public Policy Practice Needs

One innovative, consumer-directed model that has shown promise is "cash and counseling," in which cash allowances, coupled with information services are paid directly to elderly persons or those with disabilities, allowing them to purchase the services they feel best meet their needs. The program began as a demonstration and evaluation program in three states: Arkansas, Florida, and New Jersey. Due to the success of those programs, cash and counseling programs have recently expanded to eleven states: Alabama, Iowa, Kentucky, Michigan, Minnesota, New Mexico, Pennsylvania, Rhode Island, Vermont, Washington, and Pennsylvania. Additionally, Illinois has been funded by the Retirement Research Foundation to implement their own cash and counseling program.

Education/Training Needs in Caregiving Public Policy

Education and training for direct care workers as well as family caregivers remains a concern for some policymakers. Similar to health professionals, the majority of direct care worker have no formal training specific to geriatrics. As the population ages, legislation for geriatric education and training programs in the U.S. Department of Health and Human Services, Health Resources and Services Administration, Bureau of Health Professions, should be expanded to include direct care workers and family caregivers. This policy and legislative change would provide support toward building an infrastructure that is prepared to respond to the growth of the aging population and the expansion of home and community-based services.

Research Needs in Caregiving Public Policy

Although the movement toward home and community-based care and consumer direction has been largely welcomed by beneficiaries and their families, it raises some important research questions. A key question being debated in policy circles has been around whether or not home- and community-based care actually saves money relative to institutional care. Although it is impossible to argue that nursing homes are not more efficient for larger groups of individuals, one may buy smaller increments of care in community-based settings. In addition, often there are waiting lists for HCBS programs, which can sometimes make the comparisons between nursing homes costs unfair. Similarly, it is difficult to fully predict the long-term implications of consumer direction on delivery, workforce, and costs.

In general, there has been no sustained funding to study long-term care, which has made research in this area patchy. Long-term care is not the domain of any single foundation. It does live in any single government agency. As a result, researchers have not made a substantial amount of progress in the study of its delivery.

Conclusion

The role of informal or family caregivers has become increasingly important as the population continues to age and patients receive less institutionalized care. Based on data from the Commonwealth Fund Biennial Health Insurance Survey, in 2003, nearly one in ten working-age adults aged 19–16 cared for a sick or disabled family member, for a total of 16 million caregivers (Ho et al. 2005). Other studies (NAC/AARP; National Center on Caregiving) have approximated the numbers of caregivers in the nation to be substantially higher.

Yet, policymakers have been slow to adopt policies to support caregivers. Most legislation introduced at the federal level has not been enacted. As the Medicare and Medicaid programs move into more performance-based purchasing, policymakers must make certain that patients and their families are supported or they may end up just paying more for services in the long-run. However, we have yet to see how the Obama Affordable Care Act will address caregivers' and care recipients needs. We do know, however, that American is facing a crisis in long-term care and that caregiving is going to become, if it is not already, an issue of great importance to almost every American.

References

Alliance for Aging Research. (2002). *Ten reasons why America is not ready for the coming of the age boom*. Washington, DC: Alliance for Aging Research.

Anderson, G. F. (2005). Medicare and chronic condition. *New England Journal of Medicine, 353*(3), 305–309.

Association of American Medical Colleges. (2003). *Medical school graduation questionnaire: All schools report*. http://www.aamc.org/data/gq/.

Congressional Budget Office. (2004). *Financing long-term care for the elderly*. Washington, DC: Congressional Budget Office. http://www.cbo.gov/ftpdocs/54xx/doc5400/04-26-LongTerm Care.pdf.

Cubanski, J., Voris, M., Kitchman, M., Neuman, T., & Potetz, L. (2005). *Medicare chartbook* (3rd ed.). Menlo Park: The Henry J. Kaiser Family Foundation. http://www.kff.org/medicare/7284.cfm.

Epstein, A. E., Lee, T. H., & Hamel, M. B. (2004). Paying physicians for high-quality care. *New England Journal of Medicine, 350,* 406–410.

Fisher, E. S., Wennberg, D. E., Stukel, T. A., Gottlieb, D. J., Lucas, F. L., & Pinder, E. L. (2003). The implications of regional variations in Medicare spending, Part 1: The content, quality, and accessibility of care. *Annals of Internal Medicine, 138*(4), 288–298.

Foley, K. M., Smith, T. J., Gelband, H., & Lunney, J. R. (Eds.). (2003). *Describing death in America: What we need to know*. Washington, DC: National Academies Press, Institute of Medicine

Friedland, R. B., & Summer, L. (2005). *Demography is not destiny, revisited*. http://www.cmwf.org.

Harrow, B. (2005). Health care utilization and cost and the aging society. *Public Policy & Aging Report, 15*(3), 12–15.

Ho, A., Collins, S., Davis, K., & Doty, M. (2005). *A look at working-age caregivers' roles, health concerns, and need for support* (Publication #854). New York: The Commonwealth Fund.

Long, S. K., Liu, K., Black, K., O'Keefe J., & Molony, S. (2005). Getting by in the community: Lessons from frail elders. *Journal of Aging and Social Policy, 17*(1), 19–44.

Manton, K. G., & Gu, X. (2001, May 22). Changes in the prevalence of chronic disability in the United States black and nonblack population above age 65 from 1982–1999. *Proceedings from the National Academy of Sciences, 98*(11), 6354–6359.

Miller, M. E. (2005, July 25). *Paying for performance under the Medicare program*. Statement of Executive Director of Medicare Payment Advisory Commission before the Committee on Finance, U.S. Senate.

Morrison, R. S., & Meier, D. E. (2004). Palliative care. *New England Journal of Medicine, 350*, 2582–2590.

Morrison, R. S., Maroney-Galin, C., Kralovec, P. D., & Meier, D. E. (2005). The growth of palliative care programs in United States hospitals. *Journal of Palliative Medicine, 8*(6), 1127–1134.

National Family Caregivers Association. (n.d.). *Caregiving statistics*. Kensington: Author. http://www.thefamilycaregiver.org/who/stats.cfm.

O'Brien, E. (2005). *Long-term care: Understanding Medicaid's role for the elderly and disabled*. Washington, DC: Kaiser Commission on Medicaid and the Uninsured. http://www.kff.org/medicaid/7428.cfm.

Shirey, L., & Summer, L. (2000, May). *Caregiving: Helping the elderly with activity limitations* (No. 7). Washington, DC: National Academy on an Aging Society, 2, 5.

Shirey, L., & Summer, L. (2003). *Obesity among older Americans* (Data Profile No. 10). Washington, DC: Center on an Aging Society. http://hpi.georgetown.edu/agingsociety/pubhtml/obesity2/obesity2.html.

Super, N. (2002). *Who will be there to care? The growing gap between caregiver supply and demand* (Background paper). Washington, DC: National Health Policy Forum. http://www.nhpf.org/pdfs_bp/BP_Caregivers_1-02.pdf.

Super, N. (2005) *Medicare physician payment: How to build a more efficient payment system*. Statement before the House Committee on Energy and Commerce Subcommittee on Health.

The White House. (2013). Disabilities. Retrieved 30 October, 2013. http://www.whitehouse.gov/issues/disabilities.

U. S. Census Bureau (2004). *U.S. Interim projections by age, sex, race, and Hispanic origin*. http://www.census.gov/ipc/usinterimproj/.

U. S. Census Bureau (2005). *Families and living arrangement, historical time series* (Tables UC1, HH-4, MS-2, & FM-2). http://www.census.gov/population/www/socdemo/hh-fam/cps2005.html(UC1)&http://www.census.gov/population/www/socdemo/hh-fam.html(HH-4,MS-2, &FM-2).

U.S. Congressional Budget Office. (2005). *High-cost Medicare beneficiaries*. http://www.cbo.gov.

U.S. Department of Health and Human Services, Centers for Medicare & Medicaid Services. (2005). *Medicare to award contracts for demonstration projects to improve care for beneficiaries with high medical costs*. http://www.cms.hhs.gov.

Yarnall, K. (2005, October). Not enough time. In L. Sprague (Chair), *Medicare health support: Working with physicians*. Presentation at the meeting of the National Health Policy Forum, Washington, DC.

Part IV
Conclusions

Professional Caregiving: Working Together to Provide Quality, Comprehensive, Coordinated Care—A Call to Action

Ronda C. Talley and Shirley S. Travis

In the introductory chapter, we encouraged readers to critique the individual chapters by thinking about the contributions each discipline has made to caregiving and the potential for continued maturation, leadership, and innovation over time. We suspect this was not an easy task because of the vastly different conceptual lenses used by each author to report the activity of his or her discipline and the freedom each author was given to develop the chapters. Thus, our call to action in this concluding chapter has two parts. First, we used themes gleaned from the chapters in each section to construct a framework for describing disciplinary participation in caregiving related activity, as presented by the authors in their chapters. Second, we used this framework to identify strengths across the disciplinary activities that are desirable and are likely to be maintained and areas that need attention in order to move forward with quality, comprehensive, coordinated care in the twenty-first century.

Our framework has three parts: Knowledge, Functions, and Positioning for the Future. First, did the author provide evidence that the discipline contributes specialized knowledge to support caregiving research, education, advocacy, policy, and/or practice? This knowledge may to varying degrees: (a) be central to the science of the discipline, and/or (b) include constructs that enjoy protected status from the discipline in which they originated (e.g., stress and coping from psychology). Second, how involved are the members of discipline, relative to other disciplines in the book, in key functions related to caregiving activity? In the chapters, these functions included: (a) direct care provider, (b) advocate/policy maker, and (c) researcher. The researcher category included methodologists, theorists, and policy analysts. In other

R. C. Talley (✉)
Department of Psychology, College of Education and Behavioral Sciences
Western Kentucky University, 1906 College Heights Boulevard,
GRH 3023, Bowling Green, KY 42101, USA
e-mail: Ronda.Talley@wku.edu

S. S. Travis
College of Health and Human Services, George Mason University,
CHHS Dean's Office, MSN: 2G7, 4400 University Drive,
Fairfax, VA 22030–4444, USA

R. C. Talley, S. S. Travis (eds.), *Multidisciplinary Coordinated Caregiving*,
Caregiving: Research • Practice • Policy, DOI 10.1007/978-1-4614-8973-3_13,

Table 1 Score Card for Each of the Disciplines

I. Specialized Knowledge
(1 = minimal contributions to 10 = highest contributions among the disciplines)

A. Central to the science of the discipline
1 2 3 4 5 6 7 8 9 10

B. Include constructs that enjoy "protected status" from the discipline
1 2 3 4 5 6 7 8 9 10

II. Involvement in Key Functions
(1 = minimal involvement to 10 = highest involvement relative to other disciplines)

A. Direct care
1 2 3 4 5 6 7 8 9 10

B. Advocacy/Policy
1 2 3 4 5 6 7 8 9 10

C. Researcher (includes methodologist, theorist, policy analyist)
1 2 3 4 5 6 7 8 9 10

III. Positioned for Significant Collaborative Work
(1 = little activity/history to 10 = high activity/history)

A. History of contributions to caregiving
1 2 3 4 5 6 7 8 9 10

B. Discipline known and respected for collaborative work
1 2 3 4 5 6 7 8 9 10

words, some disciplines appear to be more heavily involved in caregiving activity than others. Finally, is the discipline well positioned for significant collaborative work in the future? Does the discipline have a respectable history of contributions to caregiving or is the discipline new to the field and still developing involvement? Is the discipline respected for collaborative work? Table 1 provides a score card for these elements of caregiving related activity, for those who wish to quantify their own impressions of the content in each of the chapters.

Knowledge

The vast amount of disciplinary knowledge presented in the chapters provides an important foundation on which to build caregiving activity in the future. As you might expect, because of the ways in which we selected disciplines for inclusion in the book, all the authors provide evidence of specific knowledge related to caregiving activity that falls within their disciplinary interests. In other words, all the authors were able to make a case for their disciplines to have a place in the text. About half of the authors also offered convincing evidence that their disciplinary engagement in caregiving activity was central to the science of the discipline. On our score card, these disciplines would score on the higher end for the specialized knowledge they provide to the discipline. These disciplines also tend to develop constructs that enjoyed "protected status." On our score card, these disciplines would again score in the moderate to high levels on this aspect of specialized knowledge. As we discuss later, this combination of moderate to high scores on disciplinary knowledge (e.g., centrality to the discipline and protected status constructs) is the beginning of a hierarchical pattern of contributions to caregiving by the disciplines that may be useful in creating a collective call to action. Those disciplines whose caregiving activity falls within broad discipline interests that are not considered central to the science of the discipline or are relatively new or have unknown contributors will need a different action plan for collaborative work in the future.

Before we leave this section, a few words about "protected status" constructs is in order. We introduced this idea in the introductory chapter. The reader will recall our example of stress and coping as protected constructs within psychology. The advantage of these powerful constructs is that others can use the construct in research, policy, and practice; however, the definition of the construct is expected to remain as originally developed by and for a particular discipline. Thus, these are ideas that researchers, educators, clinicians, and others can depend on to survive over time and for which many disciplines can have a shared understanding of their meaning. If you are the creator of a construct that others find useful, does that make you a more significant collaborator in the future? We will return to this question at the end of the chapter.

Functions

The members of disciplines that are involved in all key functions listed on our score card (direct care, advocacy/policy, and researcher) tend to be those groups for whom caregiving knowledge is central to the science of the discipline. In reviewing the chapter discussions, there is at least one function, and often more than one, that fits the expertise and interests of all members of the discipline. These disciplines are important contributors to the scientific literature on caregiving, actively engage in advocacy and policy analysis, and either provide direct care or assist and educate those who do. Chapter authors for the disciplines of education, gerontology, human development, nursing, occupational therapy, psychology, and social work make very sound presentations about the engagement of their respective disciplines across all of these key functions.

In contrast, authors of chapters about disciplines that are primarily involved in research and/or advocacy/policy functions provide narratives that place caregiving activity within broader interests of the discipline. This set of chapters includes anthropology, communication, public health and public policy. On our score card, these disciplines would score in the low to moderate ranges on the two specialized knowledge items and some combination of high and low scores on the three key function items, with lower scores most likely on direct care and higher scores on advocacy/policy and research.

Positioning for Collaborative Work

Returning to our notion of a hierarchical ordering of disciplines engaged in caregiving activity, we can now demonstrate why some disciplines seem such obvious choices for collaborative work and others are often overlooked when collaborative models are discussed. Disciplines whose contributions are most central to the science of a particular discipline, whose work has contributed relevant constructs that enjoy protected status by the discipline, and whose members are highly engaged in all three key functions on the score card are likely to score high on their history of contributions to caregiving and high on how well known and respected the discipline members are among other disciplines with respect to caregiving activity. The quality, quantity, and applicability of the disciplinary work likely has a direct effect on these last two score card items.

We are now ready to use our score card to discuss how the results might be used to place two hypothetical disciplines in a hierarchy of disciplines with caregiving activity. Discipline A has been in existence for over a century. It scores high on specialized knowledge with a combined score of 18 on the two knowledge items. The members of the discipline fulfill all three key functions on the score card with direct care scoring highest and closely followed by advocacy/policy, and research, in that order. The total score on the three functions items is 26. The age of the discipline and the centrality of caregiving to the science of the discipline contribute heavily to high scores on significant collaborative work. These two items result in a combined score of 18. The total score on the score card across all three categories is 62.

Discipline B has been recognized in academic circles for a little less than 30 years. Caregiving activity falls broadly within the disciplines interests, especially as they relate to research and theory development. Some applications have begun to emerge in the past 30 years that hold promise for making substantial contributions to educational interventions for caregivers. The discipline scores 15 on the items for specialized knowledge and 16 on the items for key functions. Because of the history of contributions and respect for the limited amount of collaborative work to date, this discipline scores 10 on the collaborative work items. The total score on the score card across all three categories is 41.

Collective Call to Action

The score card for the disciplines emerged from the chapters we were provided. The fact that we were able to make up a score card suggests that, despite our disciplinary differences, most of our authors think about and write about disciplinary contributions in these broad categories of disciplinary knowledge, function, and collaboration. To be clear, in this concluding chapter we are not suggesting that one discipline is better than another at caregiving activities, as determined by our score card. Rather, we use the score card approach to explain why valued contributions to caregiving are more heavily attributed to certain disciplines than to others.

Earlier we asked if being the creator of a construct that others find useful makes a discipline a more significant collaborator in the future than a discipline that is still developing its scientific basis for caregiving activity. At this point, our position is "yes and no." Leaders in a field need to continue to lead. However, being a new member of collaborative work with fresh views, new ideas, and innovative approaches to existing problems also carries a great deal of importance in this complex new century. What we do not know about caregiving is probably much more voluminous and perplexing than what we have already discovered across the professions.

Our call to the action for the professions is this. Seek out those who are unfamiliar to you and listen to their disciplinary perspectives. Where constructs are familiar, comfortable, and applicable, use them. Where they do not adequately meet your needs, find new colleagues who will help you describe the unfamiliar, uncomfortable, and abstract ideas you are encountering. Finding collaborative partners who are new to caregiving activity does not mean a lesser partner in your collaborative work. Finally, if you knew caregiving 10 years ago, you do not know caregiving today. Those of us who are interested in and engaged in caregiving activity are chasing a moving target. Direct care, policy, advocacy, research, and education are changing so rapidly that it is nearly impossible to stay ahead of the trends and issues.

We believe the authors of our chapters produced exemplary work that addresses their discipline-specific contributions to caregiving. They provided the necessary foundations on which to think about and act on opportunities for collaborative work in the future. It is now up to the will of the disciplines to fully understand and appreciate what each group has to offer and to create opportunities for exciting and important work in this century. With increasing demands and needs for coordinated, multidisciplinary care from both caregivers and care recipients alike, and with the advent of the Affordable Care Act, the importance of professional caregivers working across disciplines as team members has never been more important.

Index

R. C. Talley, S. S. Travis (eds.), *Multidisciplinary Coordinated Caregiving*, Caregiving: Research • Practice • Policy, DOI 10.1007/978-1-4614-8973-3,

MIX
Papier aus verantwortungsvollen Quellen
Paper from responsible sources
FSC® C105338

If you have any concerns about our products,
you can contact us on
ProductSafety@springernature.com

In case Publisher is established outside the EU,
the EU authorized representative is:
Springer Nature Customer Service Center GmbH
Europaplatz 3, 69115 Heidelberg, Germany

Printed by Libri Plureos GmbH
in Hamburg, Germany